Visceral and Obstetr

For Elsevier:

Senior Commissioning Editor: Sarena Wolfaard
Associate Editor: Claire Wilson
Project Manager: Gail Wright
Design Direction: George Ajayi
Illustrations Buyer: Merlyn Harvey

Visceral and Obstetric Osteopathy

Caroline A Stone DO(Hons) MSc(Ost) MEd
Mount Lawley Medical Centre, Mount Lawley, Australia

Forewords by
Jean-Pierre Barral DO MROF (France)
Chairman, Department of Visceral Manipulation,
Faculty of Medicine, Paris-Nord University,
Bobigny, France; pioneer of visceral manipulation, who
has published in many languages and lectures worldwide
and
Michael L Kuchera DO FAAO (United States)
Professor, Department of Osteopathic Manipulative Medicine
Director, Center for Chronic Disorders of Aging
Director, Human Performance and Biomechanics Laboratory,
Philadelphia College of Osteopathic Medicine,
Philadelphia, USA

Illustrations by
Amanda Williams

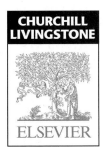

CHURCHILL LIVINGSTONE

ELSEVIER

EDINBURGH LONDON NEW YORK OXFORD PHILADELPHIA ST LOUIS SYDNEY TORONTO 2007

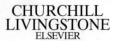

ISBN-13: 978-0-443-10202-8
ISBN-10: 0 443 10202 3

British Library Cataloguing in Publication Data
A catalogue record for this book is available from the British Library

Library of Congress Cataloging in Publication Data
A catalog record for this book is available from the Library of Congress

Notice
Neither the Publisher nor the Author assumes any responsibility for any loss or injury and/or damage to persons or property arising out of or related to any use of the material contained in this book. It is the responsibility of the treating practitioner, relying on independent expertise and knowledge of the patient, to determine the best treatment and method of application for the patient.

The Publisher

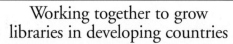

your source for books, journals and multimedia in the health sciences

www.elsevierhealth.com

The publisher's policy is to use **paper manufactured from sustainable forests**

Printed in China

Contents

Forewords

I have known Caroline for 20 years, initially as a postgraduate osteopath learning visceral manipulation, and later as someone who has enabled many other osteopaths to grow and develop. I have seen her evolve as a practitioner and as a teacher of visceral work and the osteopathic approach in general; in bringing this to the broader profession, she has made an indispensable contribution to osteopathy.

As soon as we met, I felt she had very good hands and that she would do something special in the visceral field; indeed, she has made many important contributions to the profession's understanding and appreciation of visceral manipulations within osteopathy, and how to help patients on many different levels, accordingly.

In her teaching, Caroline integrates many different components and brings alive the concepts of three-dimensional biomechanics in her inclusion of visceral tensions, torsions and dysfunctions. Just as importantly, she reveals the interaction between anatomy and physiology, thereby illustrating how soft tissue, organ, fascial and other tissue tensions can impact on homeostasis, function and recovery from pathology and injury. This helps osteopaths to approach the management, not only of patients with musculoskeletal symptoms, but also those with more complex visceral dysfunctions and disorders. This book is important for all those wishing to appreciate and incorporate work within the visceral field to their osteopathic practice. It will also help to guide those outside the profession towards an understanding of the osteopathic approach to patient care.

Visceral manipulation permits patients to feel better in their life and it is something that osteopaths must include in their evaluation of patients and their dysfunctions. In particular, osteopaths have a special contribution to make in the field of gynaecology and obstetrics. To help a woman to have a child and for her to achieve this in the best conditions is a chance that should be open to all. We have certain unique keys to improve factors around fertility, pregnancy and delivery, and it is our duty to do it, as health and function can be subtly but powerfully influenced by the osteopath's gentle, and knowing, 'listening' touch.

I commend this book to anyone wanting a deeper understanding of the osteopathic approach to healthcare, and applaud Caroline on her continuing dedication and contribution to osteopathy.

Grenoble 2006   *Jean-Pierre Barral*

Churchill said, 'I always avoid prophesying beforehand, because it is a much better policy to prophesy after the event has already taken place.' I wish hindsight were my assigned task; however, I was asked to write a 'foreword' and not a 'backword'. In concluding this foreword, therefore, I decided to be somewhat bold in my assessment of this book. Please read on to understand why.

My global foreword is simply this: *Visceral and Obstetric Osteopathy* is a valuable, clinically applicable text written without pretence. In it, the author easily communicates her clinical expertise by translating static anatomy into a palpable experience. Techniques are clearly and concisely written and follow directly from their anatomical descriptions. The elegance of the technique presentation in this book lies in the simplicity of the diagrams used to summarise them.

Chapter details in this foreword could be broadly painted because there is a clarity in the overall structure of the book. There are three parts to this book: (1) The Introduction and first three chapters are basically overview materials; (2) Chapters 4–8 are visceral-system specific and literally constitute the heart of this text; and (3) Chapters 9–10 contain the author's clinical application perspective.

- *Introduction and Chapters 1–3.* Don't judge the value of this text by its overview alone. Aware of the impossibility of writing overview materials to please everyone, the author wisely and simply states her perspective. The result is an interesting synopsis of concepts and clinical-approach models as understood and/or postulated in her training as an osteopathic professional. There is little attempt to convince any healthcare practitioner (osteopathic or otherwise) with outcome studies about the value of upcoming techniques … but then that was never her stated purpose. Note that the Introduction is clearly written from the perspective of a practitioner whose medical education and permitted scope-of-practice are more limited in her own country than in the USA. I therefore felt occasional reservations about the historical or clinical perspectives presented. There are significant differences in American and non-American applications of osteopathic care in part because 'osteopathic medicine' in the United States is practised by more than 60,000[1] complete physicians, including D.O. obstetricians and gynaecologists, internists, and family medicine specialists. Osteopathic medicine is therefore a much less 'contentious' word in the United States, where residencies exist in these and other fields, including NMM/OMM (neuromusculoskeletal medicine/osteopathic manipulative medicine) where many of the visceral and homeostatic concepts noted in her text

are taught and valued. Interestingly, these reservations were not felt outside of the Introduction. My overall summary: this part of the book is of an easily read, simplified discussion of commonly and less-commonly used osteopathic approaches constituting a nice background for the rest of the text.

- *Overview of individual systems (Chapters 4–8).* This is the essence of the text and the reason to own it! Building on clear anatomic descriptions, the simple-yet-elegant diagrams facilitate acquisition of these often under-appreciated clinical techniques. These are not chapters written to validate the approach, rather they are careful, clear descriptions of how to manually contact and balance anatomy. For practitioners wishing to learn for themselves the value of integrating such techniques, this is the place to start. While the sections are not exhaustive in their overall scope to influence visceral function (e.g., sternal techniques were absent and viscerosomatic approaches were superficially addressed), the author's intent was fully met. The text excels in presenting the manual approach to the viscera themselves in an unambiguous and complete fashion. Finally, I would also be remiss if I did not praise the author for including arterial, venous and lymphatic vasculature as approachable visceral structures.
- *Patient management: visceral and obstetric.* The last two chapters of the textbook were clinically delightful and particularly appealing. Some patient management scenarios suggested much more care than I currently provide (or would have been willing to have considered prior to reading this text); some scenarios suggested much less osteopathic care than I thought could be done and her description didn't change my opinion about what I would do for my patients; and many scenarios I secretly applauded because I felt we would have managed that patient with that condition in exactly the same fashion. As a clinical educator, the key appeal to this section is that the scenarios that I interpreted as too much, too little or 'just right' are unlikely to be the same ones that the reader identifies. Such food for thought can only serve to help us to 'dig on' in our clinical understanding

and to evolve in our respective arts and practices.

That brings me back to my foreword's 'brave' prophecy that this text has the potential to positively reform the healthcare we provide our patients.

- *'Reform must come from within, not without.'* As an osteopathic practitioner, I thank Caroline Stone for this contribution to the osteopathic profession.
- *'Reform, that you may preserve.'* As someone who has had a successful practice for over 25 years, I thank this book for continuing to remind me to integrate new (and/or rediscovered) science, philosophy and art into my practice.
- *'If you try to make a big reform you are told you are doing too much, and if you make a modest contribution you are told you are only tinkering with the problem.'* I don't believe reform was on the author's mind at all. Nonetheless, intentionally or not, as an outside reviewer and educator I want to go on record as saying that this book strikes a happy balance to do so.

In conclusion and in my opinion, *Visceral and Obstetric Osteopathy* has the potential to be an instrument of reformation ... if not of a profession, at least of one practice at a time.

Osteopathic founder, A. T. Still, M.D., D.O. said, 'Know you are right and do your work accordingly.' In sharing anatomic fact and her clinical perspective, Caroline Stone has constructed a text that empowers the reader to consider that possibility.

Michael L. Kuchera,
Philadelphia 2006   *D.O., FAAO*[2]

---

[1]2006 figures. Osteopathic medicine is the fastest growing segment of healthcare providers in the USA so numbers will increase significantly after publication of this text.

[2]Dr Michael Kuchera and his father, William Kuchera, are also the authors of *Osteopathic Principles in Practice* and of *Osteopathic Considerations in Systemic Dysfunction* (Greyden Press).

Preface

Osteopathy is a great profession, and I have been very happy to help actively promote and develop it over the past 20 years. Establishing a firm basis and enthusiasm for the practice of visceral osteopathy has been a huge part of my professional life; of this I am very proud. Osteopathic care for pregnant women and patients suffering from a wide variety of 'visceral' problems need not be complex or confusing. This book aims to help all practitioners, regardless of their individual approaches to patient care, to appreciate a range of basic, advanced, subtle and integrated approaches in the visceral and obstetric fields of osteopathic healthcare.

Some of the techniques and approaches discussed in Chapter 10 'Osteopathy and obstetrics' may be subject to practice restrictions in the UK. Readers and practitioners are advised to check current legal boundaries for practice in their region/location. Their inclusion in this book does not in itself infer practice rights.

Mount Lawley 2006   *Caroline Stone*

Acknowledgements

In writing this book, I would like to thank the following people who have all helped in a number of ways: Ray and Catherine Power for help with illustrations; Julie Peipers for support; Amanda Heyes for lots of care, comments and treatment; and other colleagues who have attended recent courses and offered great feedback. I would also like to thank Anne Cooper and Jenni Paul for their insights and helpful comments. Thanks also to Claire Wilson and Gail Wright at Elsevier for their efficient and friendly work on this book.

I would most like to thank my husband, Brad, for his love and enthusiasm for this project, and our beautiful daughter Jasmine for her self-sufficiency and patience! Love also to our second child, who will arrive as this book nears publication.

Introduction

The field of visceral and obstetric osteopathy is not new but is increasingly popular and relevant in current patient-oriented healthcare systems in which the body's inherent self-regulating and self-healing mechanisms are increasingly recognized and valued therapeutically.

Osteopaths themselves are also keen to maintain and develop their scope of practice and as general and professional awareness of the potential of osteopathic care is reawakened, practitioners are more enthusiastic than ever to explore the human dynamic in increasingly three-dimensional and integrative ways.

Osteopaths see a variety of patients complaining of many problems, including but not limited to:

- low back and neck pain
- repetitive work-related injuries or strain
- effects of trauma such as whiplash
- asthma and other breathing problems
- colic and irritable bowel syndrome
- postoperative pain and adhesion problems
- back, joint and soft tissue pain during pregnancy

- postpartum pelvic problems, including pelvic floor injuries
- headaches and TMJ pain
- ENT problems
- developmental, feeding, sleeping and other problems in babies and children.

Any or all of the above problems may benefit from the application of visceral osteopathy, even if the symptoms arise within the musculoskeletal system (and the patient has no accompanying visceral symptoms or disorders). In other words, although a visceral approach can be used when patients present with visceral symptoms, it is also helpful when there are only musculoskeletal symptoms of biomechanical origin.

BASIC CONCEPTS OF VISCERAL AND OBSTETRIC OSTEOPATHY

Visceral osteopathy is a way of exploring those tensions of the body that reside within the organs and associated tissues, with the aim of improving overall movement, lessening any barriers to better function and allowing the body's own self-healing and self-regulating mechanisms to function more optimally. Any problem within the body may have a visceral component.

These types of factors can be present in people with no symptoms of visceral disease, in much the same way that many of the biomechanical/musculoskeletal tensions and restrictions present in someone with, for example, low back pain are not in themselves always symptomatic.

Obstetric care by osteopaths centres around allowing the woman to accommodate her pregnancy as comfortably and physiologically as possible, with the aim of reducing or removing stress and strain not only for the mother and for labour, but for the developing baby as well.

Osteopathy in these contexts is an understanding of how three-dimensional anatomy relates to physiological function and how manual treatments can help restore optimum functioning and improve healing.

VISCERAL OSTEOPATHY

Visceral osteopathy is a field concerned with:

- the three-dimensional dynamics of body biomechanics (including musculoskeletal, myofascial, connective tissue and organ structures)
- reflex activity in the central and peripheral nervous systems
- neuroemotional–immune links
- effective circulation and drainage of all the body fluid systems and tissues.

A patient does not need to present with a visceral problem (e.g. irritable bowel or hiatus hernia) for a visceral approach to be relevant. Many cases of musculoskeletal pain can be helped by releasing asymptomatic problems within various organs and body tissues. Also, just because someone has presented with some sort of visceral symptom does not mean that the primary treatment is applied to those organs. It could be equally if not more important to consider the surrounding or related musculoskeletal system components. Visceral approaches within osteopathy are merely another tool for the osteopath to utilize when managing a whole variety of patient presentations.

For most patients and presentations, a variety of tensions, torsions, stresses and strains are apparent throughout the whole of the body and the osteopath often applies a combination of treatment to 'old injuries' or sites of infection/inflammation and fresh or recent problems and traumas. Osteopaths are aiming to interact with the physiological functions within the body and to promote health and better function by removing irritating factors and barriers to the homeostatic self-regulating mechanisms of the body. *Better movement is considered the key to this process, and visceral osteopathy is at its simplest the study of movement within the visceral systems and related tissues and structures.*

OBSTETRIC OSTEOPATHY

Many women and many health practitioners consider that much of the pain and discomfort associated with pregnancy and birth is 'part of one's lot' and not really amenable to treatment. Most women experience physical problems and often the majority wait for the end of pregnancy to bring relief to their suffering. This does not have to be the case, as many of the problems associated with pregnancy can be managed or alleviated using an osteopathic approach.

Osteopathic care for pregnant women, pre- and postnatally, focuses on helping the mother's structure (spine, joints and soft tissues) to cope with the increasing demands of the pregnancy. It helps to alleviate some of the pains and problems associated with changes in posture, weight bearing, and the stretching of various ligaments and tissues that support the uterus. It also helps to prepare the body and pelvis for labour and delivery, may have a role to play during labour and helps the woman recover from the traumas and strains imposed during the birth process (be that 'natural' delivery or 'caesarean'). Osteopaths can help in managing existing spinal and joint problems during pregnancy, aiming to reduce the impact that the pregnancy has on the disc disease or ligamentous and muscular strain problems, for example.

Obstetric osteopathy also aims to make the space available for the developing baby as 'comfortable' as possible, thus potentially reducing mechanical stress on the baby during pregnancy. This may have many effects, including giving space for the baby to freely rotate and move around within the uterus, and get into an optimum position for labour and birth. Improving the mechanics of the joints and muscles of the pelvis in particular is also thought to help ensure that the birth canal is as accommodating as naturally possible. This is thought to reduce the risk of injury not only to the mother but also to the baby. There is also a large field of study called paediatric osteopathy which is concerned with the osteopathic management of problems from birth through infancy and childhood to early adulthood, which is not fully addressed in this book.

Intrapartum care is also an area of practice in osteopathy. Here, the osteopath is legally a 'birth partner' to the labouring woman and does not have medical control of the situation. Their role is to support the mother and offer whatever osteopathic services all parties (including the midwifery and obstetric carers) agree upon, with the aim of reducing strain in labour and potentially improving birth processes and outcomes for the mother and child. This is an area of special interest and not one that all osteopaths would routinely offer.

OSTEOPATHIC MEDICINE

Using osteopathy as part of a management system for the very sick, the diseased or those with a weakened immune system is not contraindicated, nor is (as mentioned above) its use in natural conditions such as pregnancy or during labour.

Osteopathic medicine is a term used to describe how osteopaths view health and disease, and how they consider that effective and efficient movement in *all* body tissues, structures and fluid circulations contributes to health and balanced homeostatic function. Osteopaths consider that irritations in tissues and nerves and barriers to effective fluid circulations are all related (in part) to movement and biomechanical restrictions in the body tissues (including muscles, joints, connective tissues, organs, blood vessels and so on).

Osteopaths consider that there is a biomechanical component to pathological processes and disease, and that examination of the body's tissues for movement disorders should form part of any general medical screening procedure.

Consequently, osteopaths consider that a normal part of medical management of pathology and disease should be restoring or improving movement in all body tissues where possible, as they believe that this will aid physiological recovery.

If movement is restored, communication between parts is more efficient, fluid circulation and drainage improve, irritating signals are reduced and the body's homeostatic and immune mechanisms can operate more effectively, thus restoring health and better function.

The term 'osteopathic medicine' is a contentious one, as it has often been interpreted as meaning that osteopaths are working outside their scope of practice. Osteopaths have historically defended the use of their principles in the management of health and disease issues, as supplementary care, complementary care or alternative care, depending on the situation. Providing the pathological nature of conditions is understood and appropriate considerations made, for example in terms of techniques used, forces applied and ethics and legalities observed, then osteopathic management can provide sometimes quite marked relief of symptoms associated with those conditions. Not only that, but the impact on physiological processes may enable the body to utilize its own self-regulating and healing mechanisms more effectively, and thus may contribute in some way to the resolution of ill health. Osteopaths contend that treating the person, rather than the disease, leads to improved outcomes on more levels than simple application of disease-oriented therapy alone.

Whilst part of their work is aimed at symptom management, through the link between movement and physiology and the way that osteopaths consider that movement restrictions impact on physiology and hence reduce tissue health and functioning, there is some consideration of the potential aetiological impact of the movement restrictions on pathological development and progression. Hence osteopaths also theorize that some of their management addresses pathological change. This is an area where the evidence base for osteopathic concepts is currently small.

Ethics, risk/benefit equations, evidence-based medicine, diagnostic rights, consumer (patient) protection, regulatory issues, safety and medicolegal considerations, research options and patient-centred care are all important topics for any practitioner to be aware of. The osteopath and patient negotiate between them a contract of care that enables them both to contribute to the patient's health management, with the aim of reducing symptoms and suffering. Osteopaths respect pathological and tissue state changes, meaning that if appropriately applied, there are very few absolute contraindications to practice. Consequently, osteopaths become engaged in the management of people with cancer, immune insufficiency, genetic disorders, in postoperative care and many other situations. Osteopaths bring their principles to bear so that relative contraindications (for example, to mode of technique applied at a certain time) can be identified and management adjusted accordingly.

Pathology creates tissue change, including protective spasm, rebound, pain and tenderness, oedema and congestion, which reacts upon palpation. When these factors are placed in context with case history and other examination components such as special tests and imaging, the osteopath can tailor their application of therapeutic manipulations and mobilizations accordingly, in a safe manner with low risk. Awareness of tissues states and pathological processes forms part of the safety net for patient and practitioner.

DEFINITIVE OSTEOPATHIC TENETS

Osteopathy is not a two-dimensional mechanistic approach; viewing the body as a complex Meccano set is not what osteopaths are about. Osteopaths see the body as something where mind, body and spirit interact and are reciprocally related, and where the building blocks of the body (its *tissues*) interact and both influence and are influenced by internal physiology and homeostasis. Note that the word 'tissues' has been used, as most observers erroneously consider that osteopaths are interested only in bones, ligaments, muscles and tendons. Osteopaths work with *all* body tissues and fluids, even though they may sometimes use the musculoskeletal tissues as a 'handle' into deeper, less accessible structures, tissues and circulatory pathways.

Structure and function are reciprocally related

Things function in a certain way as a result of how they are made and structured. If the structure alters, then so will the function. This concept informs osteopathic practice in the following way.

- Anatomy governs physiology.
- Soft tissue dynamics relate to physiological efficiency and effective homeostatic balance.
- Altered soft tissue mobility both reflects and contributes to poor physiological function and pathological change.
- Improvement of mobility and restoration or normalization of movement patterns improve the self-regulatory and self-healing functions of the body, thus promoting better function, health and well-being.
- Osteopaths therefore examine the body to identify areas of altered or poor movement, and make attempts at restoring that movement, to improve function and therefore reduce symptoms.

The rule of the artery is supreme

Circulation is immensely important to health and without adequate nutrition, tissues cannot perform efficiently. At a cellular level, the dynamics of the extracellular matrix (ECM) and the micro-circulation are important to function and immunity where movement of cells and fluid through the ECM plays a key role. Drainage is also important, as without effective lymphatic and venous drainage, the appropriate 'chemical' homeostatic balance is not maintained and waste removal is inefficient.

In identifying the 'rule of the artery' as supreme, osteopathy's founder, Dr AT Still, focused on nutrition and felt a lot of manual treatment should be directed at 'irrigation of withering fields'. Although the language may be somewhat old-fashioned, the physiological implication is clear.

Osteopaths are also particularly interested in the role of the autonomic nervous system. Historically, the functioning of the sympathetic nervous system and its influence on circulation through vasoconstriction mechanisms was an area of considerable osteopathic interest and research. Increased sympatheticotonia was attributed to a variety of mechanical disturbances and other stressors in the body, with resultant ischaemia and other physiological changes in the end organ or target tissue. Adapting sympathetic outflow in some way would presumably affect these aspects and influence nutrition in the end tissue or field (and therefore impact on tissue health and healing). Today, osteopaths continue to work with all parts of the autonomic and somatic nervous systems, in order to interact with the body's physiology in general, and circulation and fluid movement in particular.

The body has self-healing and self-regulatory mechanisms

Communication is vital to health and good function. The body has built up some amazing methods of communication between its diverse parts and tissues, which are still being investigated and discovered. Osteopaths consider that movement restrictions negatively impact on communication (be it chemical, neural, mechanical or otherwise), thus affecting homeostatic balance. Remove or reduce these movement barriers and the body will naturally reorient itself towards health and better functioning.

The musculoskeletal system is the primary machinery of life

The musculoskeletal system is more than a framework to carry our internal organs around. It is the means by which we express ourselves, how we perform tasks and care for others, and by which we can recognize in others their actions and feelings. Without an effectively functioning and coordinated musculoskeletal system, the way we live our life is indeed compromised.

Through its contact with and acknowledgement of these factors, and the subsequent manual therapy applied to the body, osteopathy is uniquely placed to interact with the patient's prime motives, emotions and functions, on all levels.

The whole is more than the sum of its parts

Integration within and between parts is essential for effective body function. We are more than just a collection of cells; there is something about the way all those cells work together that summates and enables life as we know it to be expressed. Osteopaths accordingly never consider how any particular joint, muscle tissue or organ works in isolation, and do not look at body systems separately. The concept of 'specialisms' within practice,

as exist within the orthodox medical model, is anathema to osteopaths. Vitalistic concepts apply.

Motion is life

Whether it be an electrical current passing along a nerve, blood circulating through the body or muscles twitching and joints articulating, motion is an absolute characteristic of life. For an osteopath, assessing quality of motion is like assessing someone's quality of life: poor movement not only indicates that the person is not able to physically live their lives to the full or express themselves with ease, but also that their body systems are not functioning optimally and that their health and immunity are compromised as a result.

Find it, fix it and leave it alone

The aim is to find the main focus of distress or dysfunction in the body, address that as far as possible and then leave the body to carry on sorting itself out from that input. Osteopaths work on the concept that the body knows what is good for it, and will always aim to bring itself into a healthy state wherever possible. If it can be given the right sort of helping hand, it will 'run with that impetus' and shift its function away from dis-ease and towards health and better function.

As Dr Still said: 'To find health is the mission of any doctor – anyone can find disease'.

It is the osteopathic ability to tune into the body's needs and integrated functioning that creates a different approach to other manual therapy practitioners. The ability of osteopaths to utilize a highly refined palpatory awareness to work on many levels of bodily and human function at once is a special skill, and one that enables a deeper understanding of health and disease to emerge.

CONSIDERING THE WHOLE

Figure I.1 shows a typical patient, one who presents with a variety of biomechanical and soft tissue restrictions. The actual torsion pattern is not important – we all recognize that patients have restrictions throughout their bodies; it is the practitioner's job to interpret those tension patterns with respect to the presenting symptoms and underlying physiological processes.

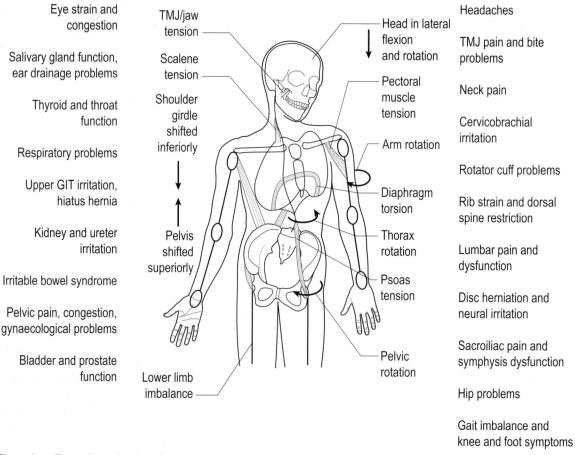

Eye strain and congestion

Salivary gland function, ear drainage problems

Thyroid and throat function

Respiratory problems

Upper GIT irritation, hiatus hernia

Kidney and ureter irritation

Irritable bowel syndrome

Pelvic pain, congestion, gynaecological problems

Bladder and prostate function

TMJ/jaw tension

Scalene tension

Shoulder girdle shifted inferiorly

Pelvis shifted superiorly

Lower limb imbalance

Head in lateral flexion and rotation

Pectoral muscle tension

Arm rotation

Diaphragm torsion

Thorax rotation

Psoas tension

Pelvic rotation

Headaches

TMJ pain and bite problems

Neck pain

Cervicobrachial irritation

Rotator cuff problems

Rib strain and dorsal spine restriction

Lumbar pain and dysfunction

Disc herniation and neural irritation

Sacroiliac pain and symphysis dysfunction

Hip problems

Gait imbalance and knee and foot symptoms

Figure I.1   Three-dimensional torsion pattern.

This 'typical' patient could be presenting with a variety of symptoms, which may be manifesting within the musculoskeletal field or the visceral field (or both!).

- The torsion at the head, with some side-bending/lateral flexion and rotation, may present with pain and aches in the temporomandibular joint (TMJ) or with headaches or, because of the way the torsion affects the jaw, tongue and throat tissues, may be presenting with chronic ear infections and congestion.
- The torsion within the chest may be related to dorsal spine aches and rib strains or may be related to respiratory symptoms, lung and chest wall stiffness and decreased lung volume, for example.

- The torsion within the chest may have spread through to the mediastinum and be creating tension in the central tendon of the diaphragm. This may be contributing to mechanical aches and pains in the ribs, costal margin or crurae and upper lumbar spine or may be affecting the gastro-oesophageal junction and contributing to symptoms of gastric reflux or indigestion.
- The pelvic torsion may be consequent to lower limb problems but could also be related to the pelvic floor and hence prostate or bladder, for example.
- Coccygeal torsions could be related to the cranial base and cervical restriction pattern (through dural links) and could be involved in uterine or vaginal problems from pelvic fascial tension from the coccyx.

WHERE IS THE PROBLEM?

This is the biggest question in any management scenario – where to apply the therapeutic input in the most beneficial, least stressful and most economic way, meeting the needs of both the patient and the ethics, principles and constraints of the healthcare system being utilized. It depends on your diagnostic and healthcare belief systems, and any individual practitioner's hypotheses all have a certain risk/benefit equation attached to them. In other words, your beliefs determine how you examine someone, how you interpret those findings, what other information you take into consideration and what you think will be a beneficial therapeutic intervention. The anticipated beneficial effects of any management applied have to be weighed against the risks imposed through its application.

As indicated by the figure and previous discussions, finding the primary cause of a problem or the underlying main restriction or tension pattern is not easy, as the body works in so many reciprocally integrated ways; it is a bit like asking the chicken and egg question. The patient does not have to have any particular symptoms in the visceral tissues for the organs to be participating in the overall biomechanical problem that is contributing to the patient's presentation. The organs and associated tissues may be tight, scarred, tense or irritated subclinically – they may just be moving awkwardly. This could be sufficient to physically constrain certain parts of the musculoskeletal system (through anatomical links) or may be reflexly irritating the musculoskeletal system (through shared/segmentally related parts of the nervous system).

This means that the visceral system must be examined generally as part of any overall assessment, to evaluate its relevance in that particular patient. The osteopath could then eventually treat asymptomatic areas of the patient's body in order to resolve symptoms elsewhere. Of course, if the patient does have visceral symptoms (either currently or in the past) then the osteopath already has indicators that various organs should be explored for signs that they are maintaining poor or restricted movement within the musculoskeletal system, or are in part maintaining the visceral dysfunction itself. To requote one of the basic tenets: 'You can't fix it till you've found it, and you can't find it until you look'.

Working in the visceral and obstetric osteopathic fields simply means the practitioner increases their ability to work three-dimensionally within the body.

TISSUE AWARENESS AND INTERPRETATION

Diagnosing any visceral component means that the practitioner must explore those tissues carefully and whilst there are some basic screening techniques designed to give an overview. there is no substitute for a sensitive, thorough and thoughtful evaluation. (Note: 'diagnosing' in this context means identifying and describing in osteopathic terms a movement change in or around a particular organ or related structure). Adding visceral osteopathy to one's repertoire will mean that additional time has to be set aside when evaluating a problem but this should lead to more effective management of the patient's problem through a more refined overall working hypothesis and diagnosis.

Invariably, in all cases there are some tensions found within the musculoskeletal system and some within the visceral, vascular or nervous systems of the body. It is the practitioner's job to interpret the relevance and importance of the different components of a patient's presentation and how they all fit together, before formulating a management plan based on that working hypothesis.

Visceral osteopaths utilize a variety of techniques to explore the organs and related tissues, to interpret findings and to treat what they find. As one is exploring tissues that may be scarred, inflamed, irritated or have some sort of pathological process going on, tissue awareness and medical knowledge must be part of the practitioner's training prior to examining the visceral field. That said, there are several components that can easily form a general examination of the visceral system and associated musculoskeletal components, which are listed below (the list is not exclusive). With experience, some or all of these may be incorporated into an individual's practice.

Overview of patient assessment

The following types of routines are widely used and may form part of global assessment of the patient when making an initial diagnosis or hypothesis, as well as part of an ongoing review of progress. They can be individualized according to situation and need and represent an averaged style of approach.

Case history taking

Includes the use of analytical questioning, a range of communication and observation tools, differential diagnostic sieving, development and exploration of working hypotheses.

Use of special tests

According to case needs, general screening of several body systems may be required. Osteopaths can utilize various basic medical screening tests such as manual neurological testing, percussion and auscultation, and can be aware of the need for blood and urine tests, x-rays, ultrasound and other imaging techniques. Where medical diagnosis is required or may be advisable, the osteopath will refer on for further care, often whilst continuing to manage the patient in a way that does not compromise them receiving the necessary tests or treatment and is not detrimental to any possible potential condition awaiting diagnosis.

Standing assessment

- When assessing a person, do not look just at their spinal mechanics using a posterior view. View the person from all sides, *and in particular*, don't forget your patient has a front.
- The objective is to identify areas of the body which are affecting overall posture and standing balance.
- Passive observation can be used, as well as active movements by the patient, to identify general body parts or sections that are not partaking in normal posture and movement.
- General listening techniques can be utilized. Listening techniques make use of fascial and connective tissue tensions and torsion patterns that are created through restrictions in organs, muscles, joints or other body tissues, to identify significant problems. This concept is discussed later.

Sitting assessment

- Removing the influence of the lower limbs can often reveal more specific patterns of restriction within the torso, neck and head.

- Practitioner observation of the patient, active movement by the patient, and passive examination of the patient can all be used.
- Special tests such as orthopaedic, respiratory or cranial nerve testing can be used, as required.
- General listening techniques can be utilized.
- Evaluation of spinally located reflex fields can be performed.

Supine (and sometimes sidelying or prone) assessment of the body

- Passive exploration of the tissues, be they musculoskeletal, vascular, neural, visceral or fascial, is undertaken.
- Mobility and motility tests can be performed. *Mobility* tests include testing articulations of the organs, testing sliding surfaces, examining the elasticity, compliance or stretch within an organ or its attachments/supporting tissues. *Motility* in this context is not peristalsis of the hollow/tubular organs such as the gut, but an osteopathic term relating to inherent movement within the structure being evaluated. Both these concepts are discussed later.
- Local listening techniques can be utilized.
- Soft tissue and dermatome reflex zones can be explored.

Passive examinations require sensitivity, especially in the presence of any particular pathological process within the tissues being examined. Medical diagnostic indicators from the case history and physical appearance of the patient can all point to certain pathological processes, of which the practitioner must be aware. On palpation of the abdomen, for example, there are various conditions that require consideration. The presence of aortic aneurysm, oesophageal varices, ulcers, carcinoma and infection, to name but a few, all involve particular changes within the tissues which render them weak, easily damaged and irritated. Overforceful palpation can further damage and injure the tissues, sometimes with serious consequences, and there is a risk of further spread of the pathological condition. Hence the practitioner cannot physically examine the patient without an awareness of underlying conditions and associated risks.

Medical diagnosis is the remit of orthodox doctors, consultants and specialists but all allied health professionals must have training in this area, for the above reasons. That said, visceral palpation is possible in many cases, by using gentle direct techniques or indirect techniques; there are few absolute contraindications. Note: 'direct' and 'indirect' are osteopathic technical terms for styles of physical examination and treatment and will be discussed later.

BASIC COMPONENTS OF VISCERAL OSTEOPATHY

'Organs move'... and that movement (both gross and internal to the organ) contributes to physiological function.

'Visceral mobility' can be:

- between adjacent organs, such as the liver and right kidney, lobes of the lungs, bladder and uterus, etc.
- between organs and adjacent somatic structures, such as the lungs and the ribs/intercostals, the kidney and psoas, stomach and diaphragm, etc.
- organs can express movement such as peristalsis of the gut tube, fallopian tube or ureters, and be motile, such as the heart and its rhythmic pumping, and the expansion and deflation of the lungs.

'Visceral motility' can be:

- an expression of its embryological derivation or migration
- an expression of its vitality
- this is not the same as 'peristalsis'. Note: visceral motility is discussed in a later chapter.

Both mobility and motility can be explored and evaluated by osteopaths, and both can be improved through a variety of manual techniques (both direct and indirect).

Organ manipulation can consist of:

- articulation
- stretching
- inhibition
- general mobilization*
- recoil techniques*

---

*These terms will be explored in later chapters.

- functional, listening and 'involuntary' manipulations*

in order to evaluate all components of visceral movement.

Manual treatments are applied to:

- change the way the musculoskeletal system is responding
- change the way the organs are responding
- affect circulation and fluid drainage
- affect neural reflexes and input (and other forms of communication within the body)

and are aimed at improving function and reducing symptoms.

Organ manipulation is:

- about improving movement, locally to the organ or at a distant point
- aimed at changing function and physiology/homeostasis. Knowing the effects of reduced/altered mobility helps you critically appraise your treatment protocol.

The protocol for osteopathic intervention is simple.

- Reflect on the nature of the condition.
- Explore for tissue barriers to circulation, immune function and effective neural and other communication.
- Analyse impact of physical touch on the pathologically adapted tissue.
- Understand implications of altered blood flow, immune function and neural communication on the pathological processes or condition.
- Rationalize the impact and aim of the intended therapeutic input and consider the risk/benefit equation.
- Be able to justify and communicate actions in osteopathic as well as medical/scientific terms where possible.
- Practise ethically and safely, with informed consent.

POINTS TO REMEMBER IN VISCERAL OSTEOPATHY

- The patient does not need to be complaining of any visceral symptoms (objective or subjective) in order for their organs to require 'treatment'.

- Osteopathy has a role to play in the management of various pathological states and disease processes.
- Not all treatment to help resolve visceral dysfunction is applied to the organs.
- There are very few contraindications to osteopathy – just to how it is applied.
- Differential diagnostic medical knowledge is required in order to rationalize patient care and to manage people appropriately, including referral to other medical specialties as indicated.
- It is not possible to identify everything by feel alone. Palpatory quality may give much interesting information but it is not a replacement for diagnostic imaging or other types of tests.
- A few manual techniques applied to the organs are not going to reverse severe tissue changes such as deep ulceration, scarring and fibrosis.
- Mobilizing the organs in the presence of conditions such as bacterial infection, haematoma and carcinoma is contentious.
- General osteopathic care of patients with the above types of condition is not contentious, when used as a supportive or complementary (as opposed to alternative) care regime.
- What an osteopath may mean by mobilization of an organ may not be immediately clear to patients, medical professionals and others with no osteopathic training. Confusion often arises when discussing the issue.
- The scope of osteopathic practice as perceived outside the profession is quite limited; for example, that it mostly deals with back pain, various sporting injuries and general biomechanical problems.
- The scope of practice as perceived within the profession is much broader, even though the current evidence base is insufficient to define best practice.
- Expanding one's scope of practice means that the onus for illustrating competence rests with the osteopath (or practitioner) concerned.

ABOUT THIS BOOK

The following chapters introduce the range of anatomical (and therefore physiological and biomechanical) inter-relationships between the different body systems and how the body functions in an integrated manner. Various examination and treatment techniques are introduced, and discussions on patient management in various situations are included. Some case histories are given to illustrate how the approaches discussed throughout the book are applied in practice.

Chapter 1

General principles

VISCERAL SUPPORT

The organs are supported and contained by the efficient biomechanical couplings of the musculo-skeletal system, without which the organs would not function effectively. There are various muscular and fascial supports to the visceral systems and these help to hold the viscera in a vertically oriented stack or column. The thoracic and pelvic cavities are bounded by skeletal components, making their internal mechanics more constrained than those of the abdominal cavity, which is mostly bounded by various muscles. The thoracic and abdominal cavities also have differing pressures, which are balanced against each other, so that the overall relationship between the two cavities is in equilibrium.

BODY CAVITY DYNAMICS

The body cavities house the viscera, with a few exceptions (notably the thyroid and parathyroid glands, oropharyngeal glands and the testes).

The body cavities include the cranium and spinal column (bounded by the dura); the thoracic cavity bounded by the pleura, pericardium and cervical fasciae superiorly and the thoracic diaphragm inferiorly; and the abdominopelvic cavity bounded by the thoracic diaphragm above and the pelvic floor muscles below.

As will be explored in detail later, the mechanics of the muscles and articulations of the somatic body cavities are reciprocally related to the viscera and their fascial and serous membrane attachments. In order to appreciate this relationship, its three-dimensional (3D) movement dynamics must be recognized. Clinical work is much more effective once a 3D picture of the person and their movement patterns has been built up. This makes their management much easier to rationalize and tailor individually.

All the body cavities are interconnected and movement in one area will be transmitted to another. For example, respiratory movements from the thoracic diaphragm cause tissue movement in the cervical as well as the pelvic regions, and any weakness or damage to the diaphragm will lead to herniation of abdominal contents into the thorax as a result of the differing pressures between the two cavities. Osteopaths believe that the biomechanical relationships between the cavities are more complex than these simple examples, and much of the transference of movement is via fascial and connective tissue structures, which link the viscera to each other and to various musculoskeletal system structures. The body cavities should not in fact be viewed as separate but are continuous with various 'transverse stabilizing' structures such as the diaphragm and peritoneal mesenteries to give support, anchorage and, sometimes, motion. Embryologically, the body cavities are initially continuous and only become artificially divided by the further development of other structures such as the diaphragm.

CORE-LINKS OF FASCIA AND THEIR 'TRANSVERSE' ATTACHMENTS

One of the reasons why the mechanics of the body are so integrated is the way in which all the structures are linked. There is a connection from the brain along the spinal cord and out to the peripheral nerves, which is formed by the dura, which links the central nervous system as one continuous organ. The dura connects various cranial bones and vertebrae running along the length of the spine, through to the coccyx. This has been labelled as the 'core-link' of fascia, in osteopathic concepts.[1] There is also a connection between many organs and structures which runs from its attachments at the cranial base, through the cervical region, down into the mediastinum, onto the diaphragm and then from below that, down through the abdominal cavity and into the pelvic bowl. This can be thought of as a 'visceral core-link' as opposed to the above 'neural core-link'.

These fascial cores of the body run longitudinally and are traversed horizontally by various structures which help to separate the body cavities or divide them into subsections. The neural core-link is traversed by the tentorium and denticulate ligaments and the visceral core-link is traversed by the thoracic diaphragm, the vertebropericardial ligament, the broad ligament and the pelvic floor. These are shown in Figure 1.1.

Osteopaths do not limit their understanding of body cavities to the 'traditional' descriptions of 'thorax, abdomen and pelvis'. For them, a body cavity is any space which is bounded by fascia (connective tissue), including vascular space, muscle sheaths, individual cell membranes, the extracellular matrix surrounding the interstitial spaces containing interstitial fluid, muscle fasciculi, and so on. All these body cavities are interconnected through the microscopic cytoskeleton, extracellular matrix and generalized fascial sheaths to larger structures such as the mesenteries, ligaments, tendons and ultimately bones and muscles. The fascial structures not only support structures but allow movement and reduce friction and tissue stress.

Fascial structures run continuously through the body and osteopaths do not favour the artificial breakdown into separate structures given different names by various anatomists over the centuries (www.osteodoc.com/fascia.htm). This confuses any understanding of how these fascial structures are functionally linked. Osteopaths are very interested in the 'unity of function', which is a way of thinking that tries to understand how all parts of the body work together as a unit. As such, fascia is intimately involved in all body mechanics and is part of the structural dynamic of the person.[2]

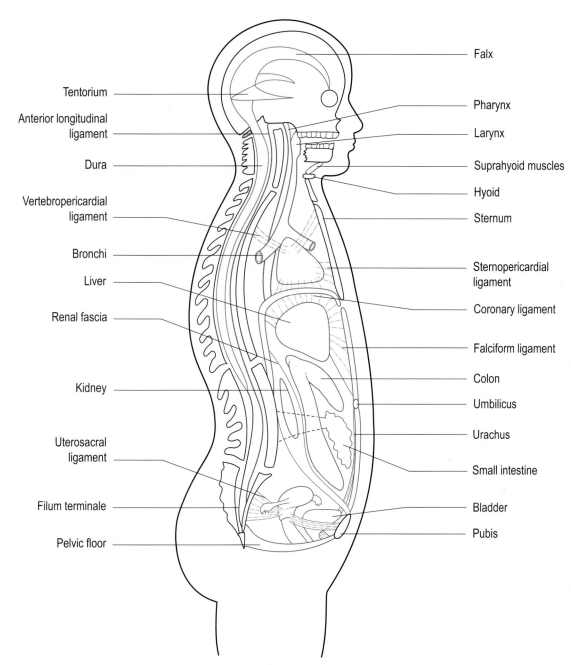

Falx

Tentorium

Anterior longitudinal ligament

Dura

Vertebropericardial ligament

Bronchi

Liver

Renal fascia

Kidney

Uterosacral ligament

Filum terminale

Pelvic floor

Pharynx

Larynx

Suprahyoid muscles

Hyoid

Sternum

Sternopericardial ligament

Coronary ligament

Falciform ligament

Colon

Umbilicus

Urachus

Small intestine

Bladder

Pubis

Figure 1.1   Neural and visceral fascial core-links.

Tensegrity and reciprocal tension membranes

Core-links of fascia connect all the body cavities, from the macro- to the microscopic. Movement can be transmitted almost simultaneously from one area to another, through the tensile properties of the fascial structures. Practically, osteopaths will feel through these fascial structures and can identify tension patterns that spread diversely throughout the body, by contacting and moving one or two distant parts and appreciating the way the movement passes through all the body's structures, on a gross level and even down to a cellular level.[2]

Tensegrity is a biomechanical term used to describe structures which are held together by tension rather than compression.[3] Forces within a tensegrity structure are dissipated evenly, with each part having to bear minimal strain, whilst the structure as a whole is very strong and resistant to stress. Tensegrity structures contain some elements which are under tension (being 'stretched') and some elements which are under compression (being 'squeezed'). In the human body, soft tissues such as muscles, ligaments and tendons represent the tensile components and bones represent the compression components.

A model of a tensegrity structure can be made using sticks and elastic, as shown in Figure 1.2. All the sticks are 'suspended' in space, by tension in the elastic. The sticks are very stable and very little energy is required to maintain the structure in place. For the human body, this is good news as, being a tensegrity structure, little muscle activity is required to hold the bones (skeletal framework) in place. With a little imagination, various 'spaces' or 'cavities' can be seen, bounded by either the sticks or the elastic, or both.

In the body, muscles span from one bone to another (within the model, from one stick to another). When these contract, they will shift the position of one stick relative to the others. All the relative positions of the sticks will change, as all

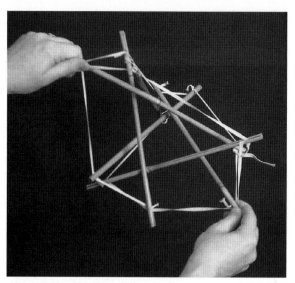

Figure 1.3 Structure torsioned one way opens out some 'spaces'.

the sticks are connected together by the elastic 'tension' components. Figure 1.3 shows the hands changing the position of the sticks, as though by a muscle contraction. This shift in the whole structure will open out some spaces within the model and close some down.

If the same sticks are pulled another way, then the whole structure shifts into a different 3D arrangement, so closing down the previously open spaces and opening up new ones. This is shown in Figure 1.4.

In the body, there is a continual shifting and relative 'repositioning' going on within the body tissues as they accommodate changes in posture and various movements. To appreciate the full dynamic picture, the effects of this shifting of stick and elastic positions must be considered with respect to the body cavities. Figure 1.5 shows a balloon in amongst the sticks and elastic to represent the organs of the body, which are relatively non-compressible. Hence every time the structure as a whole shifts and twists, the space taken up by the balloon is either compressed or torsioned. This change in its 'cavity dimensions' must be able to be absorbed by the balloon (i.e. the organs of the body).

Other spaces are not 'filled', as such, but are 'bridged' by various sheets of muscle or fascial layers, which are represented by the tissue

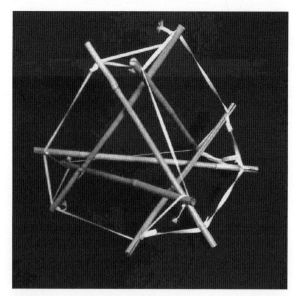

Figure 1.2 Basic tensegrity structure.

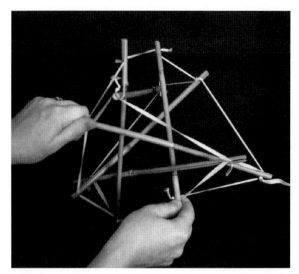

Figure 1.4 Structure torsioned another way closes those 'spaces' and opens others.

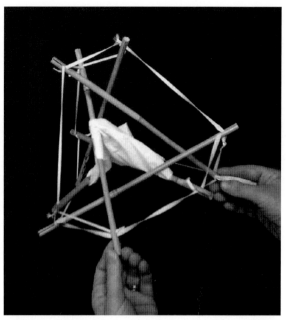

Figure 1.6 Other spaces are bridged with layers or sheets of 'muscle or fascia'.

between the sticks in Figure 1.6. Every time the structure as a whole distorts, the sheets must be able to flex and 'go with' that movement, in order not to restrict the flexibility of the overall structure.

Whenever there is a movement disorder or an alteration in tension of one 'elastic' structure or another (i.e. some muscle, tendon or other soft tissue structure), this will 'preset' the tensegrity structure (i.e. the body) to adopt a subtly distorted resting posture. Not only that, but when the body comes to move, the way in which the structure will now spring and twist 'around' this tension will be different from before. Thus areas of strain and stress will develop at various points in the structure where before none existed as the 'non-distorted' tensegrity structure dissipated load evenly, to all parts simultaneously.

As stated above, the sticks represent the compression components, i.e. the bones; the elastic represents the tensile components, i.e. tendons, ligaments and some fascial 'bands' or structures; the balloon represents the body cavities filled with organs; and the white tissue represents such things as the diaphragm, peritoneal or other fascial layers, that divide or surround the body cavities. In this context, visceral osteopathy is merely ensuring that none of the organs, fascial layers or other structures interfere with the global elasticity, flexibility and absorbability of the body as a whole.

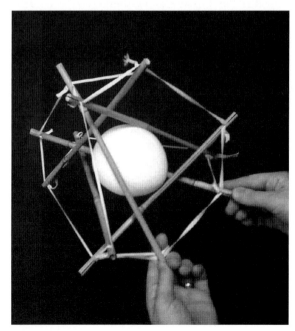

Figure 1.5 Some spaces are filled with non-compressible 'organs'.

FLUID DYNAMICS

Fascial sheaths, planes and cavities also form conduits for the passage of vessels and nerves. In this way, body cavity dynamics become involved in gross fluid movement throughout the body. The shifting layers illustrated by the tensegrity model demonstrate that there is the potential for much compressing and releasing of tissues and vessels in order to passively help the pumping and mobilizing of fluids.

Fluid, and in particular water, makes up a large part of each person. Body water content can change over time; for example, infants have low body fat and low bone mass and are 73% or more water whereas in old age, only about 45% of body weight is water. Healthy adult males are about 60% water while healthy adult females are around 50%. This difference reflects females' higher body fat and smaller amount of skeletal muscle.

Water occupies two main fluid compartments: intracellular and extracellular. Extracellular fluid consists of two major subdivisions: plasma, the fluid portion of the blood, and interstitial fluid in spaces between cells. A small proportion of extracellular fluid is also found in lymph, cerebrospinal fluid, eye humours, synovial fluid, serous fluid and gastrointestinal secretions.

Each fluid compartment of the body has a distinctive pattern of electrolytes. Extracellular fluids are similar (except for the high protein content of plasma) where sodium is the chief cation and chloride is the major anion. Intracellular fluids have low sodium and chloride where potassium is the chief cation and phosphate is the chief anion.

There is continual fluid movement amongst compartments, regulated by osmotic and hydrostatic pressures. Net leakage of fluid from the blood is picked up by lymphatic vessels and returned to the bloodstream. Exchanges between interstitial and intracellular fluids are complex due to the selective permeability of the cellular membranes. Two-way water flow is substantial.

Mechanical influences on fluid movement

Although the vast majority of the above-mentioned fluid movement is chemically and osmotically controlled, there is some passive influence arising from the physical squeezing and compressing of vessels and fluid spaces by various parts of the musculoskeletal system, and through the change in pressures caused by respiration.

The best known of these are the actions of the thoracic diaphragm and the calf pump mechanism. Both increase venous and lymphatic return to the heart on a gross scale.[4] Both inspiration and expiration will increase venous flow, depending on which vessels are observed. Subdiaphragmatic venous flow increases with inspiration, whereas pelvic or lower limb venous flow slows with inspiration.[5] As mentioned above, mechanical effects are also thought to operate on a cellular or interstitial fluid level, sometimes with relatively powerful effects[6] mediated through the mechanics of the extracellular matrix. Any and all body movement would engage the fascia and connective tissues (right down to the extracellular matrix) and create tiny mechanical shifts, torsions and mobilizations within it, causing tiny compressions and relaxations that help to move fluid and aid circulation and drainage. Hence body cavity movement helps with fluid dynamics on many levels.

This is a passive mobilizing force but one that can be affected by the tension states within the soft tissues and fascia of the body. Any trauma, torsion or irritation of the tissue will affect its elasticity and biomechanical properties and will therefore have a knock-on effect on the tissues' ability to promote fluid movement. As fluid dynamics in the microcirculation are very important to tissue health, any impairment of fluid flow would impede efficient homeostatic balance and physiological function. Osteopaths consider that this would form part of disease aetiology and pathological change within any affected tissue.[7]

Osteopaths would consider that they are aiding fluid movement by improving respiratory mechanics; by improving diaphragm function through mobilizing related anatomical and articulatory structures; by improving fascial and general connective tissue elasticity and mobility; and by releasing tension deep within the body, hypothesizing that this helps the extracellular matrix of tissue to be more flexible and therefore more accommodating to fluid movement. Fluid dynamics and lymphatic flow are discussed in further detail in a later chapter, where neural reflexes related to circulation are reviewed.

VISCERAL MOVEMENT, POSTURE AND TENSION RECEPTORS

All of the above-mentioned fascia, of course, surrounds and embeds the viscera, and the organs are simply a part of the movement continuum within the body cavities. Mobility of the organs will help promote serous fluid movement between peritoneal, dural, pericardial and pleural membranes, as well as within the muscular and mucosal layers of the organs themselves. As the movement passes through the organs, the mesenteries will be slightly distorted and will stretch and accommodate this movement, as well as the shifting pressures and stretches caused by changing volumes in the hollow organs (through digestion, bladder filling and so on), as well as respiratory movements.

The mesenteries, peritoneal ligaments and muscle walls of the organs have various receptors that are sensitive to a range of stimuli, both physical and chemical.[8] It seems that the fascial attachments of the organs can act as tension monitors, detecting the amount and possibly direction of forces acting upon the organs.[9] Factors that stimulate these receptors are not completely understood but it is being recognized that they might play a role in whole-body balance mechanisms through potential links with the vestibular system.[10] This takes the concept of visceral movement to a level beyond mere nutrition and into general body functioning and balance.

Osteopaths incorporate these concepts into their general biomechanical assessment of the body and these theories partly underpin their approach to three-dimensional movement disorders, where asymptomatic visceral restrictions are related to musculoskeletal system restrictions, strains and symptoms.

VISCERO–PTOSIS

Given the above discussion, osteopaths consider visceral function is related to efficient support, good circulation and drainage, and efficient movement patterns. In such circumstances visceral physiology should be optimum. Poor posture affects the integrity of the body cavity balance, leads to muscular imbalance, relaxation in some areas and tension in others. This affects visceral support and often leads to viscero-ptosis.

The weight of the abdominal cavity is normally supported through the pubis and is spread over the 'dome' of the pelvic organs. This helps to spread pressure away from the pelvic organs themselves. The viscera are held in a vertically oriented 'stack' or column, which is maintained by the abdominal muscles. The viscera literally support themselves and are effectively arranged in layers, supported by adjacent organs and by their mesenteric attachments. Any change in cavity dynamics or poor posture will lead to altered visceral position, and possibly viscero-ptosis. Viscero-ptosis can be clinically relevant in a variety of situations.

MECHANICAL EFFECTS OF POOR ORGAN SUPPORT

Poor visceral support can lead to viscero-ptosis or organ prolapse. This commonly affects the pelvic organs, as a result of pelvic floor weakness, or the gastrointestinal organs through a weakened lower abdominal wall (herniation).

Generalized changes in body posture seem to be related to alteration in visceral support mechanisms. Body cavity alignment and organ position do seem to change as people age, usually with the result that organs shift inferiorly over time. A number of changes have been noted through research. Hyoid position lowers as people age, which leads to changes in position of the mandible and descent of oropharyngeal structures.[11] The diaphragm descends slightly, which is related to a decrease in thoracic cage diameters.[12] Spinal changes, especially loss of lumbar lordosis, are related to pelvic organ prolapse,[13] and the pelvic floor lowers with age.[14] Organ prolapse is known to be multifactorial, with debate about the role of collagen and the smooth muscle content of local tissues, for example.[15] Little research has investigated the role of general postural change but osteopaths historically attribute to it many cases of prolapse.

Osteopaths would manage someone complaining of the physical effects of ptosis by first working on their posture and general body bio-mechanics in an attempt to reverse or alter to some degree the changes to the body cavities. They would consider that there is little point in only working locally (for example, by exercising the pelvic floor to strengthen it and so lift the pelvic organs) if the other areas of the body and body cavities were still in the adverse or ptosed posture. Osteopaths would start most cephalically, working to lift the sternum, raise the diaphragm and then lift the general visceral column by treating the abdominal region before finally coming to the pelvic region and addressing whatever local factors are present there.[16]

PHYSIOLOGICAL EFFECTS OF POOR ORGAN SUPPORT

Apart from mechanical distortion and prolapse of organs giving rise to various physical symptoms, cases of viscero-ptosis are also thought to lead to actual visceral dysfunction and disease. For many years, the role of viscero-ptosis in organ disease has been prominent in osteopathic philosophy. As far back as the late 19th and early 20th centuries, medical authors discussed the 'new' disease concept of viscero-ptosis, which struck a chord with many osteopaths (www.meridianinstitute.com/eamt/files/contents.htm). One such author was Byron Robinson, whose work *The abdominal and pelvic brain* (1907) was widely read (www.meridianinstitute.com/eamt/files/robinson/Rob1ch39.htm). He had the following to say on viscero-ptosis:

Splanchnoptosia though a single unit is a general disease of the thoracic and abdominal viscera accompanied by relaxation of the thoracic and abdominal muscular walls. In short splanchnoptosia prevails wherever the nerves of respiration innervate. In splanchnoptosia not only several viscera are simultaneously affected but also the thoracic and abdominal walls are relaxed. From an erroneous and limited view of the founder of splanchnoptosia (Glenard) and the acceptation of the error by numerous followers the idea has prevailed that ptosis of single viscera occur and to them numerous pathological symptoms have been attributed. Hence a stately literature has arisen from nephroptosia, stomachoptosia, coloptosia

(transverse), enteroptosia, etc., etc. On this error of single visceral ptosis has been founded the irrational surgery of so-called visceral pexies. One viscus may be afflicted with a greater degree of ptosis than another, however, splanchnoptosia is a general process affecting the thoracic and abdominal walls, the visceral mesenteries and visceral shelves.

He went on to say:

The abdominal viscera are maintained in their normal physiologic position by: (a) nerves and vessels; (b) peritoneum; (c) ligaments; (d) visceral pressure; (e) ligaments; (f) visceral shelves; (g) abdominal walls (muscular and osseous). The first idea of importance is that no organ is absolutely or immovably fixed but that each viscus is endowed with a certain degree of movement, hence, the irrational surgical fixation (pexies) of organs is obvious. The mobility of organs is due to various factors as: (a), attitude (prone or erect); (b), respiration; (c), material within the tractus intestinalis (ingesta, gas); (d), material within the tractus urinarius (urine); (e), muscular movement of viscera (rhythm) and abdominal wall; (f), gestation (material within the tractus genitalis). Hence the abdomen should be viewed as occupied with viscera capable of more or less mobility – that fixation of abdominal viscera is abnormal, as e.g. peritoneal bands and visceral pexies.

In general, in splanchnoptosia, canalization is compromised, nerve periphery traumatized, common visceral function (peristalsis, secretion, absorption, sensation) deranged; circulation (blood, and lymph) disordered; respiration disturbed – ending in malnutrition and neurosis. The symptoms of the splanchnoptotic are complex and numerous. Each cause in splanchnoptosia produces a vicious circle of – pathological physiology – pathological effects on the visceral tracts – digestive, genital, urinary, lymphatic, vascular, nervous, respiratory – impairing nourishment. Splanchnoptosia is often mistaken and wrongly diagnosed as neurasthenia, nervous exhaustion, hysteria, spinal anaemia, menopause, nervous dyspepsia, and neurosis.

Other problems of visceral mobility and consequent function were also discussed at length in the same era. One of the most popular was autointoxication: namely, being slowly poisoned by stagnation in the viscera and inappropriate absorption of matter into the body from luminal contents. This was considered to cause many irritating and debilitating disorders. Constipation was the most common disorder that was related to autointoxication, which has been associated with bodily ailments for millennia.[17] Autointoxication, like viscero-ptosis, was also a popular theme amongst early osteopathic practitioners.

In modern medical communities, both of these concepts have fallen out of favour and many now consider them thoroughly demoted to folklore. There are very few modern clinicians who would still consider them distinct disease entities, with set diagnostic criteria.[18] As medical fashions change over time, it is possible that many current concepts will be similarly derided when retrospectively reviewed. One such current 'catch-all' disorder which is commonly diagnosed and associated with a whole host of symptoms and systemic disorders (quite similar to those caused by viscero-ptosis, in fact) is fibromyalgia. In this disorder, postural misalignment or poor spinal or musculoskeletal movement is also related to the onset of the fibromyalgia syndrome,[19] which incorporates a whole host of generalized symptoms including pelvic pain, constipation, hypotension, thyroid problems, coccyx pain and tiredness.[20]

Osteopathic philosophy does on occasion still make reference to the idea of viscero-ptosis and autointoxication and still orients some aspects of management around these concepts. For the most part, though, visceral osteopathy makes more use of the mechanical components of viscero-ptosis, namely visceral prolapse, than it does of the disorder-as-disease component. That said, the influence of general body posture on organ orientation, mobility and function is still very important to osteopaths, and whenever the organs need to be addressed for whatever reason, that treatment must be 'contextualized' by considering what influences the general body is having on that organ dynamic. Some influences that general posture has on the viscera are illustrated in Figure 1.7.

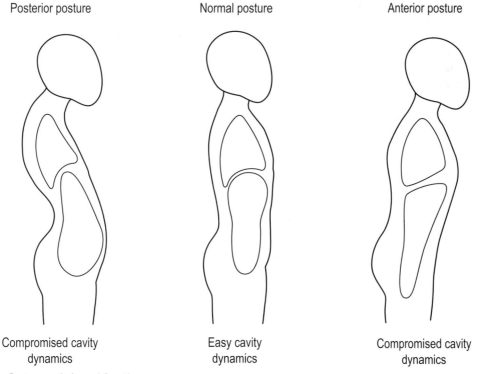

Posterior posture   Normal posture   Anterior posture

Compromised cavity dynamics   Easy cavity dynamics   Compromised cavity dynamics

Figure 1.7 Posture and visceral function.

When dealing with cases of prolapse, osteopaths would literally start from the top. It is not thought useful only to address organ prolapse, say, in the lower pelvic bowl, without first 'relieving pressure' on the whole visceral stack and fascial systems of the body by raising all the tissues from the head and throat, and then moving onto the thorax to lift the diaphragm, which will then engage the abdominal organs, supporting them superiorly, and finally taking pressure off the pelvic organs, allowing them to settle into a new position. This can then be maintained by re-strengthening the pelvic floor and lower abdominal muscles, and by ensuring that the postural adjustments do not revert, if possible.

VISCERAL MOTION

The osteopathic management of visceral problems and the use of visceral techniques within the management of musculoskeletal problems involve more than just knowing a few techniques to mobilize the organs. AT Still, the founder of osteopathy, was reported never to teach technique at all; he only ever demonstrated treatments and students had to sort out for themselves what was being done on an individual basis. There is great merit in this approach, as describing a technique in isolation cannot represent what is meant by a treatment. It is virtually impossible to describe a sensation in print; in other words, it is difficult to teach someone without them receiving direct feedback regarding their palpatory experiences as they explore the visceral field. However, even the best hands-on instructors cannot impart everything at one sitting and so a reference text discussing how osteopaths approach the treatment of viscera is of value. In this chapter, the underlying concepts of visceral movement are introduced (acting as preparation on how to evaluate and potentially treat patients with visceral factors).

The study of visceral movement dynamics has long been part of the osteopathic approach to patient care.[21] Its study outside osteopathy is also now becoming more relevant to orthodox medicine, and there is increasing research into measuring the normal physiological patterns of visceral movement.[22]

As discussed before, visceral osteopathy involves the use of various types of mobilization applied directly to the organs through the body wall, or indirectly through movements applied to body sections or segments that are attached physically or reflexly related to the organs within the body cavities.[16,23]

In addition to gross movements, all tissues, including the organs, will bend, be deformed and undergo stretch and compression during general body movements and respiration. The quality or quantity of such dynamics depends upon the physical properties of tissues such as viscoelasticity, creep and hysteresis, which describe the behaviour of the tissue under loading, stress and strain. Osteopaths consider that these physical characteristics give each organ a unique 'feel' which can help to identify it and its degree of health. Altered physical properties arising from inflammation and other pathological processes will affect palpable visceral characteristics such as stretch, deformation and compressibility. In this way, osteopaths can distinguish to some degree whether a tissue is normal or not normal (although, of course, one cannot diagnose any individual condition or state by feel alone).

Discussion on the osteopathic interest in visceral motion therefore includes not only gross movements of the organs but also their 'internal' physical properties such as compliance, stretch, deformity and so on, as well as any physiological movements such as peristalsis or other 'pacemaker' activities. Osteopaths are also interested in what they term 'motility'. Unfortunately for matters such as interprofessional communication and scientific comparisons and research, this does not mean what others would understand it to be: namely peristalsis, contractility and smooth muscle myogenic or neurogenic activity. Osteopaths use the term to refer to the natural rhythmic vitality of the tissues and organs, which is being expressed through a cyclic repetition of the embryological movement and migration patterns that the tissues and organs followed during development. Osteopaths also call this movement 'inherent motion' and believe it can be evaluated and compared to 'normal' and also 'treated', in the sense that the body or tissue can be encouraged through touch and certain types of mobilizations to return to expressing its natural and normal rhythmic pattern of 'motility'. These movements are further discussed below.

GROSS VISCERAL MOBILITY

Osteopathic visceral mobility testing involves trying to replicate 'normal' movement and see if the organs and tissues allow that or if the movement appears adapted/restricted or altered in some way. In order to appreciate the various aspects of visceral movement and how osteopaths may examine and ultimately treat organs for a variety of 'disorders', it is necessary to consider further those factors that would influence the gross movements of organs.

SLIDING SURFACES

Peritoneal, pleural, pericardial, capsular, dural and other fascial/connective tissues coverings, wrappings and layers form surfaces along which the organs can slide or move. The above tissues are mostly serous membranes, which secrete fluids, such as peritoneal fluid, pleural fluid and so on, that buffer contact between membranes (sliding surfaces), creating easy movement of one organ on another or of an organ against part of the body wall or musculoskeletal structure.[24] The lubricating action of the fluids is normally independent of such things as changes in force and direction of movement.[25]

Gross movement of the organs (rather than simple peristalsis) is often described as 'visceral slide' by the orthodox medical profession. Its physiological importance is not currently recognized or explored, however. Note: the term 'visceral slide' is usually confined to the normal, longitudinal movement of the intraabdominal viscera caused by respiratory excursions of the diaphragm. Beyond recognizing that organs move as a result of external forces acting upon them, such as diaphragmatic excursion and torsion through the ribcage or muscular abdominal wall, little study seems to have been done regarding the physiological importance of that movement for most of the organs, except perhaps for the pelvic organs.[26]

The sliding and movement of various organs are being increasing well mapped through ultrasound imaging or cine mode magnetic resonance imaging.

These imaging techniques can help in various surgical approaches or to avoid various complications. For example, ultrasound imaging is often used prior to laparoscopic surgery, to prevent trocar (cannular) penetration of the greater omentum or other adhered organs and hence further subsequent adhesion formation.[27] The presence of restrictions on ultrasound images has also been found to be a reliable indicator of the presence of actual adhesions, on subsequent surgical exploration.[28] These adhesions are often between the anterior abdominal wall and the greater omentum, which arises from the greater curvature of the stomach and has connections with the transverse colon and the posterior abdominal wall. Adhesions can alter the normal visceral mobility and sometimes even the position of the organs. Note: osteopathic management of adhesions and painful sequelae is discussed later.

The above types of imaging have given rise to the study of visceral kinematics within orthodox medicine. These studies are now so sophisticated that they can show such things as uterine peristalsis in real time and the presence of many types of intraabdominal adhesions.[24] These imaging processes would clearly be of great value in monitoring the effect of visceral manipulation on adhesion flexibility and visceral mobility, and would be very useful research tools.

The physiological and clinical relevance of all this movement of the organs, through respiratory diaphragm excursion, general body movement and changing volumes of the hollow organs, is not fully understood or acknowledged. Nor is the potential for any alteration, reduction or cessation of that movement to contribute to pathological change recognized as particularly important. To reiterate, osteopaths consider that reduction in motion (be it amplitude, direction or timing) is highly relevant to an organ's ability to function appropriately, and that manipulating or mobilizing the organ in some way would help to restore more appropriate physiological function, thus promoting health.

Examples of this passive mobility of organs would include the elongation of the heart with diaphragmatic descent; mobilization of the prostate with pelvic floor contraction; movement of the cervix and uterus during intercourse; stretching of the pharyngeal lymphoid tissue in speech and neck movements; deformation of the eustachian tube in swallowing and jaw movements; descent of the sub-diaphragmatic organs during respiration and movement of the bladder with pelvic floor relaxation. If these global organ movements are not possible, then some physiological impairment is thought to follow.

Visceral mobility testing involves trying to replicate 'normal' movement and see if organs allow that or if the movement appears adapted, restricted or altered in some way. The distortion from normal forms part of the diagnostic description and guides treatment protocols. It also gives a comparison of 'before and after' treatment to help assess change and monitor treatment outcomes.

ARTICULATIONS

The physical anatomy of visceral and other structures gives rise to movement patterns that are effectively 'predetermined' by the shape of the organ, the orientation of its blood vessels and supportive tissues or 'ligaments', and the proximity and consistency of adjacent structures. These movement patterns are generally predictable and can be thought of as 'articulations' of the organs. Examples of visceral articulations are given in Table 1.1.

The organ articulations can thus be examined much as one would those of a musculoskeletal joint. Normal range of movement, end feel, midrange

Table 1.1   Examples of visceral articulations

Visceral structure	Sliding surface	Posterior articulations	Anterior articulations	Lateral articulations	Superior articulations	Inferior articulations
Kidney	Slides within renal fascia	Moves over psoas, quadratus lumborum and 12th ribs, cysterna chyli and lymphatic duct	Duodenum on right, tail of pancreas, and splenic flexure on left	Spleen and descending colon on left, ascending colon on right	Adrenal gland and liver	Ureter
Uterus	Broad ligament, retrovesical pouch and pouch of Douglas	Small intestine and rectum	Small intestine	Parametrium and fallopian tubes	Small intestine and sigmoid	Bladder
Liver	Bare area of liver	Diaphragm	Diaphragm and upper abdominal wall muscles	Diaphragm and ribcage	Diaphragm	Kidney, stomach, duodenum, colon
Stomach	Lesser sac (omental bursa)	Pancreas	Diaphragm and upper abdominal wall muscles	Spleen	Diaphragm	Transverse colon, small intestine
Upper lobe of lung	Oblique fissure on left, horizontal fissure on right	Ribcage via parietal pleura	Ribcage via parietal pleura	Ribcage via parietal pleura	Scalenes and cervicobrachial structures via pleural dome and Sibson's fascia	Diaphragm via parietal pleura
Heart	Pericardium	Broncho-pulmonary ligament	Sternum, via sterno-pericardial ligament	Lungs, via mediastinal pleural	Hilum of lungs and great vessels	Diaphragm, via pericardial sac

quality, amplitude and so on can be identified and compared to physical findings. Changes to the expected norm are then considered and rationalized with respect to such things as any pathological process, surgical intervention, general body tension pattern or reflex phenomenon. Clearly, congenital malformations, anomalies, extra or missing organs, surgical alteration or scarring and adhesions can all alter the relative position or movement of an organ. Careful attention should be paid to the case history for indications of the above and accurate palpation, where the osteopath tries to be objective and open-minded during assessment, usually means that most gross anomalies are identified (or at least suspected) during examination.

AXES OF MOVEMENT

Each organ will naturally move in a particular manner, direction and amplitude through the influence of various supports, surrounding structures and physical attachments to the body walls or blood vessels, for example. Despite some inevitable 'margin of error' caused through normal anatomical variation, visceral movements can be reasonably accurately and consistently described.

Influence of 'ligaments'

Many organs have so-called 'ligaments' or mesenteries supporting them. These are made from pleural, peritoneal and other fascial/connective tissue sheets or structures and the term is not synonymous with that used to describe the dense arrangement of fibres that make up the connecting structures between bones. Some authors consider that use of the term 'ligament' in describing visceral anatomical structures is unwarranted and causes confusion[29] but this is unlikely to change in practice.

The ligaments or mesenteries not only influence the directions of the movement but also provide routes for the passage of nerves, blood and lymph vessels. Figure 1.8 shows some of the ligaments supporting and guiding the ascending colon: Toldt's fascia fixes the ascending colon posteriorly whilst the mesocolon allows the transverse colon some movement, thereby creating a 'hinge' between the 'fixed' ascending colon and the 'mobile' transverse colon. The hepatic flexure is kept suspended superiorly by the phrenicocolic ligament.

Influence of vascular pedicles

Many organs are not only nourished by blood vessels but are also supported by them, such as the kidneys, ovaries and testes, liver, heart and lungs. In the case of the kidneys, the vascular supports give slightly different movement patterns on either side. The left kidney has a relatively shorter artery than vein, and the right kidney has a relatively longer artery than vein (due to the position of the aorta being left of the inferior vena cava), as shown in Figure 1.9. This means the right kidney is slightly less well supported by its longer artery than the left.

As another example, the left renal vein is the tributary for the drainage of the left testicular or ovarian vein (whereas on the right, these veins drain directly into the inferior vena cava). This means that the left ovarian or testicular vein has a longer and more vertical drainage route than the right, and is draining into a more mobile (and therefore more easily compromised) left renal vein, due to the slightly different renal mobility on this side). Hence left testicular or ovarian varicosities are more common than on the right.

Influence of surrounding structures

The posterior abdominal wall, the pelvic bowl, the respiratory diaphragm, tentorium, pelvic floor or ribcage are all examples of anatomical non-visceral structures that can influence visceral position, movement and function.

Facet influence on cavity dynamics

The differing shapes of the vertebral facets create different dynamics for cavity movements which, coupled with basic fascial arrangements, means various sections of the vertebral column have interesting functional links with various body cavities, and the organs therein.

- Upper cervicals control throat and into head.
- Midcervical spine down to upper dorsal spine controls upper mediastinum.
- Midthoracic spine controls lower mediastinal and peridiaphragmatic areas.
- Lower thoracic spine down to midlumbar spine controls abdomen.

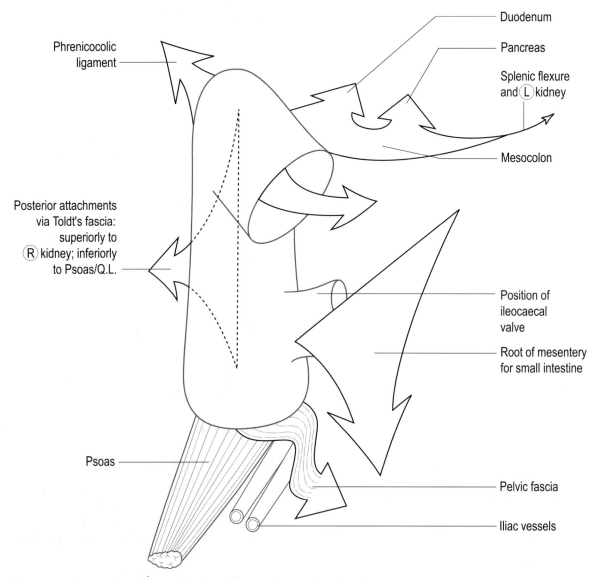

Figure 1.8 Some peritoneal/connective tissue 'ligaments' supporting the colon.

- Lower lumbar spine and sacrum controls pelvis.

Interestingly, these facet analogies also correlate with neural relationships via the sympathetic nervous system.

- Upper cervicals link with superior cervical ganglia to affect head and throat structures.
- Mid to lower cervicals, to D4 region via stellate, middle cervical ganglia and the first four paravertebral chain ganglia affect mediastinal organs (anything remaining above diaphragm).
- Below D4 region to dorsolumbar region affects subdiaphragmatic and abdominal organs.
- Upper lumbar spine down to pelvis affects pelvic organs, via hypogastric plexus.

Neural relationships are discussed in more detail in a later chapter.

Figure 1.10 shows the facet orientations of some of the vertebrae. In the upper cervicals, the

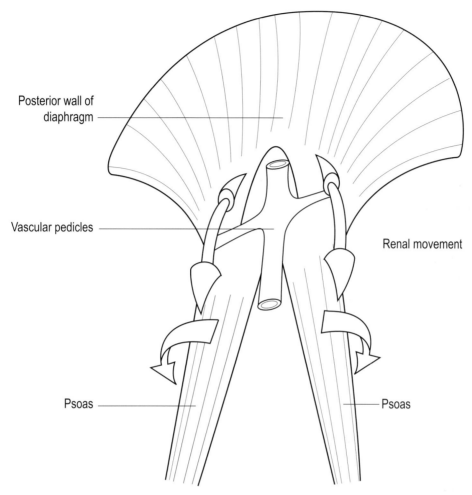

Figure 1.9 Support of the kidney and renal fascia and 'vascular pedicles'.

facets face either superiorly or directly anteriorly, giving the unique rotatory and tilting motions of the upper neck. In the rest of the cervical spine, the facets are slightly concave posteriorly above C5 and slightly convex posteriorly below C5. The lower cervical facets are similar in orientation to the dorsal facets, above D4. The lower cervicals effectively work with the upper dorsals and as the facets curve slightly posteriorly, the axis of rotation of this area of the spine is slightly behind the vertebral bodies. On rotation of the head, the throat area and anterior upper ribcage will move more than the posterior components of the neck (being near the circumference of the turning circle of the cervical spine).

From the lower cervical spine, there are a number of fascial attachments, linking the lungs and other mediastinal contents to the spine. Thus, when the neck rotates, the upper parts of the lungs and mediastinal contents follow as they are engaged by their fascial attachments. Below D4 and above the lower dorsal spine, the facets curve slightly anteriorly, giving an axis of rotation of the spine anterior to the vertebral bodies. The visceral fascial links in this section of the body pass from the D4–5 region anteriorly to the sternum, and link together the spine, bronchi, posterior wall of the heart and the anterior pericardium with the sternum. When the thorax rotates, this section of the body will follow the facet orientation,

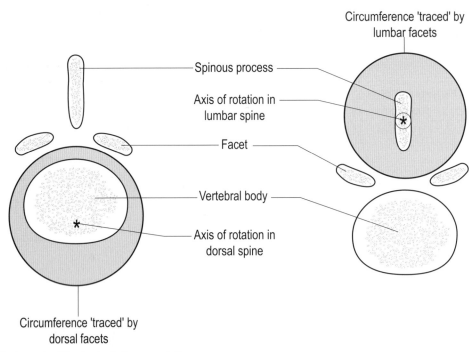

Figure 1.10 Impact of facet orientation on rotation.

with the posterior part moving more than in the cervical region. Now, as the organs move with the dorsal spine, the organs are in a relatively 'static' position, with the bony components moving around them (being near the axis of rotation of the thoracic spine). The other cavity rotation patterns are also shown in Figure 1.11.

From the lower dorsal spine, the facets are oriented more with the upper lumbars, with the facets now facing more posteriorly again. The fascial attachments in this region guide the subdiaphragmatic organs and the upper gastrointestinal tract. Now, these organs again move nearer the circumference of the turning circle of the spine, and rotate in a similar manner to the throat structures. Continuing down the spine, the lower lumbars and the sacrum are fascially attached to the pelvic organs (sigmoid, rectum, urogenital organs). The facets again change direction slightly and are now oriented more inferiorly. This gives a turning circle with the axis slightly within the pelvic bowl. Coupled with the fascial attachments linking the organs to the sacrum and low lumbars, this means that those organs should rotate anterior to the spine. However, in practice, because of the closed bony circle of the pelvis, this rotation is

adapted to a superior and inferior 'spiralling' movement.

> In practice, this means that the organs are used to operating in a particular mobile environment, each with its own basic axes of movement, as shown in Figure 1.11. In a global visceral assessment, these basic patterns can be helpful in appreciating the level of distortion from normal, in much the same way as a global spinal assessment.

Diaphragmatic recesses

The junction between the cervicodorsal-controlled cavity zone (thoracic organs) and the lower dorsal–upper lumbar-controlled cavity zone (abdominal organs) is interesting, as the organs here are in a transition movement pattern. Coupled with the anatomical configuration of the costodiaphragmatic pleural recesses and the renal fascia, this means that the lower lobes of the lungs and the kidneys move more in a superior inferior direction than a rotatory pattern. Again, any conflict between the cavity dynamics and this transition zone will manifest in visceral restrictions

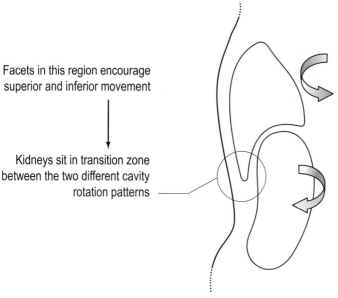

Facets in this region encourage superior and inferior movement

Kidneys sit in transition zone between the two different cavity rotation patterns

Thoracic/chest movement is 'anterior', as facets in this region encourage 'anterior' movement

Lumbar/abdominal cavity movement is 'posterior', as facets in this region encourage posterior movement

Figure 1.11   Differing rotation in cavities in relation to facet shapes.

and dysfunction. The transitional zone movements are shown in Figure 1.12.

Psoas shelves

Other architectural arrangements of the body's anatomy can affect movement patterns. For example, the psoas muscles form a 'shelf' upon which the kidneys move up and down (as per their transition zone movements). However, the psoas muscles are curved and as the kidneys move down, they also rotate externally and have a slightly lateral pendular movement, as they 'roll over' the curved belly of the psoas. This renal movement is illustrated in Figure 1.9, where the kidneys can slide up and down the 'shelves' of the psoas muscles, guided by their vascular pedicles.

Curve of posterior abdominal wall

The anterior curve of the posterior abdominal wall reinforces the rotation dynamic of the abdominal cavity, exaggerating the way the small intestine in particular swings from side to side during spinal movement.

Funnel of pelvic floor and curve of the pubis

The pelvic floor muscles create a very interesting movement dynamic within the pelvic bowl.

Coupled with the enclosed bony shape of the pelvis, the muscles will adapt the pelvic organ motion to a superior and inferior moving spiral. This superior and inferior movement moves the pelvic organs upwards into the zone of the lower abdomen, where they meet the lateral rotatory movements of the lower abdominal zone. The spiral motion develops as a transition between the abdominal lateral rotation, the curve of the pubis and the funnel shape of the pelvic floor muscles that induce the superior and inferior motion. Again, any conflict between the cavity dynamics and this transition zone will manifest in visceral restrictions and dysfunction.

ORGAN FLEXIBILITY, DEFORMITY AND COMPLIANCE – 'INTERNAL MOBILITY'

Stretch, compliance and elasticity of an organ or tissue are natural components depending on the histology and internal anatomy of that tissue ('structure governs function'). As such, each will have its own biomechanical properties and physical consistency, which can be appreciated to varying degrees during palpatory examination. The osteopathic examination of visceral slide and

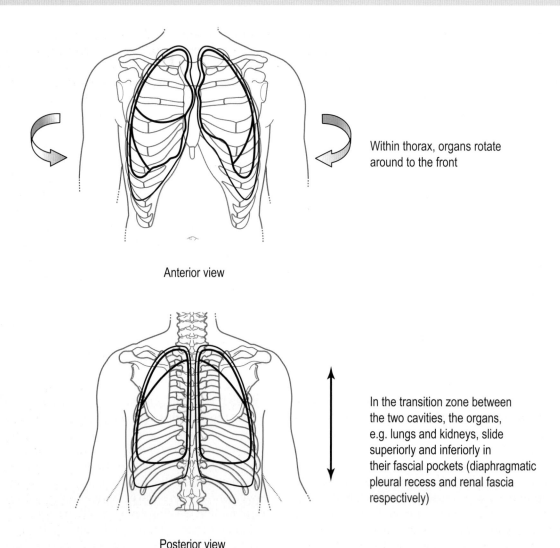

Within thorax, organs rotate around to the front

Anterior view

In the transition zone between the two cavities, the organs, e.g. lungs and kidneys, slide superiorly and inferiorly in their fascial pockets (diaphragmatic pleural recess and renal fascia respectively)

Posterior view

Figure 1.12   Different directions of slide in regional cavity dynamics.

organ mobility consists of evaluating these factors as well, and incorporating them alongside other physical examinations and standard medical test results (if applicable) to formulate a working diagnosis for patient management.

MOTION CHANGES IN RELATION TO FUNCTION OR PATHOLOGY

Restriction of mobility is a consequence of many pathological processes. Inflammation, for example, will alter the consistency of the serous fluid, in essence making it sticky, contributing to reduced movement and decreased slide between organs. Surgery and scarring or adhesions can also reduce visceral slide,[30] as can muscular spasm and contraction within an organ. Osteopaths can carefully examine the body in order to explore the movement possibilities created by the natural sliding surfaces of the organs, so determining whether the movement of the organ is 'normal' or 'abnormal'.

Tissues adapt and remodel themselves constantly. In somatic tissues (skeletal muscle, for example), this phenomenon is well known, where muscle fibres will modify their internal anatomy to adapt to differing strains caused by immobilization, eccentric exercise or surgical tendon transfer.[31] The same is thought to be true of visceral hollow organs and smooth muscle structures where, for example, smooth muscles adapt to loads such as intestinal obstruction, which causes hypertrophy and other changes.[32]

There is a whole bioengineering field of study, looking at the links between biological structure and function. Its 'founder', YC Fung, suggests that biomechanics is the 'middle name' between biological structure and function.[33] The study of the biomechanics of human tissues seeks to explain their function on the basis of structure and mechanics. A central research goal in the study of tissue mechanics is understanding (and thus better controlling) the mechanics in relation to the structure of any biological tissue, how mechanical information is transduced by the cells, and how changes in the cellular and molecular structure of tissues thereby affect function.

The structure–function relations in skeletal muscle, for example, are well recognized and the changes to muscle fibre arrangements in response to mechanical force are well documented. Muscles can change their internal architecture in response to immobilization, eccentric exercise and surgical tendon transfer. Stress and strain acting upon a tissue induces change so that the tissue is more suitably adapted to its new biomechanical environment.[31]

The same appears true of many visceral hollow organs and smooth muscle structures. Smooth muscles do adapt to loads such as intestinal obstruction, which causes hypertrophy and other changes.[32] The function of the bladder is dependent on its underlying structure. Change in the ratio of connective tissue to smooth muscle components, for example, can significantly alter compliance and functional capacity, structurally impairing the bladder's ability to empty fully.[34]

The mere fact of motion passing through all tissues is intimately linked with how the cells communicate and therefore function. All tissues are linked by a fascial web and at a cellular level, integrins connect the extracellular matrix to the internal cell skeleton, via the membrane. Integrins are known to act as mechanoreceptors.[3] Mechanotransduction engages the cytoskeleton through to the DNA, and this vibratory motion passes through the cell in a dynamic, harmonic manner.

Cellular events such as membrane ruffling, changes in shape and motility, and signal transduction occur within spatial and temporal harmonics that have potential regulatory importance, and these vibrations can be altered by growth factors and carcinogenesis, for example, indicating that they are linked with pathogenesis and altered function.[35] Even fluid circulation is dependent on movement[36] and any changes in microcirculation at a cellular level (including capillary permeability) resulting in interstitial compositional changes may play an important role in disease development.[37] Within lymphatic vessels (coupled with a spontaneous contractility), expansion and compression of the initial lymphatics depend on deformation of the tissue in which they are embedded, indicating that mechanical factors influence fluid movement.[38] Also, within organs bounded by serous membranes (peritoneum, pleura and pericardium), the gross movement of the organs helps with cavity dynamics and fluid circulation.[39,40]

If the tissues' biomechanical architecture is changed (due to stress, injury, torsions or tension, for example) then microcirculation, initial lymphatic flow, mechanical signalling and cellular communication all become altered, and this could have significant effects on tissue function. This concept underpins much of the osteopathic clinical philosophy. Improving mobility and changing motion patterns will readapt the internal architecture of tissues over time, thus influencing the physiological (mechanical and fluidic) properties of that structure with the aim of improving health and immunity. Tissue remodelling through application of manual techniques in pathological situations is considered important for disease progression.

Fung's efforts could be summarized as trying to wed engineering science with biology. Accompanying research could aim to evaluate and categorize the changes in tissue mechanics that various pathological processes and states induce in the tissues. This would then be a scientific expression of something osteopaths as yet are only able to describe in lay terms, as a result of what they are feeling during palpation.

PERISTALSIS AND PACEMAKER ACTIVITY IN SMOOTH MUSCLE ORGANS

The smooth muscles of the organs and other cells within the organ structure appear responsible for internal motion of an organ, such as intestinal peristalsis.[41] Peristalsis is not just a rhythmic phenomenon that is unique to the gut, as a way of 'unconsciously' moving digested products from one section to another. Peristalsis occurs in all hollow organs, such as the bladder,[42] stomach,[43] bile duct,[44] ureter,[45] uterus[46] and vas deferens.[47] It also occurs within the 'solid' organs such as the prostate[48] and liver,[49] where there are peristaltic-like waves within the organs and their ducts or 'exits' (although it is not always clear whether neurogenic or myogenic properties are operating). These peristaltic waves often appear to be coordinated and not just random; in other words, they appear to be under some sort of pacemaker activity.[50] Peristaltic waves also appear in other visceral-related structures such as the lymphatic channels in the mesenteries.[30]

Pathological function in all of the above organs is related to or associated with changes to peristaltic activity within their smooth muscle components. Pharmacological approaches are commonly used to address these peristaltic aberrations but the osteopathic approach would be to mobilize and stretch or physically work with the tissue in a particular way, with the aim of influencing smooth muscle reactivity and feedback reflex loops within the nervous system influencing that activity, to normalize the peristaltic and pacemaker activities of those tissues and organs. This concept underpins much of the 'visceral osteopathy' management protocols in various diseases and pathological situations.

VISCERAL 'MOTILITY' AND EMBRYOLOGY

Embryology is fundamental to understanding function in practice. Osteopaths use embryology in many contexts during patient management and do not confine themselves to using it as a descriptive mechanism for understanding congenital malformation.

One embryological concept that osteopaths use is their belief that all tissues from the same embryological derivations and basic tissue types remain 'functionally' related during life. All mesenchymal structures have a similar vitality and interrelatedness, as do all ectoderm structures and so on. Even though the tissues have differentiated into many seemingly totally unrelated structures in the adult, they can still be 'recognized through touch' as being in communication with each other, and with their embryological roots.

Another concept is derived from the way in which tissues are moulded by the motive forces created by the emerging functionality within the embryo. All cells within the embryo have a metabolic field; even before recognizable blood vessels have begun to form, structures must be nourished and metabolic waste removed. Each cell will be oriented around its metabolic field in such a way that it can be enabled to function and further differentiate. The differentiation of cells will happen at various rates, causing a range of kinetic forces to be produced which in themselves will compress some tissues and stretch others. The physicality of differentiation promotes further development and change, each in accordance with the metabolic needs of the cells or tissue concerned. The embryo's living cells exert biodynamic stresses against each other which spatially orient and direct ongoing growth and movement.

This spatial awareness and integration within and between the tissues leaves a palpable trace within the body, even as an adult. One branch of osteopathy considers that health is organized around the directional and spatial lines of development which were oriented around the metabolic needs of those tissues. In order for tissue health to be maintained, tissues must be helped to organize themselves around their original metabolic fields and midline development. This is done through applying very gentle palpatory exploration of the tissues to allow them to reorganize themselves towards better function.

Much of the underlying theory for these concepts was developed by Blechschmidt[51] who used the term 'biodynamics' to describe the movements of these metabolic fields in the developing embryo.

He felt that these dynamic fields of activity seemed to arise from the very geometry of the cellular foundations of life and produced distinct patterns of movement. Those migration patterns within the developing embryo (observed and described by Blechschmidt) appear to be identical to the movement patterns observed and described by William Sutherland in the process of osteopathic treatment. In essence, the 'generative' forces of the developing embryo are identical to the 'regenerative' forces used for healing in all of us (www.osteodoc.com/ biodynamics.htm). How this feels in practice is beyond the scope of this book but it is sufficient to state that this concept is used by many osteopaths in their daily practice and can be applied to the examination and treatment of visceral dysfunction.

A more easily discussed embryological-palpatory concept is that of 'visceral motility' which was introduced in the introduction. Visceral motility represents the remnants of the motive forces created and utilized during development, in a more generalized way than the biodynamic approach above. For example, the gut tube elongates, twists and then migrates, part of it in an anticlockwise direction when viewed from the front and part of it in a clockwise direction when viewed from above. Another example is the heart, which starts as a straight tube and then twists on itself into a figure of eight, before merging and developing into four distinct chambers.

In development, then, the organs have each undergone a particular rotatory, spiral migration to reach their adult destination, shape and form. Through adult life, it is as though the organs are still trying to continue that spiralling pattern – they express the same 'momentum of direction' that they grew with. As the organs clearly do not continue to change position in adult life, the organs are felt to express a cyclical motion which is akin to an initiation of motion into their embryological orientation, followed by a pendular or cyclical return to a neutral 'starting' position. This cyclical movement is small and represents the vital forces still being expressed within the body. It is an involuntary or inherent motion or motility. This motility can be palpated, and the osteopath can help it restore itself to a better rhythm and pattern if this is somehow disturbed. Disturbance or distortion of this inherent motion is thought to be related to poor function, inefficient physiology,

and ill health within the tissues. Restoring effective and normal motility is felt to improve health and better function.

The patterns and expressions of visceral motility were originally described by Jean-Pierre Barral,[23] building on the work of William Garner Sutherland.[52]

BASIC VISCERAL MOTILITY

Readers should refer to the appendix for an illustration of each organ's motility, as per Barral's descriptions.

TESTS

The visceral motility is a pendular movement that occurs around a neutral point. Each organ will have its own axes of movement, its own amplitude, quality and symmetry. One direction of swing of the pendular motion is referred to as 'inspir' and the returning direction is referred to as 'expir'. The organs should express their motility in a rhythmic and balanced way. If there are any restrictions, scars, tension, spasm, emotional problems or other irritations, then the motility of the organ can be altered in some way. Usually there is more emphasis of the motion either in expir or inspir (the organ moves well one way but doesn't return easily). Visceral motility is not quite a 'virtual movement' but it is subtle and the movements within are very small (unlike mobility, which can be quite large, depending on organ ligaments, or peristalsis, which can be measured easily on ultrasounds or real-time MRI). Objective measurement of motility is still being explored.

That said, the aim in treatment is to restore motility to the affected organ. This is usually done with a technique called 'induction'. The motility of the organ is 'listened' to passively, to determine the alteration from normal of its motility pattern. During induction, the hand will slightly accentuate or exaggerate the larger motion (be it inspir or expir) or the motion with the better quality (if the amplitude is not too altered). On the return motion, do not block this but do not encourage it either. There is a very small component of 'resistance' which is more as though the practitioner is 'ignoring' the return motion rather than actually following it. Keep 'encouraging' the larger motion until the induced motility matches the expected normal motility for that organ. The motility may reach a 'still point' or neutral, where there is no movement occurring for a while. Often this lasts a few seconds or a minute or two, after which the organs will restart their restored motility (in the 'proper' or optimal direction). The practitioner should not force the tissues and if the wait appears quite long, sometimes this is because the technique has been incorrectly applied, the still point has been missed or the practitioner is working in the wrong place (and has therefore misdiagnosed the motility problem).

An addition to Barral's approach would include the use of a direct technique to first isolate or reduce the influence of surrounding ligamentous or soft tissue irritations acting upon the organ, to see if those irritations are the cause of the reduction in motility observed. In this instance, the organ will be contacted and lifted gently into a direction that relaxes or eases tension in surrounding soft tissues. The movement here is one of mobility, into a pathway of least resistance

(not into a direction that engages any tissue barrier). Once the organ is suitably 'supported' in its optimal position (by the practitioner remaining in contact with the tissues), the organ's motility can be observed again. If the surrounding tissues are adversely affecting the motility, it will return or improve whilst the organ is being physically supported/relieved of the pressure of surrounding tissue tension. This indicates that the motility change was secondary to the primary articular or ligamentous restriction of the surrounding tissues. If the motility is unchanged during this process then the tissue should be released and the above-described technique of induction applied, as this time the problem is a primary one of motility.

The concept of motility can be used just as a monitoring tool or a primary mode of treatment. For those who do not use it in practice at all, there are still many aspects of visceral work that can be done, utilizing a whole variety of mobility tests and treatments, and a beneficial patient outcome should be achieved.

References

1. Frymann VM. The core-link and the three diaphragms. A unit for respiratory function. In: The collected papers of Viola M Frymann DO, 2nd edn. Michigan: Edward Brothers; 2000:134-40.
2. Cathie D. The fascia of the body in relation to function and manipulative therapy. Indianapolis: American Academy of Osteopathy Year Book; 1974:81-4.
3. Wang N, Butler JP, Ingber DE. Mechanotransduction across the cell surface and through the cytoskeleton. Science 1993;260(5111):1124-7.
4. Miller JD, Pegelow DF, Jacques AJ, Dempsey JA. Skeletal muscle pump versus respiratory muscle pump: modulation of venous return from the locomotor limb in humans. J Physiol Online 2005; 563(3):925-43.
5. Willeput R, Rondeux C, De Troyer A. Breathing affects venous return from legs in humans. J Appl Physiol 1984;57(4):971-6.
6. Schmid-Schonbein GW. Microlymphatics and lymph flow. Physiol Rev 1990;70(4):987-1028.
7. Northop T. Role of connective tissue in acute and chronic disease. Paper presented at the Annual Meeting of the Academy of Applied Osteopathy, Atlantic City, 1952:67-9.
8. Grundy D. What activates visceral afferents? Gut 2004;53(Suppl 2):ii5-8.
9. Grundy D. Speculations on the structure/function relationship for vagal and splanchnic afferent endings supplying the gastrointestinal tract. J Auton Nervous System 1988;22:175-80.
10. von Gierke HE, Parker DE. Differences in otolith and abdominal viscera graviceptor dynamics: implications for motion sickness and perceived body position. Aviat Space Environ Med 1994;65(8):747-51.
11. Kollias I, Krogstad O. Adult craniocervical and pharyngeal changes – a longitudinal cephalometric study between 22 and 42 years of age. Part II: Morphological uvulo-glossopharyngeal changes. Eur J Orthodont 1999;21(4): 345-55.

12. Suwatanapongched T, Gierada DS, Slone RM, Pilgram TK, Tuteur PG. Variation in diaphragm position and shape in adults with normal pulmonary function. Chest 2003;123(6):2019-27.

13. Mattox TF, Lucente V, McIntyre P, Miklos JR, Tomezsko J. Abnormal spinal curvature and its relationship to pelvic organ prolapse. Am J Obstet Gynecol 2000;183(6):1381-4; discussion 1384.

14. Pinho M, Yoshioka K, Ortiz J, Oya M, Keighley MR. The effect of age on pelvic floor dynamics. Int J Colorectal Dis 1990;5(4):207-8.

15. Goh JT. Biomechanical and biochemical assessments for pelvic organ prolapse. Curr Opin Obstet Gynecol 2003;15(5):391-4.

16. Stone C. Science in the art of osteopathy. Cheltenham: Nelson Thornes; 1999.

17. Chen TS, Chen PS. Intestinal autointoxication: a medical leitmotif. J Clin Gastroenterol 1989;11(4):434-1.

18. Baron JH, Sonnenberg A. The wax and wane of intestinal autointoxication and visceroptosis – historical trends of real versus apparent new digestive diseases. Am J Gastroenterol 2002;97(11): 2695-9.

19. Muller W, Kelemen J, Stratz T. Spinal factors in the generation of fibromyalgia syndrome. Z Rheumatol 1998;57(Suppl 2):36-42.

20. Waylonis GW, Heck W. Fibromyalgia syndrome. New associations. Am J Phys Med Rehabil 1992; 71(6):343-8.

21. Barber ED. Osteopathy complete. Virginia Beach: LifeLine Press; 1898.

22. Fujiwara T, Togashi K, Yamaoka T, et al. Kinematics of the uterus: cine mode MR imaging. Radiographics 2004;24(1):e19.

23. Barral J-P, Mercier P. Visceral manipulation. Seattle, Washington: Eastland Press; 1988.

24. Lienemann A, Sprenger D, Steitz HO, Korell M, Reiser M. Detection and mapping of intraabdominal adhesions by using functional cine MR imaging: preliminary results. Radiology 2000;217(2):421-5.

25. D'Angelo E, Loring SH, Gioia ME, Pecchiari M, Moscheni C. Friction and lubrication of pleural tissues. Respir Physiol Neurobiol 2004;142(1):55-68.

26. Petros PE, Ulmsten UI. An integral theory of female urinary incontinence. Experimental and clinical considerations. Acta Obstet Gynecol Scand 1990;153(Suppl):7-31.

27. Kolecki RV, Golub RM, Sigel B, et al. Accuracy of viscera slide detection of abdominal wall adhesions by ultrasound. Surg Endosc 1994;8(8): 871-4.

28. Tan HL, Shankar KR, Ade-Ajayi N, et al. Reduction in visceral slide is a good sign of underlying postoperative viscero-parietal adhesions in children. J Pediatr Surg 2003;38(5):714-6.

29. Mirilas P, Skandalakis JE. Benign anatomical mistakes: right and left coronary ligaments. Am Surg 2002;68(9):832-5.

30. Van Helden DF. Pacemaker potentials in lymphatic smooth muscle of the guinea-pig mesentery. J Physiol 1993;471:465-79.

31. Lieber RL, Friden J. Functional and clinical significance of skeletal muscle architecture. Muscle Nerve 2000;23(11):1647-66.

32. Gabella G. Hypertrophy of visceral smooth muscle. Anat Embryol (Berl) 1990;182(5):409-24.

33. Fung YC. Biomechanics. Mechanical properties of living tissues, 2nd edn. New York: Springer; 1993.

34. Levin RM, Haugaard N, Levin SS, Buttyan R, Chen MW, Monson FC, Wein AJ. Bladder function in experimental outlet obstruction: pharmacologic responses to alterations in innervation, energetics, calcium mobilization, and genetics. Adv Exp Med Biol 1995;385:7-19; discussion 75-9.

35. Pienta KJ, Coffey DS. Cellular harmonic information transfer through a tissue tensegrity-matrix system. Med Hypoth 1991;34(1):88-95.

36. Secomb TW. Mechanics of blood flow in the microcirculation. Symposia Soc Exp Biol 1995;49: 305-21.

37. Plante GE, Chakir M, Lehoux S, Lortie M. Disorders of body fluid balance: a new look into the mechanisms of disease. Can J Cardiol 1995;11(9):788-802.

38. Schmid-Schonbein GW. Mechanisms causing initial lymphatics to expand and compress to promote lymph flow. Arch Histol Cytol 1990;53(Suppl): 107-14.

39. Lai-Fook SJ. Mechanics of the pleural space: fundamental concepts. Lung 1987;165(5):249-67.

40. Healy JC, Reznek RH. The peritoneum, mesenteries and omenta: normal anatomy and pathological processes. Eur Radiol 1998;8(6):886-900.

41. Huizinga JD, Robinson TL, Thomsen L. The search for the origin of rhythmicity in intestinal contraction; from tissue to single cells. Neurogastroenterol Motil 2000;12(1):3-9.

42. Wellner MC, Isenberg G. Stretch-activated nonselective cation channels in urinary bladder myocytes: importance for pacemaker potentials and myogenic response. Experientia 1993;66:93-9.

43. Suzuki H. Cellular mechanisms of myogenic activity in gastric smooth muscle. Jpn J Physiol 2000;50(3): 289-301.

44. Lonovics J, Madacsy L, Szepes A, Szilvassy Z, Velosy B, Varro V. Humoral mechanisms and clinical aspects of biliary tract motility. Scand J Gastroenterol 1998;228(Suppl):73-89.

45. Vereecken RL. The physiology and pathophysiology of the ureter. Eur Urol 1976;2(1):4-7.
46. Kunz G, Beil D, Deiniger H, Einspanier A, Mall G, Leyendecker G. The uterine peristaltic pump. Normal and impeded sperm transport within the female genital tract. Adv Exp Med Biol 1997;424:267-77.
47. Kimura Y, Adachi K, Kisaki N, Ise K. On the transportation of spermatozoa in the vas deferens. Andrologia 1975;7(1):55-61.
48. Exintaris B, Klemm MF, Lang RJ. Spontaneous slow wave and contractile activity of the guinea pig prostate. J Urol 2002;168(1):315-22.
49. Ueno T, Tanikawa K. Intralobular innervation and lipocyte contractility in the liver. Nutrition 1997;13(2):141-8.
50. Lang RJ, Exintaris B, Teele ME, Harvey J, Klemm MF. Electrical basis of peristalsis in the mammalian upper urinary tract. Clin Exp Pharmacol Physiol 1998;25(5):310-21.
51. Blechschmidt E, Gasser RF. Biokinetics and biodynamics of human differentiation. Principles and applications. Springfield:Charles C Thomas; 1978.
52. Sutherland WG. Teachings in the science of osteopathy (ed. Wales A). Forth Worth, TX: Rudra Press; 1990.

Chapter 2

Neural links and reflex relationships

'FACILITATED SEGMENTS' AND THE SOMATIC COMPONENT TO DISEASE

One of the main historical hypotheses under-pinning the osteopathic management of various visceral problems is the theory that manipulating or somehow mobilizing the body, usually parts of the spinal vertebral column, will have an effect on visceral function through reflexes to segmentally related organs. This phenomenon is thought to be mediated through the central nervous system and spinal cord, and is a belief system for which the evidence base is not complete.

The visceral and somatic nervous systems are anatomically linked together at the spinal cord and central nervous system levels and normal function allows the two to communicate, share various 'staging posts' in the nervous system communication network, and pass signals through these which do not get misinterpreted. Normal reflex arcs operate, for example, between one organ and another, between one somatic structure and another, and between various organs and somatic structures. Health depends on appropriately functioning spinal reflexes and feedback loops. A normal spinal reflex arc is shown in Figure 2.1.

IN LAY TERMS

The osteopathic concept is that something interferes with the normal operation of spinal reflexes, and with the normal threshold levels of stimulation required to trigger off other neural responses and efferent signals to distant parts of the body. That 'something' means that signals which would previously not have triggered a response now do, or that signals get amplified to a level out of proportion with the original stimulus. It also means that somatic irritation can be interpreted as coming from the viscera and visceral irritation or dysfunction can be interpreted as arising within the soma. If somatic irritation is interpreted as arising from the viscera, the central nervous system imagines that the viscera is damaged, infected or otherwise functioning adversely and so needs 'fixing'. Somatic irritation (such as inflammation and altered mechanical function in various tissues), if sufficient or long-lasting enough, is thought to provoke such changes in the nervous system, giving rise to altered efferent signals to the viscera, inducing, for example, vasoconstriction, altered visceral

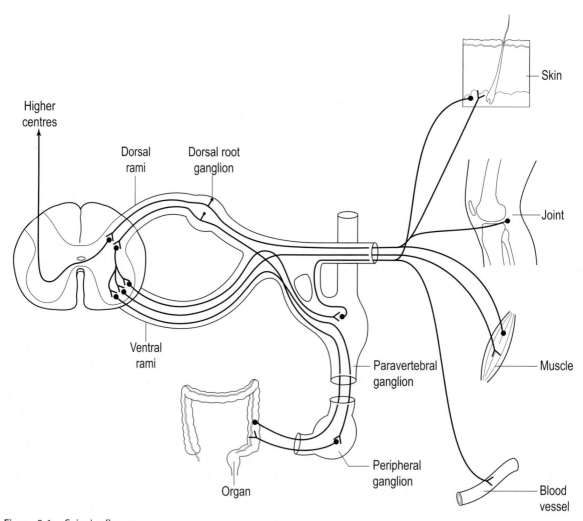

Figure 2.1   Spinal reflex arc.

function and peristalsis, and so on, which are contrary to the organ's actual needs. This is perceived to adversely affect visceral function, limit tissue health and immunity, and potentially contribute to pathological development within the organ.

This phenomenon is called *somatic dysfunction*. It indicates a state in the somatic tissues (such as vertebral soft tissues and articulations) that can ultimately influence visceral and vascular function, and hence homeostasis, immunity and health. The state of the nervous system induced by this somatic dysfunction has been called by osteopaths a *facilitated segment*. In this context, somatic dysfunction is considered by osteopaths to be partly aetiological to pathological change and development of disease in segmentally related organs. This is one aspect of the theory of somatic components to disease: if the spine is dysfunctional in a particular way, the body is predisposed to disease and pathological processes. Osteopaths consider that these somatic dysfunctions should form part of standard medical diagnostic criteria. These reflexes are called *somatovisceral reflexes*.

Another aspect of the theory of a somatic component to disease is the way in which somatic tissue can become affected by irritation arising in the viscera (the opposite route to that described above). In this aspect of the theory, the spinal soft tissue and articulatory changes are considered 'indicators' of visceral disease, and are thus objective signs of visceral dysfunction. These spinal changes are often the first signs of underlying visceral dysfunction and osteopaths consider that they should form part of standard medical screening criteria. These reflexes are called *viscerosomatic reflexes*. They underlie the referred pain phenomenon (see later) and necessitate careful differential diagnosis of painful spinal conditions that may in fact be visceral in origin, to avoid misdirected treatment.

The presence of somatic dysfunction is diagnosed by palpating the spine and surrounding segmentally related soft tissues to identify certain soft tissue changes and movement restrictions, which are indicative of poor neural function arising from the associated dysfunctional segment. Particular palpable changes in the spinal vertebral soft tissues and articulations indicate the presence of '*osteopathic* lesions', which is the historical term used to describe the presence of reflex phenomenon,

linking visceral and somatic function. This term has now been replaced by 'somatic dysfunction', which is somewhat unfortunate as it implies that the tissue change is solely within the musculoskeletal tissues, whereas in the concept as a whole, visceral, fascial and vascular tissue can also give rise to 'pathological' reflex phenomena. The actual soft tissue changes involved will be discussed below.

The unifying factor between viscerosomatic and somatovisceral reflexes is that they are both thought to be perverted versions of normal spinal reflex phenomena. When the spinal cord or higher centres start to alter their function, several things can occur:

- the synapses are too responsive and pass on signals that would normally be damped down (sensitization). This was the original interpretation of the facilitated segment or 'acute osteopathic lesion'
- the synapses have become unresponsive and are not passing on signals that they normally would (habituation). Osteopaths' term for habituated segments is 'chronic osteopathic lesion'
- the synapses become confused, misinterpreting the origin of signals from either the viscera or the soma (neural cross-talk)
- the synapses 'reflect back' the irritating signals, not only stopping them from being passed on (to the efferent fibres) but somehow 'radiating' the irritation back along afferent nerve fibres, thereby irritating any tissues that send afferent nerves to that segment (neurogenic inflammation).

If the cord changes can be reversed, then so should the adverse effects. Altering (afferent) neural signals to the cord is thought to be done by relieving tissue contracture, reducing inflammation and improving circulation and drainage in the affected tissue, which should ultimately change efferent output from that section of the cord. Biomechanical changes caused by spinal manipulation are thought to have physiological consequences by means of their effects on the inflow of sensory information to the central nervous system.[1]

There are a variety of techniques that can be applied to the soft tissues and articulations with the aim of normalizing function and therefore sensory, afferent information. These include soft tissue stretch and mobilization, joint manipulative techniques, articulation and other soft tissue releases, although the evidence base for the neural effects of these techniques is small. This reflex relationship was historically utilized empirically in practice and was a major component in the application of osteopathic medicine as opposed to osteopathic mechanics.[2] As scientific research has advanced, evidence is beginning to emerge for possible underlying mechanisms to support this type of reflex phenomenon, which are briefly discussed below,[3] and although its clinical relevance is far from being rationalized, it gives a basis for continued osteopathic exploration into this potentially important field of work. However, it should be noted that the scientific community remains sceptical of the clinical relevance of such hypotheses and claims.[4]

Figure 2.2 gives some brief algorithms that osteopaths use when considering neural reflexes. Some of the terms (e.g. 'acute' and 'chronic') will be further explained throughout the remainder of this chapter. 'TART' (see below) is a mnemonic for the changes found when palpating tissues, such as the spinal column, which indicate the presence of somatic dysfunction. The changes in fact are more complex than this implies, which will be taken up later.

There have been many attempts at identifying and researching the possible underlying mechanisms to the above hypotheses and, as stated, as scientific knowledge increases, these pathways are becoming clearer. The finite actions of neurophysiological relationships are complex and this book will not attempt to discuss all current models. It will, however, indicate what use osteopaths make of such theories in practice.

SPINAL REFLEX ARCS

One of the more important aspects of the above reflex phenomenon is the convergence of visceral and somatic afferent fibres onto the same wide dynamic range cells in the dorsal horn of the spinal cord. Normally the wide dynamic range cell will filter any afferent traffic and use such phenomena as frequency modulation to categorize the origin of the signal from either visceral or somatic tissue. Any subsequent neural signals (either to higher centres or across the interneurone pool to the ventral horn of the same or adjacent segments) will be tailored accordingly, to somatic or visceral needs.

'NORMAL' SPINAL REFLEXES

As previously noted, the purpose of normally operating spinal reflexes is to communicate tissue needs or states to the central nervous system, so that it can mobilize the rest of the body's function accordingly. These reflexes operate at a local segmental level or via higher centres in order to regulate visceral and somatic function. They were historically considered to be isolated in function, with somatic reflexes controlling somatic function only and visceral reflex arcs controlling visceral function only. This is now known not to be the case, with significant communication identified between the two parts of the nervous system.

The integration of somatic and visceral nervous system components is increasingly well understood, giving a degree of somatic influence on visceral function (and vice versa). This is understandable physiologically, as internal physiology must be adapted to meet the changing demands from the somatic (musculoskeletal) system and structures.[5] Hence the presence of somatovisceral reflexes to inform this integration is logical and necessary. In this way, the somatic body and its component parts (including, but not confined to, spinal muscles, articulations and related soft tissues) are thought to be somewhat regulatory of the viscera and vasculature throughout the body.[6] Hence somatic structures are linked to homeostatic functioning and regulation.

Historically, appreciation of methods of adjusting the internal body to 'external' body needs has been simplistic and included (for example) an 'all or none' response to the 'fear, flight or fight' reaction modulated through the sympathetic nervous system. The sympathetic and parasympathetic branches of the autonomic nervous system were previously thought to 'compete' against each other and work antagonistically. These ideas are now known to be misleading and inaccurate and it is recognized that the integration between the two branches of the autonomic nervous system, and with the somatic nervous system, is sophisticated

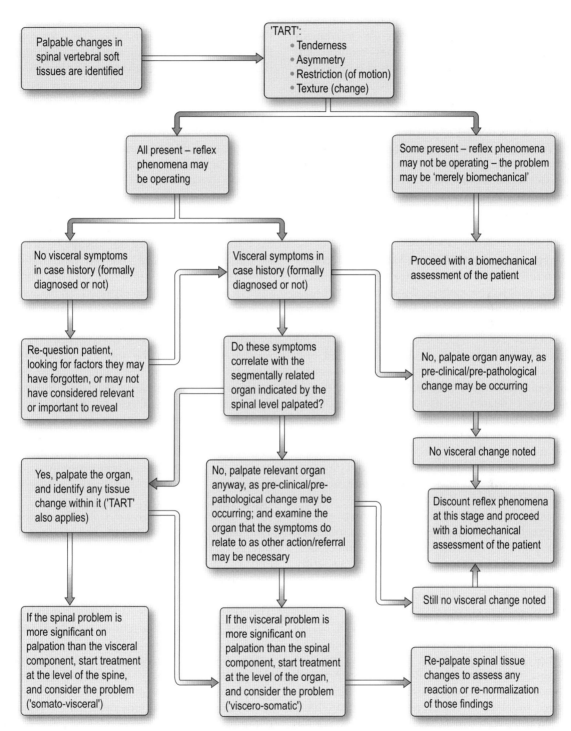

Figure 2.2   Algorithms for neural reflexes.

and subtle, mostly working in dynamic harmony with each other.[7] Even whole-body movement patterns and behaviour traits may require high levels of coordination and integration between the somatic and visceral nervous systems.[8] In other words, the convergence between autonomic and somatic nervous systems aids communication and health, if functioning appropriately.

Not only is effective communication a key outcome of normally operating neural reflexes, but so too is the important function of neurotrophism (see below).

Embryology and the spinal reflex arc

The spinal reflex arcs discussed above arise consequentially from embryological developmental relationships. The embryo develops segmentally and the emerging nervous system is surrounded by somites. Each somite will differentiate into various tissue types which then migrate to distant parts of the body. The somite will 'spread and migrate' from its central axis, 'dragging' its neural components with it. The neural segment that is ultimately related to its somite will find that somite distributed widely through the body. Similarly, neurones to developing viscera will also be 'dragged' and elongated as those end organs migrate, rotate and continue to grow and develop. Those visceral neurones from any one segment will also eventually be found in diverse parts of the body. Thus, somite and visceral maps can be constructed which represent the neurotomes of each segment.[9] The myotome, sclerotome, dermatome and viscerotome will each be in a slightly different anatomical location from its fellows, but each will be innervated from the same region of the embryological neural crest.[10]

Any efferent signal from one segment of the spinal cord may innervate quite widespread and distant parts of the body in the relevant dermatomes, myotomes, viscerotomes and sclerotomes. Conversely, the afferent signals that ultimately merge together at one cord segment can have arisen from widespread areas of the body. All the relationships are linked through their embryological roots. An example of the variation in distal location for one set of segmentally related tissues is illustrated by the spread of the C3–4–5 segment. The dermatome is over the side of the lower neck and top of the upper arm. The myotome is over the shoulder and upper back. The sclerotome is the scapula (for example), and the motor innervation also spreads to the thoracic diaphragm.

Afferent signals from those diverse parts, be they somatic or visceral, will converge on a particular spinal segment, via its dorsal horn. From there, ascending signals need to be differentiated as to origin, to enable an appropriate central response to those signals. As stated earlier, this is the job of the wide dynamic range cells in the dorsal horn.

Referred pain

Such differentiation may not always be accurate, as the phenomenon of referred pain indicates. Here, noxious stimuli (afferent signals) from the viscera are frequently interpreted by higher centres as arising from segmentally related somatic structures.[11] Hence cardiac pain can be perceived as arising from the neck or jaw, upper gastrointestinal pain from the shoulder or chest, and urogenital pain from the lower back or pelvis, as examples. This implies a relationship between the somatic and visceral systems. Beyond being an underlying mechanism of referred pain patterns, the role of this integration is not understood. The phenomenon of referred pain is usually classified as part of a 'normal spinal reflex response'.

'ABNORMAL' SPINAL REFLEXES

The osteopathic profession has always been interested in the integration between the somatic and autonomic nervous systems, with research into potentially clinically relevant phenomena dating back to the work of Luisa Burns in 1907.[12] The osteopathic profession has continuously referred to general scientific medical models regarding neural physiology, attempting to find common ground for further research. Gradually, the particular relations that may underpin the osteopathic theories are becoming increasingly interesting to the orthodox medical and scientific community.[13,14]

Current understanding of this model of somatic dysfunction indicates that restriction in somatic mobility, and autonomic, visceral, and immunological changes, are produced by pain-related sensory neurones and their reflexes.[15] This model has evolved from earlier work by Irvin Korr,[16] which proposed the muscle spindle as the origin of irritating stimuli that could summate at cord level and lead to efferent visceral signals as a result of somatic afferent input. The more recent models emphasize the nociceptor and its reflexes as a source of the connective tissue, circulatory, visceral and immunological changes associated with the somatic dysfunction.[3]

Sympatheticotonia – circulatory controls and other relationships

Regional blood flow distribution

Many early osteopathic concepts regarding the effects of reflex phenomena were focused on the perceived changes to the efferent signals passing along the sympathetic nerves to the blood vessels of various end tissues or organs. The presence of somatic dysfunction was thought to lead to specific (segmentally mediated) vasoconstriction or general (whole-body) vasoconstriction. Vasoconstriction clearly reduces blood flow into the end tissue or organ, and early osteopaths felt that the presence of various somatic dysfunctions through the spine and body would trigger sufficient reflex phenomena to cause relative tissue ischaemia, thus significantly compromising function and health, and leading to increased predisposition to disease and decreased potential for recovery from it.[16]

Reducing spinal articulatory restriction and soft tissue irritation was thought to improve tissue flow locally, and in segmentally related tissues, by reducing the reflexly induced sympatheticotonia. They also considered that if there was vasoconstriction in one part, this would create increased blood pressure in another part of the circulatory system. Peripheral vasoconstriction through sustained sympatheticotonia from chronic and multiple somatic dysfunctions would lead to a long-term increase in blood pressure, consequently adversely affecting health. They also believed that if they worked on various parts of the spine where somatic dysfunction was present, this would help to 'open or close' various parts of the circulatory system (i.e. the abdominal or gastrointestinal blood pool or the limb blood pool, for example), which would help improve overall circulatory control and 'redistribute the blood mass'. Currently, there is no clear supportive clinical evidence for

this, although the osteopathic interest in circulation persists.

Certainly there seems to be some physiological link between the autonomic nervous control of various 'blood pools' (or, more properly, blood volume distribution) and the somatic nerves, as for example lumbar skin warming causes vasoconstriction of the mesenteric (gastrointestinal) arteries, increases gastrointestinal contractility and overall blood pressure.[17] There are also many autoregulatory mechanisms by which exercise (and use of the musculoskeletal system) will alter cardiovascular function (increasing cardiac rate and, to some degree, stroke volume)[18] but again, this does not provide clinical relevance for osteopathic concepts but merely indicates the presence of underlying mechanisms that may play a role in the purported actions.

This concept relates not only to management of visceral dysfunction but also to many cases of musculoskeletal pain and dysfunction. Regional blood flow control for the upper limb is important in cases of tissue strain and injury to the wrist, elbow or shoulder, for example, and if there are spinal restrictions, osteopaths would consider that those areas may be causing reflex sympathetic blood flow variation (potentially compromising tissue health in the affected part). In order to optimize vascular control to the affected part, all other areas of sympathetic blood flow irritation must be eased, so that overall, central blood flow distribution control can normalize and therefore effectively regulate flow to needy parts. Osteopaths do not consider this type of regional blood flow variation to be as pathological as arterial occlusion but they do feel that prolonged minimally affected vascular input to an area will have an eventual poor outcome on local tissue health, healing and function.

> Osteopaths treat an area not simply because it is biomechanically related to a particular irritated tissue or structure, but because it is physiologically related to it or to structures that influence physiology in that irritated tissue. This is a major difference from a purely 'orthopaedic' approach.

Further discussion on blood flow and other fluid flow dynamics is included in Chapter 8.

Neurotrophic function

Neurotrophic function in nerves is an essential communicating mechanism and nutritional-immune regulator for the innervated tissue. The neurotrophic function of nerves is known to be disturbed after peripheral nerve injury[19] but osteopaths contend that neurotrophic behaviour can also be affected through the above-mentioned reflex phenomena.[16] Neural regeneration, nutrition and signalling mechanisms are therefore distorted, potentially severely compromising end-tissue functionality and health. This distortion in neurotrophic function is related to neurogenic inflammatory phenomena.

Neurogenic inflammation

The sympathetic nervous system may be involved in the generation of pain, hyperalgesia and inflammation under pathological conditions. Damage to a peripheral nerve alters the internal structures of the nerve, including coupling between afferent and sympathetic neurones. These changes are probably induced by neurotrophic factors and are responsible for sensitization of the afferents by the sympathetic fibres. This can ultimately mediate neurogenic inflammation and enhance (maintain) both the tissue-based inflammation as well as the sensitization (and therefore central processing) of the nociceptive afferents.[20] Neurogenic inflammation represents a type of irritation that is not only transmitted ultimately to efferent fibres from an affected segment, but also as a type of retrograde or 'reverse flow' irritation back down the afferent fibres to the original tissue. Neurogenic inflammation may play a role in many disease states and has been particularly noted in allergic bronchial asthma, for example.[21]

Osteopaths would contend that the reflex phenomena associated with somatic dysfunction and viscerosomatico-visceral reflexes could involve or be related in some way to the neurogenic inflammation mechanism(s). Osteopathic treatment applied to the relevant reflex-mediated somatic dysfunctions may play a role in reducing neurogenic inflammation, and therefore contribute to disease management.

The 'general adaptive response' and neuroendocrine immune function

The influence of the sympathetic nervous system on immune function has long been noted[22-24] and neuroendocrine integration is well researched.[25-27] In fact, the neuroendocrine mechanisms are significant mediators in the central nervous and autonomic nervous systems' influence on immunity, incorporating an emotional influence as well as a stress-based influence.[28] The effect of any particular stress on an individual will depend on the neuroendocrine environment on which it is superimposed, and can lead to individualized compromise in immune mechanisms.[29]

The 'general adaptive response' is a fully integrative model of how the body responds to stress.[30] This is a broader model incorporating whole-body responses to neural reflex irritation, on whatever level, which supersedes the rather outdated 'fear, flight or fight' analogies of previous decades. It supposes that reflex phenomena (if functioning inappropriately or overloaded or somehow disturbed) create whole-body physiology distortion away from normal, leading to disturbance in homeostatic regulatory controls and feedback loops, thereby promoting dysfunction and ill health and increasing the potential for pathological change and poor response to injury, stress and disease.

In osteopathic terms, reducing the impact of any stressor (such as those represented by varied musculoskeletal, somatic or visceral tissue tensions, torsions, spasms and restrictions) is thought to reduce load on the body's adaptive responses and give greater potential for more appropriate homeostatic and immune regulation and function. In this context, generalized osteopathic treatment (to individually noted somatic dysfunctions in a given patient) is considered to improve the person's capacity not only to fight disease and dysfunction, but to recover from existing pathology and distress.

OSTEOPATHIC CENTRES

Whether segmental reflex phenomena have actual clinical relevance or whether the real influence of osteopathic treatment is via a broader model such as the general adaptive response, osteopaths have historically defended their use of segmentally derived reflex phenomena. It is too early to say from any evidence base that these phenomena are either absent, inaccurate or clinically irrelevant, or indeed do operate as osteopaths claim. These relationships continue to form part of all undergraduate osteopathic training, and future generations of osteopaths will continue to explore and research their eventual contribution to patient management.

These relationships have given rise to various 'maps' used to easily identify which somatic level should be explored in relation to a particular viscera or body function. The autonomic nerves to and from the viscera can be mapped in several different ways. One can identify the patterns of efferent outflow from the thoracolumbar spinal cord to the organs, and also the afferent fibres (although there seems more anatomical variation in this arrangement than on the efferent side). One can also map central connections and this can give rise to varied descriptions of the anatomical arrangement of the autonomic nerves. However, further mapping may also be possible when the functionality of different sympathetic fibres and neurones is considered.[31,32]

Osteopaths have their own 'maps' which show the arrangement of relations between the spinal column and the viscera. They are based on various scientific evidence accumulated over the years and as a result are subject to a degree of variation between authors although the basic patterns are broadly agreed upon by most.[33] These maps identify various spinal segmental levels and particular organs. They identify various levels which relate to sensory and motor function of the organs, and collective or physiological centres (such as micturition, vomiting and nutrition), as well as vasomotor centres which are concerned with regional blood flow phenomena and vascular tone in various end organs or target tissues. Figure 2.3 shows some of these relationships.

> These maps indicate the above-mentioned somatoviscero-somatic relationships that are historically relevant to clinical osteopathic practice. They give guidance to the segmental levels associated with various organs, blood vessels and other structures, and particular physiological processes.

Patients presenting with various disorders and visceral problems can be assessed for the somatic dysfunction component by exploring the related somatic tissues as indicated by such maps. The presence of these somatic dysfunctions indicates to osteopaths the need to resolve the identified somatic component as part of the overall management of that patient, including medical management where necessary. These somatic dysfunctions are identified by various palpatory findings, which are discussed below.

Experienced osteopaths often state that one should 'treat what one finds', rather than trying to impose a set regime such as 'work on the ninth dorsal spinal articulation when there is liver dysfunction', as this suggests that the same treatment is given to each patient. This is most definitely not the case. The osteopath must examine the patient globally and treat what seems to be 'active' in that person, i.e. each person will have different somatic dysfunctions that combine either through segmental relationships or more globally operating mechanisms to adversely affect homeostasis and health. It is not possible to predict exact or specific outcomes from mobilization of somatic dysfunction components, purely because of the complex integration that is not currently fully understood. It is only possible to generalize.

Clinicians must work with what is not functioning appropriately for that individual patient and appreciate that the underlying reflex mechanisms will readapt in their own unique way. This is the reason why research into osteopathic outcomes is so difficult: the individualized nature of patient management makes randomized, blinded trials impossible to construct, with the added factor that any non-individually applied treatment protocols would not reflect what is done in osteopathic practice, and would therefore be clinically inapplicable. Some other valid research model must be found.

PALPATION OF SPINAL REFLEX PHENOMENA

'TART':

- Tenderness
- Asymmetry
- Restriction (of motion)
- Texture (change).

Note: in this chart, the spinal levels have been 'condensed' to their most common areas. In the tables throughout this book where reflex relationships have been listed, those latter figures give a generally slightly wider number of levels that are associated with any particular structure (as there is a degree of anatomical variation between subjects). Different authors may also quote slightly different levels as a result.

The body systems have been identified by types of shading, to make interpretation easier, and this chart does not include all structures, but considers the main elements from each system. These palpatory levels are generally found bilaterally, rather than unilaterally as indicated here.

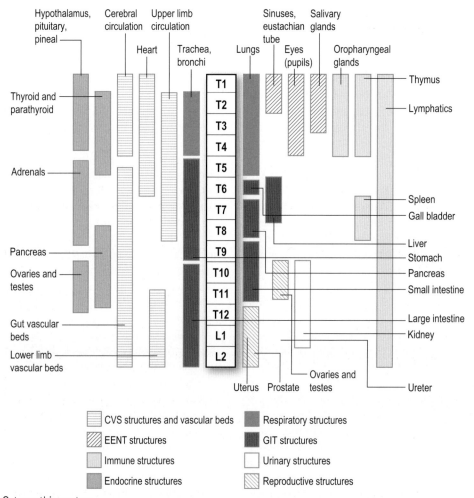

Figure 2.3   Osteopathic centres.

This mnemonic refers to some of the typical palpatory changes found when somatic dysfunction is present. The difficulty in practice lies in the fact that many of the above palpatory findings can be identified when there has been direct injury to the spine and associated tissues, and where there are no indicators of visceral disease at all. Osteopathic philosophy indicates that the longer the somatic dysfunction is present, the more neural reflex

disturbance it is likely to create, and therefore the more it is likely to be associated with secondary visceral dysfunction.

'ACUTE' VERSUS 'CHRONIC'

Palpable changes to the spinal column soft tissues and articulations have historically been labelled 'acute' or 'chronic'.[33] Clinically these terms have

Acute	Chronic
History: recent; often an injury	**History:** long-standing
Pain: acute pain, severe, cutting, sharp	**Pain:** dull, achy. Paraesthesias (crawling, itching, burning, gnawing)
Vascular: vessels injured, release of endogenous peptides = chemical vasodilation, inflammation	**Vascular:** vessels constricted due to sympathetic tone
Skin: warm, moist, red, inflamed (via vascular and chemical changes)	**Skin:** cool, pale (via chronic sympathetic vascular tone increase)
Sympathetics: systemically increased sympathetic activity but local effect overpowered by bradykinins so there is local vasodilation due to chemical effect	**Sympathetics:** has vasoconstriction due to hypersympathetic tone. Regional sympathetic hyperactivity. Systemic sympathetic tone may be reduced toward normal
Musculature: local increase in muscle tone, muscle contraction, spasm, increased tone of the muscle spindle	**Musculature:** decreased muscle tone, flaccid, mushy, limited range of motion due to contracture (see tissue changes)
Mobility: range often normal, quality is sluggish	**Mobility:** limited range, with normal quality in the motion that remains
Tissues: boggy oedema, acute congestion, fluids from vessels and from chemical reactions in tissues	**Tissues:** chronic congestion, doughy, stringy, fibrotic, ropy, thickened, increased resistance, contracted, contractures
Adnexa: (moist skin) no trophic changes	**Adnexa:** pimples, scaly skin, dry, folliculitis, pigmentation (trophic changes)
Visceral: minimal somatovisceral effects	**Visceral:** somatovisceral effects are common

Figure 2.4   Acute versus chronic palpatory findings. (is this a table? See p. 11)

been used to describe changes found after biomechanical injury that is either recent ('acute') or of long standing ('chronic'). Figure 2.4 shows the range of palpatory findings in each category.

Chronic lesions have been associated by some with somatovisceral effects, and acute lesions with few somatovisceral effects.[33] However, this does not really reflect all components often found in practice. It also implies that the neural reflex traffic is 'one way', rather than being an integrated system of multilayered reflex phenomena and feedback loops operating on many levels and directions.

Empirically, chronic biomechanical restrictions seem related to various visceral phenomena in practice. However, acute visceral irritation also seems to create soft tissue and palpatory changes in the spinal column that mimic the above-mentioned 'acute' biomechanical disorder. For example, acute gall bladder irritation seems to present not only with biliary pain and dysfunction, but also with particular spinal restrictions and soft tissue irritations, in segmentally related tissues.

As stated above, viscerosomatic reflexes form part of the mechanism in the current understanding of referred pain patterns. It seems that these reflexes invoke more than referred pain and appear to be related to irritation of somatic (e.g. muscular) structures as a response to visceral stimuli, such as inflammation and distension.[34] In several visceral conditions, part of the presenting symptomatology may be muscular tension and aching/pain in segmentally related structures. Thus the person may suffer not only from the visceral pathology or dysfunction but also from reflexly induced irritation to somatic structures, leading to painful and restricted mobility and decreased biomechanical efficiency in the affected part.[35] Manual therapy applied to those affected visceral structures may be relevant in reducing the overall somatic symptom pattern in these types of mixed visceral and somatic presentations.

In the author's experience, the longevity of the spinal changes should not be strictly attributable to whether the reflex phenomenon is somatovisceral or viscerosomatic. Clinically, the relationship is much better understood if one appreciates that the reflex disturbance affects both components and works 'both ways simultaneously'.

It seems more clinically plausible that when visceral symptoms are interfering with somatic function (and giving spinal pain as part of a visceral disease presentation), then the spinal cord segment is 'facilitated' or sensitized and has lowered thresholds that are firing abnormally. When the reflex phenomenon has been present for some time, the spinal cord will 'fatigue' or become habituated and in this case, thresholds are very high and neural reflex signals are not being communicated or 'passed' on to the higher centres or the ventral horn of the cord. To resolve this situation, the cord needs a change in stimulus and the spinal column articulations and associated soft tissue need to be 'reawakened' so that they reestablish neural reflex communication with the cord and hence trigger a normalization of neural activity, which will help to more appropriately communicate visceral information and therefore contribute to improved visceral health. This is done by applying various types of manual therapy (particularly articulation and deep soft tissue work).

A simple guide is: if the findings are 'acute', treat the viscera, and if the findings are 'chronic',

treat the spine, but make no assumptions about what is actually happening on a reflex level. Uncoordinated activity will be concurrently affecting both somatovisceral and viscerosomatic feedback loops.

This is an added layer of analysis to the points raised previously and illustrated in Figure 2.2. There it stated that if the organ felt worse than the spine, treat the organ, and vice versa. Putting these points together with the comments just made above means that the algorithm should now state that in fact the palpatory findings in the spine in the presence of visceral dysfunction are as follows.

- When an organ is chronically irritated or diseased, it is associated with long-standing soft tissue and articulatory changes in the spine. In this case, when the spinal changes are noted to be much more 'restricted', when compared to the norm, than the organ is, treat first at the level of the spine. *In this instance, the spinal cord is a maintaining factor in visceral disease.* Note: this does not imply that osteopathic care alone is required; medical intervention may well be necessary.
- If the visceral restrictions appear more significant, then treat first at the viscera.
- When an organ is chronically diseased and associated with a chronic spinal restriction, it is still possible for the viscera to become acutely irritated or for the disease to suddenly worsen. In this case, an acute response is often noted at the level of the spinal soft tissues and in fact, one can find acute spinal palpatory findings 'on top of' the chronic tissue changes. This scenario indicates that the viscera needs treating or reexamining, and any spinal work would only be symptomatic at this stage.
- When an organ is initially irritated or diseased, then it is likely to be associated with acute spinal changes. In this instance, treat the viscera and the spinal changes should revert very quickly without needing to be addressed locally. *In this instance, the spinal cord is an indicator of visceral disease.* Note: this does not imply that osteopathic care alone

PARASYMPATHETIC REFLEXES

is required; medical intervention may well be necessary.

The viscerosomatic and somatovisceral reflexes all operate via the sympathetic nervous system. However, this is not the only branch of the autonomic nervous system where neural reflex phenomena can operate.[7] It is thought by osteopaths that the parasympathetic nerves can be similarly affected by somatic-derived stimuli. The somatic components relevant to parasympathetic reflex phenomena are the upper cervical spine and sacral or pelvic regions.

The vagal ganglia link with sympathetic fibres via the superior cervical ganglia and with the upper cervical somatic rami.[36] The upper cervical spine is therefore very interesting physiologically, as these interconnections make it a very accessible place from which to interact with both branches of the autonomic nervous system, but also the somatic nervous system as well.

Upper cervical restrictions are commonly noted by osteopaths to be related to visceral dysfunction. As most of the vagal fibres are in fact sensory, restrictions in the upper cervical spine articulations and soft tissues are thought to irritate the vagal communication with the brainstem, such that the higher centres perceive visceral sensory input inappropriately (and subsequently effect an unbalanced response).

Some authors consider that vagal afferent signals may be more related to physiological function whereas sympathetic signals are more related to pain.[37] This does seem empirically so in practice, at least in the sense that vagal irritation has broad effects and is noted in many dysfunctions and different disease presentations. However, the relationship may not be as black and white as this, as mechanical stimulation and stretch to the mesenteries, for example, can lead to wide-ranging changes in other organ functions and homeostatic regulation.[38]

The author's own untested hypothesis (in partial agreement with osteopathic folklore) is that upper cervical restriction on the left is related to gastrointestinal dysfunction, on the right to respiratory function, and bilaterally to cardiovascular dysfunction, and that sacral and pelvic restrictions relate to endocrine imbalance.

ENTERIC REFLEXES

The enteric nervous system is also composed of many vitally important neural communicating networks and feedback loops, regulating gastrointestinal function. The enteric nervous system is influenced in its regulation of gut function by extrinsic neural and hormonal influences but can operate with all of these external neurones severed.[39] The subsequent functioning cannot be optimally adjusted to body needs and general homeostatic balance but the gut will nonetheless still work.

These enteric reflexes form part of the control mechanisms for peristaltic movements in all the hollow gut organs. They also play a role in regulating the transit of food from one part of the gut to another, and in preparing those advancing sections for the type of content they will be receiving. Sphincteric coordination is also part of the enteric nervous system's role. These components (peristaltic motion and pacemaker activities of visceral smooth muscle) will be discussed further in Chapter 5.

The presence of viscerosomatico-visceral reflexes is thought to be capable of distorting enteric nervous system balance and communication, thereby compromising gut function. Any tensions in the viscera, such as spasm, torsion or other mechanical distortion (for example, adhesions and scarring), are thought by osteopaths to affect the mechanoreceptors operating within the enteric neural signalling mechanisms, thereby distorting function. These visceral restrictions form a sort of 'visceral–somatic dysfunction' which should also be a diagnostic component in disease management.

The presence of mechanical torsion and tension in any hollow organ may in fact affect the compliance and mechanical communication networks within that organ, which may also disrupt the peristaltic function of other hollow organs such as the ureters, fallopian tubes and bladder, for example. In all body systems, where visceral motion in the form of compliance and peristaltic waves is a component to physiological function, the physical state of that tissue is relevant to its ongoing behaviour. This point underpins many of the visceral approaches in various patient presentations that are discussed later in the book.

ANATOMICAL RELATIONSHIPS AFFECTING NEURAL CIRCULATION AND FUNCTION

The reflex phenomena described above are not the only link between the spine (or, more correctly, various somatic structures) and the autonomic nervous system. Another major osteopathic concept is the need for the autonomic nervous system (as with all neural tissue) to have effective circulation at all times, and that somatic restriction can interfere with this circulation, thus affecting neural processing and therefore reflex phenomena.[40] The circulation problems can arise from either cerebrospinal fluid (e.g. around the spinal nerve roots in the intervertebral foramen) or the vasa nervorum. In fact, in real terms, it is difficult to separate the two mechanisms of disturbance, as both may be associated with the same location of somatic restriction.

There are various places in the body where somatic articulations of soft tissue structures can restrict or irritate the connective tissue in which various neural structures are embedded or channelled. This type of restriction may interfere with the vasa nervorum of the autonomic nerves, creating neural dysfunction and therefore poor central control of visceral function, immunity and ultimately health. Certain autonomic plexi and ganglia are most at risk from this relationship, purely as a result of their anatomical somatic relationships. These are discussed below. Clinically, when visceral dysfunction is present, it is necessary to consider not only spinal column articulatory and soft tissue changes but changes to tissues in such places as the thoracic inlet, the upper cervical spine and the rib articulations, to make sure that all the autonomic neural pathways are as undisturbed as possible and therefore not being adversely irritated by somatic input.

PARASPINAL GANGLIA

The paraspinal ganglia are where processing of modulating signals from the central nervous system to the target tissues or organs can take place.[7]

These sympathetic ganglia are located just anterior to the rib heads/costovertebral articulations and receive fibres from the spinal cord and from adjacent paravertebral ganglia. They are illustrated in Figure 2.5.

Rib restrictions stiffen and irritate the fascia and soft tissues around the rib heads, in which the ganglia are embedded. This creates tension and torsion in those soft tissues and impedes efficient circulation. This can affect the vasa nervorum of the ganglia, leading to problems with effective neural processing and communication. Rib restrictions therefore potentially interfere with neural function via a mechanical–fluidic link. This is then potentially passed on to other autonomic plexi and ultimately various organs and distant tissues. Relieving rib restrictions is an important part of the management of visceral dysfunction.

VAGAL AND SUPERIOR CERVICAL (SYMPATHETIC) GANGLIA

Restrictions in the upper cervical area are also thought to interfere with vagal function by irritating the fascia in which the nerve is embedded anterior to C1 and C2 vertebral bodies, and in the jugular foramen of the cranial base. As already indicated, the vagus nerve is a very important conveyer of visceral sensory and physiological information. Irritation at the upper cervical and jugular foramen level will potentially adversely compound this information, effectively creating a type of 'Chinese whispers' where the brainstem and higher centres get the wrong messages about what is happening systemically. Any subsequent homeostatic regulation would clearly be compromised, leading to adverse outcomes. In osteopathic concepts, upper cervical and cranial mechanics are also linked to brainstem function, which processes and passes on vagal information.

All the above mechanical considerations will also relate to the functioning of the superior cervical ganglion. In fact, there are several neural and reflex connections between the vagal ganglia, the superior cervical ganglion and the somatic nerves of C1 and C2. This makes this region a very important crossroad for somatic and autonomic reflex activity. The superior cervical ganglion itself serves the head and neck structures and is often compromised in upper respiratory, sinus, cranial,

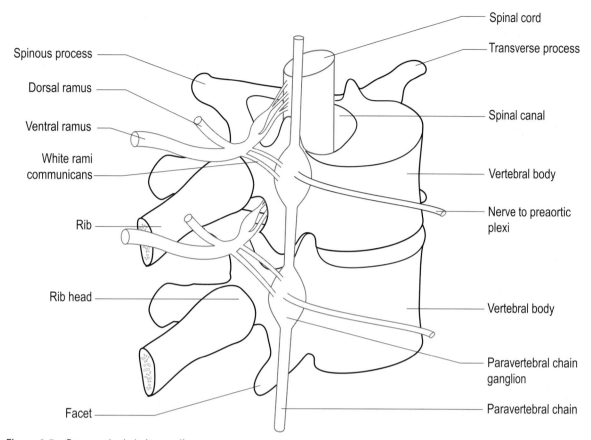

Spinous process

Dorsal ramus

Ventral ramus

White rami
communicans

Rib

Rib head

Facet

Spinal cord

Transverse process

Spinal canal

Vertebral body

Nerve to preaortic
plexi

Vertebral body

Paravertebral chain
ganglion

Paravertebral chain

Figure 2.5 Paravertebral chain ganglia.

ear and eye problems. It can be influenced by working on the upper cervical, cranial and temporomandibular mechanics.

Stellate ganglion

Figure 2.6 shows the inferior cervical or 'stellate' ganglion. This sits on top of the apex of the lung, just in front of the transverse process of the seventh cervical vertebra.

All fibres to the head and neck structures that are ultimately served by the superior and middle cervical ganglion have first to pass through the inferior cervical ganglion. This includes fibres to throat and thoracic structures (the thyroid and heart, for example) that descend from the middle cervical ganglion into the mediastinum. Any tension or torsion affecting the thoracic inlet area will compromise the fascia around the inferior cervical

ganglion, interfering with its internal circulation and causing mechanical irritation to the neural tissue, which will affect neural signals and processing to the other cervical ganglia and the various structures served by all the cervical ganglia. General osteopathic work to the upper four dorsal vertebrae and associated ribs to influence sympathetic activity in the head, neck and mediastinum will be 'wasted' if significant tension remains in the thoracic inlet area affecting the inferior cervical ganglia.

COELIAC, RENAL AND MESENTERIC PLEXI

Similar problems can affect the para-aortic ganglia, serving the abdominal and pelvic organs. These can be found nestled around various arteries that branch off from the abdominal aorta. The various

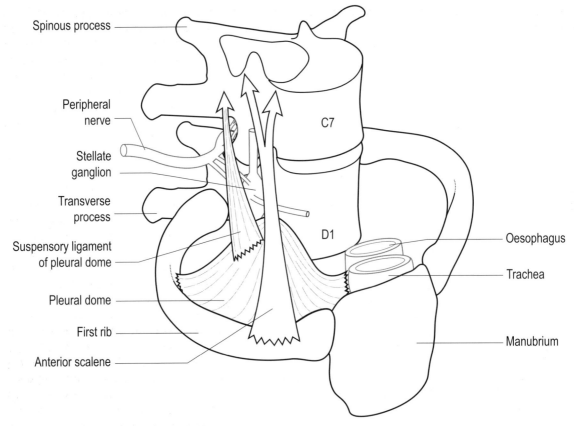

Figure 2.6 Inferior cervical 'stellate' ganglia.

(approximate) vertebral body levels where the arteries and their associated ganglia and autonomic plexi are located are listed below:

- T12 – coeliac
- L1 – renal and superior mesenteric
- L3 – inferior mesenteric.

Any mechanical restriction in the lower dorsal and lumbar regions of the spine and within the soft tissues around the face of the spinal column and central components of the posterior abdominal wall are potentially able to compromise the circulation and thereby neural activity of the above ganglia and plexi. As evidence is now emerging for neural processing and reflex activity being located at the ganglia level (in addition to spinal and higher centre reflexes), this makes the mechanics of the anterior lumbar region very influential to abdominal and pelvic visceral function.

The nerve tissue of the various ganglia and plexi is in reality a large interconnected neural mass, which is only artificially separated out into separate ganglia and plexi. The neural tissue is embedded in the fascia over the anterior lumbar vessels and region, which is also interspersed with lymph nodes and vessels. This collection of neural tissue, which also receives many vagal fibres, is referred to by osteopaths as the 'abdominal brain'. Work to the mid- and lower dorsal spinal articulations and associated ribs alone (the traditional spinal 'levels' associated with sympathetic supply to various organs) is not sufficient to explore mechanical influences on abdominal visceral function. It is also necessary to explore the lumbar spine for gastrointestinal function.

HYPOGASTRIC CORRIDOR

The hypogastric plexi of nerves commence from the inferior mesenteric plexi and pass down in front of the L4 and L5 vertebral bodies, before dividing into two at the lumbosacral junction and passing either side of the pelvic organs into the pelvic bowl.

PELVIC 'BRAIN' (PELVIC SPLANCHNIC NERVES)

When the fibres have descended into the pelvic bowl, they blend with the parasympathetic nerves from S2, S3 and S4, which are the pelvic splanchnic nerves. Together they form what osteopaths refer to as the 'pelvic brain'. Any pelvic restriction can impact on the fascia of the pelvic bowl in which the pelvic autonomic fibres and plexi are located.

OTHER REFLEX PHENOMENA

CHAPMAN'S REFLEXES

Chapman's reflexes were 'discovered' in the 1930s by an osteopath who felt that there were fascial contractures in superficial tissues which formed nodules that were reflexly linked to various organs or pathological conditions. Physical stimulation of the skin over the nodules is thought to reflexly affect the lymphatic drainage of the related organ or improve function and healing of various pathological states or diseases (by improving lymphatic drainage in affected systems or tissues).

The use of Chapman's reflexes to give a therapeutic modification of visceral dysfunction has been a controversial issue amongst osteopathic clinicians for many years.[41] These reflex areas are described by proponents as anatomically well-defined loci in fascia in superficial skin layers, which are specifically related to rather precise organ function. The Chapman's reflex centres are thought to be of value both diagnostically and therapeutically. Releasing any active Chapman's reflex point is said to benefit the immune system as a whole, to result in a favourable effect on the function of the related organ and therefore promote overall health and well-being.[33,42]

When a Chapman's reflex centre is both palpable and tender, it is said to be a 'pathological' reflex, which implies a dysfunction of the organ to which Chapman has assigned that particular reflex area. Examining the various Chapman's reflex centres by palpation for the presence of an abnormal tissue nodularity and subjective tenderness gives diagnostic indicators of underlying visceral dysfunction or pathology. Treatment of the area consists of a circular massage of the active Chapman's reflex centre (usually with the finger tip) until a palpable tissue change occurs, characterized by a lessening of the nodularity and tenderness. It is thought that this tissue change is a result of drainage of oedematous fluid from the localized pathological reflex area.

After Chapman's death another osteopath, Owens, continued his work and explored those reflexes specifically active in endocrine disorders. A specific set of reflexes linked pelvic articular mechanics with sets of nodules for the ovaries, testes and thyroid gland, as well as the adrenal gland, indicating that pelvic mechanics were influential in general endocrine imbalances.

Chapman's reflexes can be found on the posterior and anterior surfaces of the body and are located at various points along the sternum, the proximal head of the humerus, medial and lateral clavicle, occiput, cervical, dorsal and lumbar paraspinal regions, various areas of the ribcage, sacrum, coccyx and other pelvic bones including the pubis, the fibula and the tibia. They are illustrated in the appendix. Diagnosis is by location of an active anterior point, and treatment is to the corresponding posterior point, using circular soft tissue manipulation. Treatment for 30–60 seconds is usually sufficient. Care should be taken not to overstimulate the reflex point.

See Figure A3, p. 330

Relationship with trigger points and other reflex 'zones'

Some authors consider that Chapman's reflex points are part of 'trigger point' therapy as developed by Travell.[43] Chiropractic texts may refer to them as neurolymphatic points and link them with the phenomenon of 'neurovascular' points, first explored by Bennet, a chiropractor.[44]

Relationship with acupuncture points

There is also a striking degree of correspondence between Chapman's reflex centres and acupuncture points, in terms of both their specific anatomical locations and their reported effects upon precise organ or visceral function, according to Upledger, an American osteopath (www.upledger.com/ news/0000d.htm). Upledger has used both Chapman's reflex treatment and acupuncture for several years in private practice, and considers them mostly interchangeable concepts.

Whether the reflex area which influences organ function is named a Chapman's reflex centre or a Chinese acupuncture point is of little consequence clinically as long as the normalization of organ function is the result. Chapman's points can be needled in the same manner as acupuncture points, with similar positive benefit to the organ or disorder involved.

The following reflex relationships have been developed by chiropractors and are sometimes utilized in osteopathic practice.

JARRICOT'S DERMATOME REFLEXES

Jarricot determined that there were relationships between the underlying organs and the superficial tissues, which could be identified through a dermatome relationship.[45] These are indicated in Figure 2.7 and are identified by a skin-rolling technique, where the skin is picked up and rolled between finger and thumb to palpate the tissue quality. Where the skin is tender, tight and more

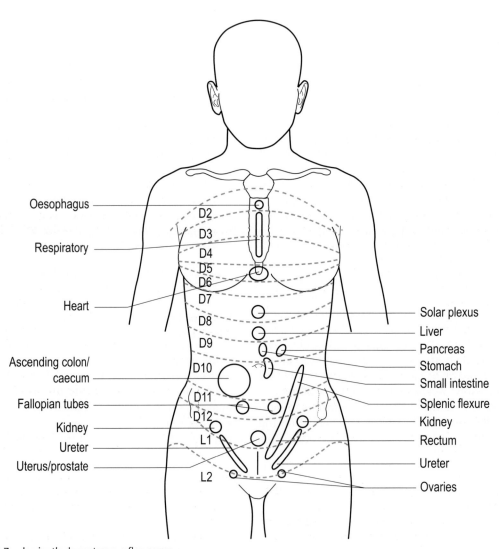

Figure 2.7   Jarricot's dermatome reflex zones.

bound down to underlying tissue than expected, the reflex zone is said to be active. Continuing to roll the skin (within the active zone) is said to reflexly improve function in the dermatome-related viscera. The zones can be usefully incorporated into practice as a 'before-and-after' evaluation for the application of other osteopathic techniques, and can help the practitioner and patient identify when change has occurred.

DE JARNETTE OCCIPITAL REFLEXES

De Jarnette identified a functional link between various points of the vertebral column, certain organs and palpable points or zones located along the occipital lines on the back of the skull.[46]

Tender and tight nodules located on particular points of the occipital lines are thought to be related to various organs through myofascial and neural links. De Jarnette prescribed a very regimented routine for the 'correction' of the reflexes, which involved work both to the occipital line nodules/fibres and to specific parts of the vertebrae (transverse processes and spinous processes) on particular vertebral levels, depending on which occipital line was involved.

Where osteopaths have become interested in general visceral reflexes or utilize the practice of applied kinesiology in their work, for example, they may incorporate De Jarnette's reflexes. Otherwise they are not often a routine part of osteopathic practice.

References

1. Pickar JG. Neurophysiological effects of spinal manipulation. Spine J 2002; 2(5):357-71.
2. Lesho EP. An overview of osteopathic medicine. Arch Fam Med 1999;8(6):477-84.
3. Patterson MM, Howell JN (eds).The central connection: somatovisceral/viscerosomatic interaction. Colorado: American Academy of Osteopathy; 1989.
4. Nansel D, Szlazak M. Somatic dysfunction and the phenomenon of visceral disease simulation: a probable explanation for the apparent effectiveness of somatic therapy in patients presumed to be suffering from true visceral disease. J Manipulative Physiol Ther 1995;18(6):379-97.
5. Sato A, Schmidt RF. The modulation of visceral functions by somatic afferent activity. Jpn J Physiol 1987;37(1):1-17.
6. Sato A. Somatovisceral reflexes. J Manipulative Physiol Ther 1995;18(9):597-602.
7. Janig W, Habler HJ. Specificity in the organization of the autonomic nervous system: a basis for precise neural regulation of homeostatic and protective body functions. Prog Brain Res 2000;122:351-67.
8. Federici A, Nocera L. The power transfer from the neuromuscular machinery to its load as a vegetative and somatic behaviour. Funct Neurol 1990;5(3):233-7.
9. McCredie J. Neural crest defects. A neuroanatomic basis for classification of multiple malformations related to phocomelia. J Neurol Sci 1976;28(3):373-87.
10. North K, McCredie J. Neurotomes and birth defects: a neuroanatomic method of interpretation of multiple congenital malformations. Am J Med Genet 1987;3(Suppl):29-42.

11. Cervero F. Visceral nociception: peripheral and central aspects of visceral nociceptive systems. Philos Trans R Soc Lond B Biol Sci 1985;308(1136):325-7.
12. Burns L. Viscero-somatic and somato-visceral spinal reflexes. 1907. J Am Osteopath Assoc 2000;100(4):249-58.
13. Koizumi K, Brooks CM. The integration of autonomic system reactions: a discussion of autonomic reflexes, their control and their association with somatic reactions. Ergeb Physiol 1972;67:1-68.
14. Sato A, Swenson DC. Sympathetic nervous system response to mechanical stress of the spinal column in rats. J Manip Physiol Ther 1984;7:141-7.
15. Van Buskirk RL. Nociceptive reflexes and the somatic dysfunction: a model. J Am Osteopath Assoc 1990;90(9):792-4,797-809.
16. Korr IM. Collected papers of Irvin M Korr (ed. B Peterson). Colorado: American Academy of Osteopathy; 1979.
17. Nagai M, Wada M, Kobayashi Y, Togawa S. Effects of lumbar skin warming on gastric motility and blood pressure in humans. Jpn J Physiol 2003;53(1):45-51.
18. Vatner SF, Pagani M. Cardiovascular adjustments to exercise: hemodynamics and mechanisms. Prog Cardiovasc Dis 1976;19(2):91-108.
19. Lundborg G, Dahlin L, Danielsen N, Zhao Q. Trophism, tropism, and specificity in nerve regeneration. J Reconstr Microsurg 1994;10(5):345-54.
20. Janig W, Levine JD, Michaelis M. Interactions of sympathetic and primary afferent neurons following

nerve injury and tissue trauma. Prog Brain Res 1996;113:161-84.

21. Renz H. Neurotrophins in bronchial asthma. Respir Res 2001;2(5):265-8.

22. Esquifino AI, Cardinali DP. Local regulation of the immune response by the autonomic nervous system. Neuroimmunomodulation 1994;1(5):265-73.

23. Bellinger DL, Lorton D, Felten SY, Felten DL. Innervation of lymphoid organs and implications in development, aging, and autoimmunity. Int J Immunopharmacol 1992;14(3):329-44.

24. Livnat S, Madden KS, Felten DL, Felten SY. Regulation of the immune system by sympathetic neural mechanisms. Progr Neuro-Psychopharmacol Biol Psychiatry 1987;11(2-3):145-52.

25. Endroczi E. Recent development in hormone research. Acta Physiol Hung 1989;73(4):417-32.

26. Tomaszewska D, Przekop F. The immune-neuro-endocrine interactions. J Physiol Pharmacol 1997;48(2):139-58.

27. Kordon C, Bihoreau C. Integrated communication between the nervous, endocrine and immune systems. Horm Res 1989;31(1-2):100-4.

28. Ballieux RE. Impact of mental stress on the immune response. J Clin Periodontol 1991;18(6):427-30.

29. Plytycz B, Seljelid R. Stress and immunity: minireview. Folia Biol (Krakow) 2002;50(3-4):181-9.

30. Carreiro J. An osteopathic approach to children. Edinburgh: Churchill Livingstone; 2003.

31. Janig W, McLachlan EM. Specialized functional pathways are the building blocks of the autonomic nervous system. J Auton Nerv Syst 1992;41(1-2):3-13.

32. Morrison SF. Differential control of sympathetic outflow. Am J Physiol Regul Integr Comp Physiol 2001 Sep;281(3):R683-98.

33. Kuchera ML, Kuchera WA. Osteopathic principles in practice. Kirksville: Greyden Press; 1994.

34. Qin C, Chandler MJ, Jou CJ, Foreman RD. Responses and afferent pathways of C1-C2 spinal neurons to cervical and thoracic esophageal stimulation in rats. J Neurophysiol 2004;91(5):2227-35.

35. Jou CJ, Farber JP, Qin C, Foreman RD. Convergent pathways for cardiac- and esophageal-somatic motor reflexes in rats. Auton Neurosci 2002;99(2):70-7.

36. Chandler MJ, Zhang J, Foreman RD. Vagal, sympathetic and somatic sensory inputs to upper cervical (C1-C3) spinothalamic tract neurons in monkeys. J Neurophysiol 1996;76(4):2555-67.

37. Grundy D. What activates visceral afferents? Gut 2004;53(Suppl 2):ii5-8.

38. Holzer-Petsche U, Brodacz B. Traction on the mesentery as a model of visceral nociception. Pain 1999;80(1-2):319-28.

39. Countee RW. Extrinsic neural influences on gastrointestinal motility. Am Surg 1977;43(9):621-6.

40. Butler DS. The sensitive nervous system. Australia: Noigroup Publications; 2001.

41. Zucker A. Chapman's reflexes: medicine or metaphysics? J Am Osteopath Assoc 1993;(3):346.

42. American Osteopathic Association. Foundations for osteopathic medicine (ed. RC Ward). Baltimore: Williams and Wilkins; 1997.

43. Simons DG, Travell JG, Simons LS, et al. Travell and Simons' myofascial pain and dysfunction: the trigger point manual, 2nd edn. Philadelphia: Lippincott, Williams and Wilkins; 1999.

44. Goodheart G, Frost R. Applied kinesiology: a training manual and reference book of basic principles and practices. California: Ronin Publishing; 2002.

45. Jarricot H. Projections viscero-cutanees. Metameres thoraco-abdominales. Torino: Minerva Medica; 1975.

46. De Jarnette B. Sacro occipital technique. Nebraska: De Jarnette; 1979.

Chapter 3

Mechanical links and global visceral screening

CHAPTER CONTENTS

RESTRICTION IN MUSCULOSKELETAL STRUCTURES LIMITS VISCERAL FUNCTION

As should now be more apparent, for osteopaths the mechanical relationship between visceral and somatic structures is quite complex. It represents more than a two-dimensional mechanistic model of how adjacent structures 'push and pull' on each other. Rather, it is how somatic movement interacts with physiology via such things as adverse mechanical influences on organ support, fluid dynamics and neural communication. It is this type of view that enables osteopaths to consider how they might be able to contribute to the management of patients suffering from a wide variety of 'visceral complaints, conditions or pathologies'.

Not all osteopaths wish to enter this area of practice on a day-to-day basis and are content with helping patients manage a wide variety of somatic complaints, such as herniated lumbar disc with sciatic radiculopathy, whiplash injuries to the neck, temporomandibular pain and headaches, sprained ankles and other sporting injuries, and workplace pain and dysfunction. For them, visceral osteopathy seems less relevant. However, as already indicated, visceral movement is simply part of the body's three-dimensional mobility-dynamic and any restriction, be it visceral or somatic, can impact on the biomechanical efficiency of the musculoskeletal system, tissues and articulations, and hence contribute to symptoms therein.

The following discussion further explores this concept and indicates how visceral osteopathic techniques and approaches can be relevant in the management of musculoskeletal system problems.

VISCERAL MOVEMENT AFFECTS MUSCULOSKELETAL MOVEMENT

Knowing the attachments and mechanical links between the viscera and the musculoskeletal system (e.g. body cavities) gives insight into how visceral restrictions can lead to tensions and poor or reduced movement in various musculoskeletal structures. Specific muscles and articulations can become affected as a result of adapted movement in the visceral field, which can then be aetiological to various musculoskeletal symptoms.

Orthopaedic biomechanical examination does not normally take into account the movement dynamics of the visceral systems and other tissues of the body, such as connective tissue planes and peritoneal ligaments. Traditional biomechanists do not consider organs to be prime movers of joints or limiters to any range of articular motion so they have no role in orthopaedic examination of articular structures. However, osteopaths *do* consider that visceral structures can affect tissue and articular function and that their assessment *should* be a part of normal biomechanical evaluation of articular and muscular/ligamentous complexes.

There are various simple mechanical links between the viscera and certain muscles and articulations. If the organs are stiff, scarred, tense or otherwise inelastic and less compliant or mobile than normal, this can physically pull or irritate the somatic tissues to which they are attached. Through this mechanism, the viscera can contribute to biomechanical adaptation within the somatic structures and possibly lead to mechanical strain and symptoms within the musculoskeletal system. The organs do not have to be suffering particular pathology at the time in order for the relationship to be significant; nor does the organ have to have

been diseased at all. It may simply be somewhat tight or tense as a result of general physiology, emotional influences or dietary imbalance.

Table 3.1 shows some of the links between the musculoskeletal system and the viscera. Often, due to the large number of visceral connections at certain parts of the skeletal framework, some areas of the body are particularly affected by the visceral system. In osteopathic practice, various vertebral restrictions are commonly associated with mechanical visceral tensions. These are different from the neural reflex links between the spinal column and the organs, which are discussed in a later chapter. Here, the links are purely physical and serve to indicate which organ should be explored when attempting to differentially diagnose the movement disorder at any particular spinal (or associated) articulation. These links are shown in Figure 3.1. Major biomechanical sites in the body are discussed below in more detail, to highlight the range of influences and interactions that visceral attachments, visceral elasticity and mobility have to mechanical function of sections of the musculoskeletal system.

CERVICODORSAL JUNCTION

The cervicodorsal area is often stressed mechanically, where the mobile cervical column articulates against the relatively rigid thoracic cage. The impact of the shoulder girdle attachments onto the manubrium and first rib (via the clavicle) also affects the forces acting through this region. Consequently, symptoms often arise through an imbalance in the mechanics of these converging forces.

Osteopaths have for many years been fascinated by the complex mechanics within the thoracic inlet and around the cervicobrachial region. They build into their biomechanical understanding concepts of how tensions in pleural, mediastinal, pharyngeal and other cervical fascial structures can affect the somatic mechanical balance at the cervicodorsal junction.

SIBSON'S FASCIA

One of the fascial structures most frequently discussed within osteopathy is Sibson's fascia, a fascial/connective tissue sheet which attaches to

Table 3.1 Some mechanical links between the viscera and the musculoskeletal system (a few examples only)

Organ	Link	Visceral/somatic structure affected
Liver	Coronary ligaments	Diaphragm
Left lobe of liver	Left triangular ligament	Pericardium, via the central tendon
Right lobe of liver	Right triangular ligament	Diaphragm, and arcuate ligaments – upper lumbar spine and 12th rib
Liver	Lesser omentum	Diaphragm
Ascending/descending colon	Toldt's fascia	Psoas and upper lumbar spine
Duodenum	Peritoneum	Upper lumbar spine
Duodenum	Ligament of Treitz	Upper lumbar spine on left, and the oesophageal hiatus/stomach
Small intestine	Root of mesentery	Coeliac and superior mesenteric plexi, cysterna chyli, and mid/upper lumbar spine
Small intestine	Articulation with pelvic organs	Uterus and sometimes the bladder
Transverse colon	Mesocolon to pancreas	Pancreas, pancreatic duct and upper lumbar spine
Kidneys	Renal fascia	Kidney, diaphragm, psoas and hips
Uterus	Uterosacral ligaments	Sacrum and piriformis
Bladder	Urachus	Anterior abdominal wall, and liver/diaphragm via falciform ligament
Bladder	Pubovesical ligaments	Obturator internus and the symphysis pubis
Pelvic floor	Muscular attachments	Ilial, sacral and coccygeal mobility
Duodenum	Ligament of Treitz	Upper lumbar spine, and diaphragm
Lung	Suspensory ligament of the pleural dome	First rib, general thoracic inlet structures, and the lower cervical spine
Lungs and bronchi	Mediastinal fascia (bronchopulmonary membrane) and the vertebropericardial ligament	Upper dorsal spine (D3–4)
Lungs and bronchi	Mediastinal fascia (bronchopulmonary membrane) and the pulmonary ligament	Central tendon, and sternal mechanics
Prostate	Fascia of Denonvilliers	Pelvic floor, sacrum and coccyx, plus gastrointestinal system
Spleen	Splenicocolic, lienorenal, and lienophrenic ligaments	Diaphragm, splenic flexure of colon, and left kidney
Pharynx/oesophagus	Hyoid and suprahyoid muscles	Temporal bones, and sphenoid/sphenobasilar symphysis

the internal edge of the first rib and passes medially to attach to the deep cervical fascia, whilst also covering the dome of the parietal pleura. It is a disputed structure and is sometimes listed as the scalenus minimus muscle, the suprapleural membrane or the costopleuro-vertebral ligament (of Zuckerlandl).[1] However, others recognize Sibson's fascia as a separate structure to the endothoracic fascia and the parietal pleura[2] which can be reinforced by one or other of the scalene muscles, and have a degree of variation in its own layout/anatomical extent. As well as the connections listed above, it attaches to the inner border of the first rib, as stated above, and extends superiorly, to attach to the transverse process of C7 (and sometimes C6). It may be implicated, along with the scalene muscles, in many cases of brachial neuritis.[3]

This fascial sheet also has a variety of attachments to the cervical fascia[4] and to other parts of the neck,[5] and can also link into the capsule of the sternoclavicular joint, the mediastinal fascia and the vascular and lymphatic vessels and neural structures (somatic and autonomic) that pass

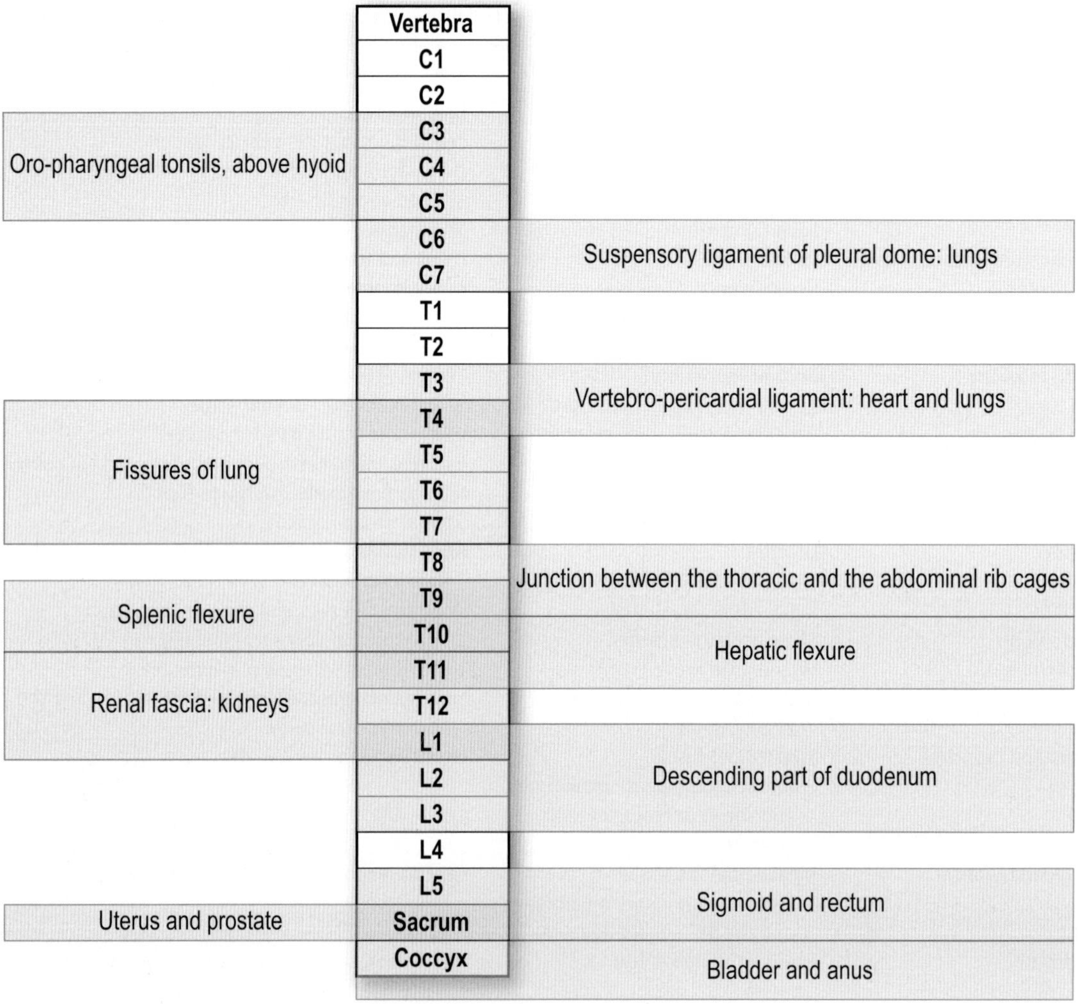

Left	Vertebra	Right
	C1	
	C2	
	C3	
Oro-pharyngeal tonsils, above hyoid	C4	
	C5	
	C6	Suspensory ligament of pleural dome: lungs
	C7	
	T1	
	T2	
	T3	Vertebro-pericardial ligament: heart and lungs
	T4	
Fissures of lung	T5	
	T6	
	T7	
	T8	Junction between the thoracic and the abdominal rib cages
Splenic flexure	T9	
	T10	Hepatic flexure
	T11	
Renal fascia: kidneys	T12	
	L1	
	L2	Descending part of duodenum
	L3	
	L4	
	L5	
Uterus and prostate	Sacrum	Sigmoid and rectum
	Coccyx	Bladder and anus

Figure 3.1 Mechanical links between the spine and the organs (some examples).

through the thoracic inlet region. All of these structures are also linked to the fascia that embeds into the periosteum of the clavicle, manubrium and first rib. These relationships are shown in Figure 3.2. It is referred to by osteopaths as the thoracic inlet 'diaphragm' and is viewed as functionally related to the thoracic diaphragm, the pelvic floor diaphragm and the tentorium (the 'cranial diaphragm'), giving the body a complex linkage pattern between four transversely operating diaphragms. These diaphragms will impact on the longitudinally running neural and visceral core links of fascia referred to previously.

As a result of these attachments, anything which causes tension or stiffening in the pleural dome (such as a variety of lung conditions or other mediastinal traumas or irritations) can lead to increasing tension in Sibson's fascia. This will be transmitted to the cervical fascia, the first rib, the clavicle and so on, with the end result that the cervicodorsal vertebral articulations can be restricted in their mechanics.

Figure 3.2 shows an oblique view of the left thoracic cavity. It shows the heart in situ, with the sternum removed. It illustrates the fascial continuity between the anterior throat and cervical region, and the mediastinal fascia and organs. The sternum and costal cartilages are initially attached to the endothoracic fascia, which then forms a connection between the anterior pericardium, the superior

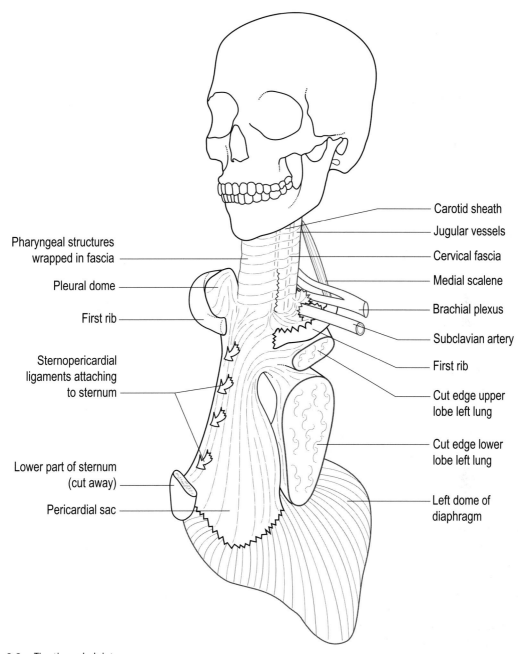

Figure 3.2   The thoracic inlet.

mediastinal fascia and the diaphragm. This connecting fascia forms what osteopaths call the sternopericardial ligament, for obvious reasons. The sternopericardial ligament links the complex mechanics of the anterior thoracic cage with the mechanics of the pericardium and heart. It creates mechanical links between the heart, mediastinum, the thoracic inlet and the cervical region, via the superior mediastinal fascia.

The superior mediastinal fascia blends with tissues and structures at the level of the thoracic inlet, biomechanically connecting all structures from the thoracic diaphragm to the thoracic inlet 'diaphragm'. From this, one can see that mechanical torsions and tensions arising within the thoracic inlet, including the clavicle and first rib (and perhaps the shoulder girdle in general), can affect the movement of the brachial plexus, the subclavian vessels and the thoracic duct. In this way, the thoracic inlet mechanics can affect vascular syndromes in the upper limb, brachial plexus irritation and lymphatic drainage of the head and neck (and body in general). Mobilization of the sternoclavicular joint may be as valuable in this respect as that of the first rib (depending on individual patient mechanics).

There is potential for a variety of biomechanical torsions which could arise from a combination of adverse movement patterns coming from the cervical spine, the first rib, the clavicle and shoulder girdle musculature[6] and also from within the mediastinum and the lung via the pleura and suspensory ligament of the pleural dome.[7] The suspensory ligament is discussed below. Thus, to relieve many pain presentations and symptoms within this region and the upper limb/chest, it may be necessary to look at many somatic *and* visceral components, in order to balance all predisposing and maintaining factors to dysfunction within this region.

SUSPENSORY LIGAMENT OF THE PLEURAL DOME

The suprapleural membrane or Sibson's fascia, which was introduced above, is a structure which is separable from the endothoracic fascia, ribs and parietal pleura.[8] The top of the parietal pleura forms a dome which rises above the first rib anteriorly such that the lung actually pushes up into the cervical region. The external surface of this parietal pleural dome is attached to the suprapleural membrane, making the mechanics of the lung and pleura inseparable from those of the thoracic inlet. The suspensory ligament of the pleural dome relates to bands or fibres which pass from the suprapleural membrane to the first rib, transverse processes and body of the lower cervical vertebrae, and is shown in Figure 3.3. In this way, the mechanics of the lung and pleura are also intimately related to those of the lower cervical spine. In fact, any mediastinal tension can pass through

to the suspensory ligament of the pleural dome, linking cervical mechanics to those of the internal chest. This can be particularly interesting in cases of whiplash or chest trauma, where internal mediastinal tissue tensions manifest in cervicobrachial pain and neurovascular presentations.

ADSON–WRIGHT TEST, MEDIASTINAL AND NEURAL TENSION TESTING

Gaining insight into the mechanics of this complex region is one matter while mechanically differentiating between structures implicated is another. The typical test for thoracic outlet syndrome is the Adson-Wright test. This has a number of variations and it is best to test in a number of different directions of arm or neck movement, with or without inspiration, as not all combinations may induce arterial compression.[9] If any of the combinations provoke arterial pulse diminution, then the test is positive. Neural tension testing as described by Butler[10] may also be very useful, and the visceral component in neural restriction in the thoracic outlet should not be forgotten.

Another useful test is the mediastinal-neck diagnostic indicator test, shown in Figure 3.4. In this test, the practitioner gently takes a subcostal contact, being careful to avoid the central epigastric region and ensuring the costal margin itself is not contacted (this is to prevent the ribcage being directly lifted during the technique). The practitioner asks the patient to perform some active neck movements, in order to assess range and symptom provocation. Then, the practitioner gently lifts up a few millimetres to slightly lift the subcostal organs and diaphragm, in order to 'take the weight' of these off the mediastinal tissues and organs to lessen the mechanical 'drag' on the cervicobrachial region. With the organs slightly lifted, the practitioner maintains this position, whilst the patient again performs the active tests that had reduced range and/or provoked symptoms. If the test results ease, then the mediastinal fascia or organ restrictions are related to the mechanics of the patient's problem. If the neck movement does not improve whilst the practitioner is supporting the mediastinal contents, then the neck problem is not immediately influenced by those tensions.

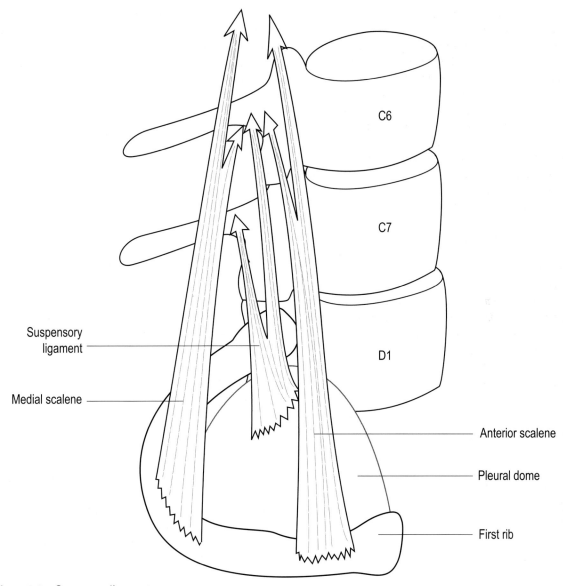

C6

C7

D1

Suspensory ligament

Medial scalene

Anterior scalene

Pleural dome

First rib

Figure 3.3   Suspensory ligament.

This is a useful test for patient education and to illustrate why chest-based treatment may be useful in the management of their acute neck symptoms. It is also a useful test to evaluate treatment outcomes, after a range of mobilizations or releases have been performed. The test itself can be adapted into a treatment approach, in which the practitioner uses the subcostal contact to release through the mediastinum, using an indirect or functional technique to unwind through to the neck region.

Another useful technique for the thoracic inlet structures such as the scalenes and the suspensory ligament of the pleural dome is the recoil technique (Fig. 3.5). Recoil techniques can in fact be used throughout the body and on many different tissue types, and are standard osteopathic manoeuvres. The aim is to find a particular tissue barrier (by gentle direct testing). Once the direction of greatest resistance is found, this becomes the direction for application of the recoil technique. The technique utilizes breathing and elastic recoil

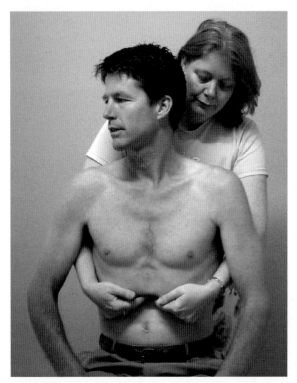

Figure 3.4   Mediastinal-neck diagnostic indicator test.

in the tissues. To set up the elastic recoil component, move the tissue into the identified barrier (greatest resistance) to the limit of tissue 'give'. Maintain that contact with the barrier whilst the patient breathes in and out. At the correct moment, release the tissue barrier and the tissue will recoil

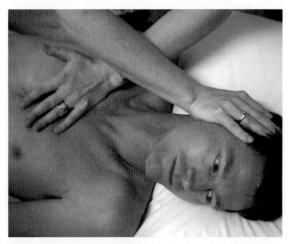

Figure 3.5   Recoil techniques for the thoracic outlet.

away from the resisted direction. There is no need to apply any last-minute 'thrust' against the tissue barrier: in fact, this is contraindicated. The correct moment to release the tissues is at a certain point in the breathing cycle.

The breathing part of the technique commences after the tissue barrier has first been engaged. Maintaining that contact, the practitioner asks the patient to breathe in (not excessively, but more than a shallow breath). It may be necessary to slightly lift the contact so as not to block the inspiration. As the patient now performs expiration, the practitioner ensures they fully engage the tissue barrier in the correct direction (against the point of greatest resistance). At the moment that the patient starts to breathe in again, the tissue must be released so that it can recoil (and ultimately rebound through the original tissue barrier, thus rebalancing the tissues and restoring more normal movement). The tissue should be released quickly – it is necessary that it springs and recoils actively. If it is allowed to just 'ease back' then the proprioceptive impetus necessary for the technique will be lost.

One caution would be to avoid using recoil techniques when there is significant inflammation or tissue irritability. As the technique requires subtlety to apply, it is easy to overstimulate already stressed tissues, so it is best to avoid such situations.

Figure 3.5 shows the contact points for the occiput and lateral skull, and the first rib, just below the clavicle. The two hands will create the tissue barrier by moving in opposing directions. When the tissues are released, it is important to ensure that the patient's head or face will not be accidentally knocked. The occipital hand must not apply pressure onto the ear or mandible, or the lateral throat. It should engage the occiput and use it to longitudinally traction the cervical column. A slight amount of rotation of the head may be required, but too much is contraindicated. Place a small pillow on the opposite side of the patient's head to limit this if necessary. The other hand contact will engage the suspensory ligament of the pleural dome indirectly by engaging the first rib, which will tension the pleural dome and then the suspensory ligament. Avoiding contact with the clavicle will direct the technique to the thoracic inlet as opposed to the shoulder girdle.

Ensure that the contact is comfortable at all times and remember that the amount of movement required to engage the tissue barrier will be no more than millimetres if applied correctly.

THE THORACIC CAGE

RESPIRATORY SYSTEM BRIDGES THE CERVICODORSAL AND DORSOLUMBAR REGIONS

The respiratory system has many links with the musculoskeletal system; indeed, the two are so interlinked that respiratory function is not possible without the actions of skeletal muscles and the movement of osseous structures. As a result, many musculoskeletal articular restrictions in the thoracic region are consequent to tension, tightness and poor function within the respiratory tissues (for example, pleura, bronchi and lungs).

The thorax isn't just to do with breathing, and it isn't just something to hang your shoulders on; it has some very interesting spiral and oscillatory biomechanics and dynamics operating during many body movements. Appreciating how the thorax moves as a unit and as part of general body mechanics will illustrate how flexible the respiratory system must be in order not to limit any of this general musculoskeletal system movement and balance.

Restrictions in the respiratory tissues will affect this movement dynamic, causing much of the rest of the body to adapt. This can ultimately lead to a whole variety of very diverse symptoms and stresses. Exploring this dynamic will give insight into why osteopaths would treat the whole body when considering respiratory function, and how management of a whole range of biomechanical dysfunctions may require treatment of the respiratory system (with or without the presence of respiratory disease and pathology).

The thorax and locomotion

In standing posture, the spinal curves should be in balance and be relative to each other.[11] The spinal curves should also function in an integrated way during walking and other body movements.

During walking and running, the pelvis rotates one way and the thorax and shoulder girdle

the other. This gives a natural longitudinal spiral torsion pattern operating along a vertical axis passing from the lower limbs, through the spine and thorax, to the upper limbs, head and neck.[12] During the gait cycle there is also a lateral inclination of the sacrum. This gives lumbar sidebending one way and then the other, leading to lateral curve development through the dorsal and cervical areas. These lateral curves also oscillate with walking. All of this oscillatory movement has to pass through the thorax. During the gait cycle the thorax also shifts anteroposteriorly with respect to the lumbar spine and pelvis with consequent adaptations in lumbar curvature and pelvic tilt.[13] As walking changes so does the interaction between the thorax and other body areas.[14] If the thorax is restricted or stiff, it will impact on the ability of the body to oscillate and will disrupt the gait cycle, possibly giving local mechanical dysfunction in, for example, the knee, feet, shoulders or pelvis. These dysfunctions could eventually strain local tissues sufficiently to give pain and other symptoms.

The thoracic cage and spine must therefore be elastic and compliant in order for general movements to pass evenly through from the lower limb and pelvis to the upper limb in a coordinated pattern, and for trunk muscle coordination to be efficient.[15] If the thorax is stiff, this reduces smooth transition of motion through the lumbar spine and between the arms and legs. Conversely, altered gait and walking patterns as a result of either upper limb, lower limb or pelvic restrictions will cause the torso oscillations to distort into a slightly different pattern. This may lead to or complicate thoracic pain presentations.

The thoracic cage, then, is part of the dynamic elastic coupling between body cavities and whole-body movements that was introduced in the previous chapter. Any changes in thoracic cavity compliance will have a large impact throughout the body (see Figure 3.6). Thoracic cage compliance is also linked to the function of the viscera contained within it, notably the respiratory system (see below).

Respiratory system coordination

It is not just walking and general thoracic cage mobility that are coordinated during walking

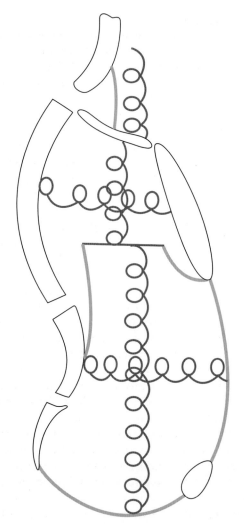

Figure 3.6   Elastic coupling through the body.

and running. Respiration must be coordinated with the overall oscillatory pattern, meaning that the thoracic movements must oscillate according to the demands of gait but also due to respiratory pressures.[16] Hence, during breathing, respiratory-thoracic movements should not conflict with the thoracic components of general body movements (for example, bending, twisting and load carrying). The chest wall should be adaptable enough to absorb these postures without greatly altering respiratory system function.[17] Respiratory action should be to 'breathe into' that locomotive and general movement pattern to retain the optimum respiratory function within any given motion pattern.

This interesting dynamic between locomotive patterns and respiratory anatomy is highlighted further when one compares the anatomy between species. Animals with different locomotive patterns have different configurations of lungs (with respect to number of lobes and bronchial tree-branching patterns), indicating a strong relationship between locomotion and respiratory development.[18]

Neural integration

To control all of this, there is quite a complex neural integration coordinating motion within the limbs, spine, pelvis and thorax to which proprioceptive information within the thoracic structures is very important.[19] The information from those proprioceptors will help to drive and coordinate upper and lower limb movement patterns, and muscular actions and interactions. Biomechanical restrictions within the thorax will impact on proprioceptive feedback, resulting in the movement becoming slightly adapted. This in turn will coordinate with neural activity throughout the rest of the body, with the result that gait patterns will be subtly changed.

The thorax in two parts

Another aspect of thoracic cage motion patterns is that the thorax appears to operate as 'two halves' within a dynamic whole. Within the thorax, there do seem to be at least two different movement 'compartments'. There is an upper section, that part of the thorax where the lungs are lining the ribcage, and a lower section, where the dome of the diaphragm is juxtaposed against the ribcage (with just small portions of lung slipping between this and the ribs). Thus there is a thoracic-pulmonary section and a diaphragmatic-abdominal section in the thoracic cage.

The 'abdominal' section of the ribcage has its actions dictated substantially by the presence of the subdiaphragmatic abdominal organs. This mechanical division between the abdominal ribcage and the pulmonary ribcage is another component where an elastic dynamic movement must operate for overall thoracic function to be effective.[20] Through this relationship, there may be general thoracic restrictions which are a consequence of poor abdominal ribcage compliance from poor mobility of the upper abdominal organs or inelasticity/scarring of the subdiaphragmatic peritoneum and other soft tissue structures. Anatomically, this division is approximately at the level of the eighth and ninth dorsal vertebrae; the thorax above is principally engaged with the respiratory system and below it is principally engaged with the gastrointestinal or urinary systems.

Articular restrictions at the D8–9 level are often associated with a disparity in movement and elasticity between the two halves of the ribcage. Problems in the respiratory system can affect the thoracic ribcage and problems in the urinary or gastrointestinal tract can affect the abdominal ribcage. More specifically, the diaphragm and the subdiaphragmatic organs such as the liver and kidneys are more usually responsible for abdominal ribcage movement disorders. However, lower lobe problems and restrictions in the costodiaphragmatic recesses are also powerful limiters of the posterior abdominal ribcage.

MEDIASTINAL INFLUENCES

The mediastinal contents are anchored to various sections of the ribcage. These fascial bands or ligaments connect various structures like the pericardium to the sternum and the transversus thoracis muscle, the pulmonary vessels to the front of the dorsal spine and the lower cervical spine, and the hilum of the lung to the central tendon of the diaphragm. These link to the cervical fascia and to the thoracic inlet, as in Figure 3.2. The sternopericardial ligament, vertebropericardial and other mediastinal ligaments will be discussed further in the chapters on respiratory function.

DORSOLUMBAR JUNCTION

The dorsolumbar junction is particularly influenced by the actions and insertions of the diaphragm. This muscle, in turn, is influenced by many visceral structures and there is a reciprocal balance between dorsolumbar function and visceral mobility, via the diaphragm.

DIAPHRAGM

The mechanics of the respiratory system are dependent upon the interaction of the lungs, the ribcage, abdomen *and* diaphragm.[21] The diaphragm itself is a fascinating structure and people have been studying its function for a very long time. Galen (129–200 AD) wrote an amazing treatise on the diaphragm and lungs and did some experiments looking at pleural mechanics and lobar movement which are actually still quite relevant today.[22]

The diaphragm is active during respiration and also other general body movements, such as lifting[23] and arm movement,[24] giving it a postural-mechanical role as well as a respiratory role. There is also quite a variation in the normal position of the diaphragm and the vertebral body height at which either dome is found: the right hemidiaphragm dome can be found between 7.4 and 11.3 vertebra below the top of T1 (average 9.7) and the left dome can be found between 8.1 and 11.8 below the top of T1 (average 10.2).[25]

When the diaphragm contracts and moves, it does so in many directions at once. There is cyclical contraction and relaxation in three dimensions, which must operate effectively in static posture and also during diverse movement of the torso and body. There is a natural regional deformation within the diaphragm[26] so that different regions move in different amounts and orientations in a variety of situations.

During the respiratory cycle, the diaphragm changes from being long and thin to being broad and thick during inspiration. There is a change of shape over the domes of the diaphragm, and altered dynamics across the central tendon. With full inspiration, the diaphragm twists and changes shape even more, with broadening in an anteroposterior direction of the inferior costal margin. The muscular domes of the diaphragm will move down about 4 cm, moving more than the central tendon, which does not tend to descend much unless there is a gross change of posture or bend within the thorax.[27]

To appreciate the movement of the diaphragm, it is useful to imagine that it 'opens' during inspiration much like an umbrella, Most of the largest changes in shape occur within the muscular domes. Accordingly, all the structures attached onto the superior and inferior surfaces of the diaphragm have to stretch to accommodate this expansion, much like the spokes of the umbrella would have to 'open' and elongate to allow the umbrella diaphragm to expand. This is particularly so with the peritoneum and all the organs attached to the underneath surface of the diaphragm, which will have to stretch out to allow the costal margin to deform, thereby allowing lung volume to change. Some of these subcostal organs are shown in Figure 3.7.

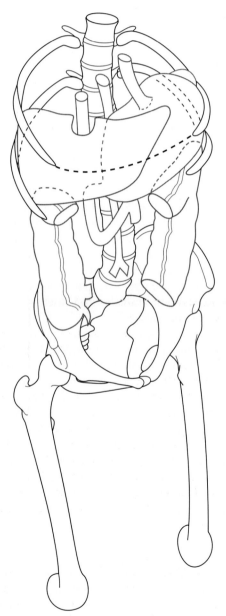

Figure 3.7   Subdiaphragmatic organs.

Subcostal scarring, for example within the gall bladder, or tension as a result of a gastric ulcer or an appendix scar that has adhesed the abdomen on one side will literally 'stick' the underneath of the diaphragm and cause it to become inelastic and poorly compliant (in the above analogy, it would prevent the diaphragm from opening out during respiration). Figure 3.8. shows which segments of the diaphragm are fixed or affected by which organs or visceral ligaments. For example, 4–5 o'clock would be left triangular ligament of liver, 3–2 would be the splenic flexure and splenic ligaments, 12–1 would be the oesophagus, 10–2 would be renal fascia and adrenals, 10–2 would be costodiaphragmatic pleural recesses, 11–1 would be the duodenum or beginning of small intestine, via the crurae, 10–11 would be right triangular ligament of liver, 9–10 would be phrenicocolic ligament of hepatic flexure, 7–8 would be falciform from liver, 6 would be linea alba from pubis or urachus. Global restriction can result from general lung or parietal pleural restrictions. Cardiac-based problems will tend to affect the left dome more than the right. Note: these are physical mechanical links and are not neurally mediated.

This type of tension pattern often leads to altered and uneven breathing patterns, using some parts of the diaphragm more or less than others. This could manifest in local subcostal or lower ribcage discomfort or may present as a culmination of mechanical adaptations elsewhere. For example, the altered breathing patterns may cause recruitment of the accessory breathing muscles, such as the scalenes. If these are utilized over a long period of time, they may become tight and tense in their own right, leading to cervicodorsal mechanical dysfunction and therefore neck pain. In order to resolve all the pain in the neck, it would be necessary to consider the mechanical chain of events within the chest through to the subdiaphragmatic region and the abdomen, where the treatment would be directed (rather than just at the neck).

Examination of the diaphragm must take into account all parts of its muscular and fascial components, as well as all its attachments, such as the costal cartilages, the upper lumbar spine and the arcuate ligaments (median, medial and lateral). The relationship between the crurae, the upper lumbar spine and the diaphragm is well known, with several techniques described for releasing

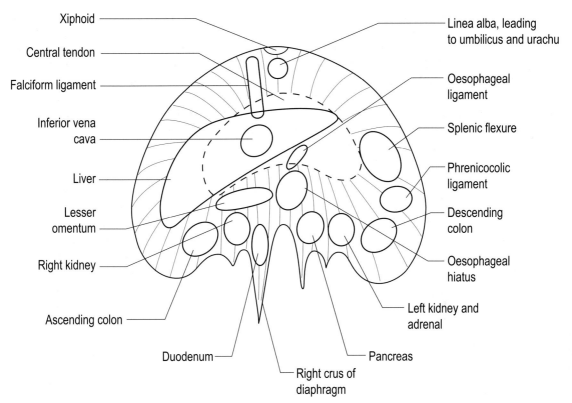

Figure 3.8 'Umbrella fixators'.

the crurae via the mechanics of the upper lumbars. There is less discussion of the relevance of the 11th and 12th ribs and the arcuate ligaments (which span between the ribs and the upper lumbar vertebrae). Most of the posterior diaphragm wall is attached to the arcuate ligaments and tension within these ligaments will affect a much larger area of the diaphragm than will tension within the crurae, which in fact only really influence the middle third of the posterior wall of the diaphragm.

The arcuate ligaments span over the aorta, psoas and quadratus lumborum, so that the diaphragm can work independently of these structures without interfering with them (and vice versa). The median arcuate ligament spans the two crura of the diaphragm; the medial arcuate ligament attaches between the crura of the diaphragm and the tip of the transverse process of L1; and the lateral arcuate ligament attaches from the tip of the transverse process of L1 to the tip of the 12th rib. They are shown in Figure 3.9.

Any organ or fascial structure which attaches to the arcuate ligaments will affect not only the diaphragm but also the mechanics of the upper lumbar spine and the lower ribs. Renal fascial problems and restrictions of the kidneys can commonly affect the arcuate ligaments, as well as the costodiaphragmatic pleural recesses. So, for mechanical problems in the upper lumbar spine and lower ribcage, these organs are particularly relevant. If the orientation and tension of the arcuate ligaments are affected, this will create inhomogeneous movement within the diaphragm which can also be passed to the lungs, other mediastinal structures, the sternum and many other musculoskeletal components.

CAVITY MOTION PATTERNS

Chapter 1 introduced the concept of different cavity dynamics which were related to vertebral facet shape and orientation. The dorsolumbar

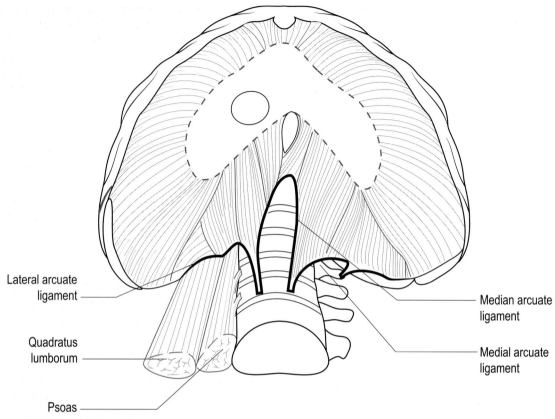

Lateral arcuate ligament

Quadratus lumborum

Psoas

Median arcuate ligament

Medial arcuate ligament

Figure 3.9 Arcuate ligaments.

junction is at the intersection of these changing cavity dynamics and is consequently affected by many and varied visceral tensions and torsions. In fact, the dorsolumbar junction, being less bound than the rest of the thoracic spine (due to the floating ribs), is more vulnerable to soft tissue torsions acting around it. In a musculoskeletal mechanical analysis, the dorsolumbar spine is often referred to as being particularly related to the functioning of the other junctional areas of the spine, including the lumbosacral joint, the cervicodorsal and the occipitoatlantoid articulation. Dysfunction at the dorsolumbar area will negatively impact on these other junctional areas, thus contributing to many biomechanical pain presentations.

When the dorsolumbar spine is affected for whatever reason, this has several consequences for visceral function. In front of this section of the spine are the coeliac and superior mesenteric autonomic plexi, the cysterna chyli and the

junction between the lumbar plexus of veins and the azygos system. If any of these are irritated, constrained or compromised then visceral function will be impaired. Consequently, the dorsolumbar region is a key segment of the spine, in that it relates to renal, gastrointestinal, endocrine, respiratory and reproductive health, and may require treatment in a wide range of presentations.

POSTERIOR WALL OF DIAPHRAGM RELEASE

One basic test for evaluating the dorsolumbar junction with respect to the above visceral and systemic crossroads is done by exploring the movement dynamics of the arcuate ligaments and associated structures.

Testing the movements of the 12th rib and arcuate ligaments often requires a little thought and care as interpreting findings can sometimes be confusing.

The medial and lateral arcuate ligaments are oriented posteriorly and slightly superiorly. Moving the 12th rib superiorly will stretch the tissues attached to its inferior border, namely the quadratus lumborum muscle.

Attaching to the rib superiorly are the intercostal muscles and the diaphragm and to test if these muscles are restricting the rib, pull caudally. If the tip of the rib is pushed anteriorly (i.e. into the body cavity), as though with the patient lying on their back the rib was lifted straight off the table, then several things can happen.

1. The rib can bend along its length, giving an impression of motion but not in fact creating any movement in its articulations at all.
2. The rib can be difficult to lift up due to tension in the quadratus and diaphragm muscles. This would give the impression that they were lying as a tight sheet over the rib and as the rib was pushed against this sheet, it would offer horizontal resistance.
3. The rib can again be restricted when it is lifted off the table, but this time it will feel as though there is a heavy weight on the ventral surface of the rib, giving a different feel to number 2. This third option would be created by tension in the organs lying adjacent to the rib, usually the kidney but sometimes the duodenum/colon, depending on which side it is and the depth/extent of the visceral tension.

In order to test out the arcuate ligament via a 12th rib contact, it would be necessary to perform a type of distraction movement of the rib away from the vertebral column. This would have to be done in a posterior and superior direction so that its elasticity is being tested along its own length (remember its oblique orientation). If the rib is lifted 'off the table', as in the tests above, then this would simply 'buckle' the ligament and not test it directly.

LUMBAR SPINE

The lumbar spine mechanics are intimately linked with various organs of the body, through their peritoneal and other fascial attachments to the psoas muscle and to various parts of the posterior abdominal wall. Figure 3.10 shows some of these organs.

The ascending and descending colons will attach to the iliopsoas muscles in the iliac fossae via Toldt's fascia, which also links these to parts of the quadratus lumborum muscle. These attachments are in fact onto the renal fascia, and from there to the muscles, but the effect is as though they were attached directly. The mesocolon for the transverse colon and the pancreas cross the upper lumbar spine around L1–2, and the root of the mesentery for the small intestine crosses the lumbar spine at the level of L3 and attaches to the structures on the face of the lumbar spine in this region (such as the aorta and inferior vena cava, the anterior longitudinal ligament, and the fascia over the front of the lumbar region).

In osteopathic circles the links between the psoas muscles and the kidneys and between L3 and the root of the mesentery are considered to be two of the most significant viscerosomatic mechanical links in the body.

There are many theories concerning the actions of the psoas muscle on the lumbar spine, but one which receives less attention is the influence on the lumbosacral junction. Any tension in psoas, whether it causes lumbar flexion or extension (with or without any sidebending or rotation), will have a tendency to compress the lumbar column against the pelvis. This will affect the lumbosacral stabilization mechanisms and lead to irritation of the iliolumbar ligaments, with a tendency to induce rotatory strains at this level. Any case where the strength and actions of the psoas muscle are important for recovery requires an examination of the fascial and visceral components that influence the muscle from within the body cavity.

PELVIS

There is a link between the mechanics of the bony pelvis and the pelvic soft tissues, including the pelvic floor. Although the pelvic floor is not considered a prime mover of the sacrum and ilia, for example, when the pelvic floor is dysfunctional there are often different bony pelvic characteristics to be found.

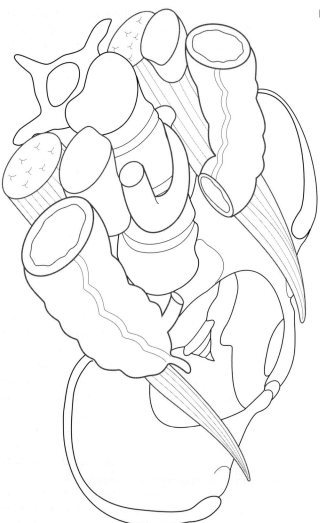

Figure 3.10   Lumbar spine organs.

Women with pelvic floor disorders tend to have a wider transverse inlet, wider intertuberous diameter, wider interspinous diameter, greater sacrococcygeal length, deeper sacral curvature and narrower anteroposterior outlet.[28] The male and female pelves are different in function and in practice, for women the problem is one of the pelvis being too open or loose and in men that of it being too closed or tight. Many cases of repetitive facet irritation and ligamentous strain and muscle spasm at the lumbosacral and sacroiliac articulations are caused or maintained by uneven tension or support in the pelvic floor musculature.

Further discussions about the mechanical influences of the pelvic floor on the movement dynamics of the sacrum and ilia are included in Chapter 10.

GLOBAL MUSCULOSKELETAL AND BODY CAVITY TESTS IN VISCERAL SCREENING

There are several forms of general osteopathic examination which can incorporate a three-dimensional perspective. This is necessary if the visceral component within the body cavities is to be assessed. These techniques are all standard osteopathic examination approaches, which will therefore not be described in detail. They include the following.

- *General osteopathic technique/examination ('GOT')*. This technique has become somewhat watered down over the years and unfortunately is not as well applied as it should be. In its original form, it is a rhythmic, oscillatory movement applied to the limbs, trunk and back, in a particular order or routine, in order to assess the way the body responds to the induced wave-like movement dynamics. Tissue responses are compared to 'normal' or expected (depending on the individual patient), and areas where the movement does not respond as expected are noted and further assessed more locally. In this type of examination routine, all the body tissues are assessed together, and the direction of restriction aids specific anatomical localization of the problem. Each person may have the same examination routine performed but this does not mean the same treatment regimen is given. The treatment is very specifically tailored depending on the tissue responses uncovered.
- *'Functional testing'*. This is where blocks of the body are tested to see how they are moving en masse in relation to each other. The body segments are slightly moved into one direction or another, and the general resistance to that motion is determined. The body is explored generally using this method, with the aim of identifying the direction of movement that offers the least resistance for each block or segment of the body tested. Treatment can in fact be applied using this technique, which follows the path of least resistance and is part of the 'indirect' technique toolkit for osteopaths. The diagnostic element is concerned with describing the movement directions which are blocked and analysing these with respect to local anatomy.
- *'Local' and 'general' listening techniques*. These techniques test widespread fascial sheets and planes running through the body as a type of roadmap to dysfunction. On the premise that 'all roads lead to Rome', a hand is gently placed over various parts of the body, one point at a time, and any fascial drag or shift is felt for. As the hand is moved around the body, 'listening' at each point of contact, the direction of any fascial drag is noted and where these points converge is the area of the body that requires attention. In some cases, all the tension patterns point to the same distant spot and sometimes there are two or three major areas of convergence of fascial drag indicators. When these are examined locally, it is usually possible to evaluate which one should be addressed first. The author tends to approach those areas where the tissue response is the most inert, as the priority. The term 'listening' is used for this as the technique requires a passive acknowledgement of tissue responses and no initiating/active motion is induced in the tissue to gain a reaction. This differs from the above techniques where motion is induced to trigger a tissue response, making those part of the 'active testing' toolkit. The term 'general listening' describes using one contact to listen for fascial tensions that permeate the whole body or across large sections. The term 'local listening' is used to describe smaller focused tissue responses, usually involving just a small area of the body. For visceral evaluation, these techniques were first described by Barral and Mercier.[29]
- *'Thermal' diagnosis*. Also introduced to osteopaths by Barral,[30] this is another type of listening technique but this time, attention is focused not on fascial drags and tissue tensions but on the heat radiating just off the body's surface. This is a very interesting dynamic, as emotional as well as pathological issues can be detected using a very minimal approach, which is extremely useful for differential diagnosis (when used in conjunction with other medical tests, where appropriate).

It is always important to put any local examination findings in context. If the organs are only examined locally or their major ligaments tested, this will not help determine the nature of the treatment, nor whether that is the best place to start treatment. Unless the practitioner is aware of how many other factors are present both locally and distally (mechanically and reflexly) then the total stressors upon the body cannot be considered and treatment is likely to be unfocused and possibly incorrectly applied.

GENERAL PALPATION INFORMATION

One key point with all palpation is: move from your feet and let your hands 'sink in'. A broader contact is more comfortable. Don't keep letting go of skin contact; this reduces tickling and other irritating signals. Keep moving – a gentle rhythmic motion seems to be the most comfortable for the organs and remember that they will tire more quickly than musculoskeletal tissues and so are prone to overhandling stress.

It takes some skill to appreciate a number of visceral restrictions and tensions. Beginners often make the mistake of carrying their expectation of 'tissue restriction feel' from their musculoskeletal experience into the visceral field. There is little point comparing the soft fluidic visceral structures to bony, muscular or tendinous ones, as the visceral ones will always feel 'all right' when compared to these harder tissues. Thus, a more sensitive approach is needed but once mastered, it can be very accurate.

Often one of the problems with visceral palpation is that insufficient skin slack is created prior to attempting the actual contact. This results in the practitioner pushing a little too firmly to get past this barrier, thereby blocking the technique. Using two hands to gently slide the skin and 'fold' the superficial abdominal tissues over each other creates easier points of entry for the palpating part. If possible, this should not be the finger tips but the sides of the fingers, the lateral palm or the length of the index finger, for example. Using the finger tips often results in a hard contact that is more uncomfortable for the patient. If the viscera are difficult to locate, it is usually best to try to 'let go' some of the depth and to relax the contact, as most people try to go too deeply as novices.

> **_i_** Many of the photographs illustrating techniques used in this book show the patient with the legs flat. It is often easier for novices to raise the knees of the patient slightly to create sufficient tissue slack. Please remember this point as the techniques are reviewed.

One important point to note is that the practitioner should not be bound by centimetres; rather, be guided by feel: contour, quality, percussion and so on. There will always be body-type variation, congenital variation and variation caused by scarring, adhesions and surgical intervention. Surface anatomy locations using measurements are only meant to be a guide and not a dictator of position.

The shape of the posterior abdominal wall is also of interest when palpating the gastrointestinal tract and urinary tract organs. The periumbilical area marks the most shallow section of the abdomen and often, very little pressure is required here to palpate down to the depth of the abdominal aorta and anterior lumbar spine. It is important to recognize that too much pressure will not aid palpation, and can be irritating to visceral and vascular structures. Also, deep palpation is contraindicated in the presence of such things as abdominal aortic aneurysm, so being able to suspect this condition (through history and evaluating pulses, for example) is necessary.

A final comment should be made regarding 'psoas' palpation. Many manual professions claim to palpate and treat the psoas muscles. They take a point of contact somewhat lateral to the border of the rectus abdominis muscle, and somewhat above the level of the anterior superior iliac spines of the pelvis. Whatever they palpate in this region is ascribed to tension in the psoas muscle, as this is how the technique was originally described. However, it is very difficult to palpate psoas directly in any place other than the inguinal region, where the psoas blends with the iliacus and runs over the brim of the pelvis. If the practitioner palpates the abdomen any more cephalically than this, they will be palpating either the colon, the ileocaecal valve, the root of the mesentery, the kidney or various duodenal structures. An accurate and in-depth anatomical knowledge is required before one embarks on visceral palpation.

GLOBAL VISCERAL SCREENING

GENERAL PRINCIPLES

Case history taking and developing a working hypothesis based on medical as well as osteopathic differential diagnosis approaches are necessary, especially to determine if the patient requires referral or other medical investigations. The risk/benefit equations for osteopathic evaluation and management must be considered and all work should be done within pain/emotional tolerance limits, with the informed consent of the patient.

Specific visceral tests are described throughout this book but one quite generalized approach can be useful, especially when global evaluation and release are sought. This approach is based on evaluating the peritoneal relations 'as one'. In other words, following embryological formation, migration and rotation, the organs become wrapped in a peritoneal 'bag' which can be evaluated as a whole structure in its own right. If the peritoneal 'bag' is functioning appropriately, it is more likely that the organs contained within will also be healthy and functioning reasonably. Treating the peritoneal bag as a unique structure also introduces a broad release through the abdominopelvic cavity and can be used to balance out several individual visceral problems. Often this approach reduces the compensation and adaptation between organs and any remaining local tensions after this type of release can be more easily and successfully managed.

PERITONEAL 'BAG' TECHNIQUES

The parietal peritoneum lines the inside of the abdominal cavity and the diaphragm and forms the roof of the pelvis. Some organs are classically described as retroperitoneal, although only the kidneys and adrenals are truly so. The pancreas and most of the duodenum and bile duct are in fact pseudo retroperitoneal. They develop as intraperitoneal structures and it is only when the folds of peritoneum move in a certain way so that the duodenum and pancreas get 'flattened' against the posterior abdominal wall and the peritoneum between them and the renal fascia 'disintegrates', that they have the final appearance of being retroperitoneal.

These relations form various retroperitoneal spaces where fluids can move across the midline and down towards the pelvis. There are in fact also 'subperitoneal' spaces and 'peri' peritoneal spaces that are of interest in visceral osteopathy (as well as for disease-spread considerations in general pathological studies), as indicated in Figure 3.11.

The subperitoneal spaces are classically defined as the broad ligament and the sigmoid mesocolon.[31] Here, the uterus and sigmoid are effectively 'wrapped' or enveloped by the parietal peritoneum, which creates various folds and spaces. The folds become the broad ligament and the mesocolon and the spaces link the sigmoid, the reproductive organs and the retroperitoneal spaces. The subperitoneal space is a large potential space in the abdominal cavity created during embryogenesis. It plays an important, although often underestimated role in the spread of intra-abdominal disease. The various mesenteric folds and ligaments serve as communicating pathways between compartments but sometimes act as barriers to the spread of disease.[32] Subperitoneal spaces also include perivesical spaces, which link superiorly with the pararenal 'retroperitoneal' spaces.[33]

The peritoneal cavity and the pleural and pericardial cavities are originally formed from one structure, the intraembryonic coelum. The coelum develops as a horseshoe-shaped structure within the embryo, with the two 'legs' passing inferiorly either side of the spine and developing gut tube, and the horizontal, curved section crossing the midline near the developing heart and lungs. The two 'legs' eventually unite to form one single peritoneal cavity and the horizontal section becomes separated from the 'legs' via the developing diaphragm, which effectively 'cuts them off', leaving the pleural and pericardial spaces seemingly separate from the peritoneal cavity. In fact, the external margins or surface of the coelum create a subserous 'layer' that persists into the adult. This subserous space is a continuum that forms an anatomical plane linking the subpleural space with the subperitoneal space, hence creating a thoracoabdominal continuum.[34] This is very useful clinically, as this continuum can still be palpated running longitudinally through the body and releases along its length can unify function and movement dynamics between the thorax and the abdomen very effectively.

In practical terms this gives several 'intersystem' relationships. The bladder is linked to the umbilicus and hence to the falciform ligament of the liver and is oriented or pulled up and down 'in front' of the peritoneal bag. In this way the liver may play a role in vesical/bladder irritability, which may give

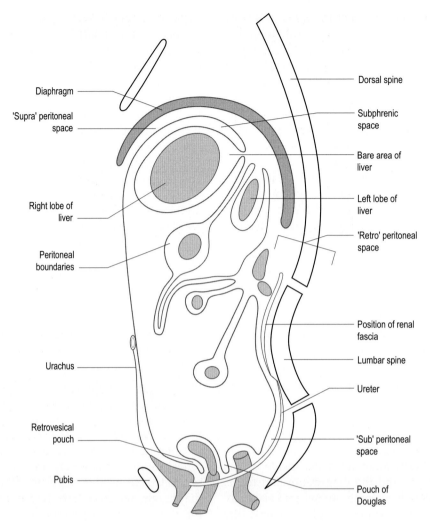

Figure 3.11   'Peri' peritoneal relations.

rise to enuresis, for example. The kidney grows upwards from the pelvis, 'stretching' the ureter as it goes. This links the posterior bladder to the retroperitoneal spaces, and the duodenum and pancreas. The kidneys and ureters move up and down 'behind' the abdominal organs/peritoneal 'bag'. The draping of the parietal peritoneum over the uterus (or posterior bladder and seminal vesicles in the male, to create the fascia of Denonvilliers) means that the reproductive tract is engaged in the motion patterns passing from the liver via the umbilicus to the bladder, and through the ureters back up to the kidneys and ultimately the liver. Effectively, there is a swinging of the urogenital tract around and underneath the abdominal organs and structures. When the peritoneal 'bag' is assessed, all these global relationships can be considered and explored. This technique is shown in Figure 3.12.

The technique involves placing the two hands around the abdomen, or sometimes one anteriorly and one posteriorly, in order to make a broad contact with the parietal peritoneum. The practitioner listens carefully for any particular movement dynamics within the fascial sheet and thoraco-abdominal continuum, and looks for an overall torsion pattern operating through the serous structures as a whole.

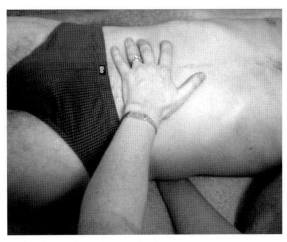

Figure 3.12   Peritoneal 'bag' release.

References

1. Bergman RA, Afifi AK, Miyauchi R. Illustrated encyclopedia of human anatomic variation: part 1: muscular system. University of Iowa; 1999. Only available online at:www.vh.org/Providers/Textbooks/Anatomic Variants/Text/S/04Scalenus.html

2. Currarino G. Cervical lung protrusions in children. Pediatr Radiol 1998;28:533-8.

3. Lawson FL, McKenzie KG. The scalenus minimus muscle. Can Med Assoc J 1951;65:358-61.

4. Williams DW. An imager's guide to normal neck anatomy. Semin Ultrasound CT MRI 1997;18(3): 157-81.

5. Ojiri H, Tada S, Ujita M, et al. Infrahyoid spread of deep neck abscess: anatomical consideration. Eur Radiol 1998;8:955-9.

6. Langley P. Scapular instability associated with brachial plexus irritation: a proposed causative relationship with treatment implications. J Hand Ther 1997;10(1):35-40.

7. Poitevin LA. Thoraco-cervico-brachial confined spaces: an anatomic study. Ann Chir Main 1988; 7(1):5-13.

8. Gaughran GRL. Suprapleural membrane and suprapleural bands. Anat Rec 1964;148:553-9.

9. Gillard J, Perez-Cousin M, Hachulla E, et al. Diagnosing thoracic outlet syndrome: contribution of provocative tests, ultrasonography, electrophysiology, and helical computed tomography in 48 patients. Joint Bone Spine 2001;68(5):416-24.

10. Butler DS, Jones MA. Mobilisation of the nervous system. Edinburgh: Churchill Livingstone; 1991.

11. Jackson RP, Hales C. Congruent spinopelvic alignment on standing lateral radiographs of adult volunteers. Spine 2000;25(21):2808-15.

12. Witte H, Preuschoft H, Recknagel S. Human body proportions explained on the basis of biomechanical principles. Z Morphol Anthropol 1991;78(3):407-23.

13. Harrison DE, Cailliet R, Harrison DD, Janik TJ. How do anterior/posterior translations of the thoracic cage affect the sagittal lumbar spine, pelvic tilt, and thoracic kyphosis? Eur Spine J 2002;11(3):287-93.

14. Van Emmerik RE, Wagenaar RC. Effects of walking velocity on relative phase dynamics in the trunk in human walking. J Biomech 1996;29:1175-84.

15. Davis KG, Marras WS. The effects of motion on trunk biomechanics. Clin Biomech (Bristol, Avon) 2000;15(10):703-17.

16. Young IS, Warren RD, Altringham JD. Some properties of the mammalian locomotory and respiratory systems in relation to body mass. J Exp Biol 1992;164:283-94.

17. Barnas GM, Green MD, Mackenzie CF, et al. Effect of posture on lung and regional chest wall mechanics. Anesthesiology 1993;78(2):251-9.

18. Simons RS. Lung morphology of cursorial and non-cursorial mammals: lagomorphs as a case study for a pneumatic stabilization hypothesis. J Morphol 1996;230(3):299-316.

19. Vernazza S, Alexandrov A, Massion J. Is the center of gravity controlled during upper trunk movements? Neurosci Lett 1996;206:77-80.

20. Cala SJ, Edyvean J, Engel LA. Abdominal compliance, parasternal activation, and chest wall motion. J Appl Physiol 1993;74(3):1398-405.

21. Lichtenstein O, Ben-Haim SA, Saidel GM, Dinnar U. Role of the diaphragm in chest wall mechanics. J Appl Physiol 1992;72:568-74.

22. Derenne JP, Debru A, Grassino AE, Whitelaw WA. History of diaphragm physiology: the achievements of Galen. Eur Respir J 1995;8:154-60.

23. Al-Bilbeisi F, McCool FD. Diaphragm recruitment during nonrespiratory activities. Am J Respir Crit Care Med 2000;162(2 Pt 1):456-9.

24. Hodges PW, Gandevia SC. Activation of the human diaphragm during a repetitive postural task. J Physiol Online 2000;522(1):165-75.

25. Suwatanapongched T, Gierada DS, Slone RM, Pilgram TK, Tuteur PG. Variation in diaphragm position and shape in adults with normal pulmonary function. Chest 2003;123(6):2019-27.

26. Pean JL, Chuong CJ, Ramanathan M, Johnson RL Jr. Regional deformation of the canine diaphragm. J Appl Physiol 1991;71:1581-8.

27. Gauthier AP, Verbanck S, Estenne M, Segebarth C, Macklem PT, Paiva M. Three-dimensional reconstruction of the in vivo human diaphragm shape at different lung volumes. J Appl Physiol 1994;76: 495-506.

28. Handa VL, Pannu HK, Siddique S, Gutman R, Van Rooyen J, Cundiff G. Architectural differences in the bony pelvis of women with and without pelvic floor disorders. Obstet Gynecol 2003;102(6): 1283-90.

29. Barral J-P, Mercier P. Visceral manipulation. Seattle, Washington: Eastland Press; 1988.

30. Barral J-P. Manual thermal diagnosis. Seattle, Washington: Eastland Press; 1996.

31. Hashimoto M, Okane K, Hirano H, Watarai J. Pictorial review: subperitoneal spaces of the broad ligament and sigmoid mesocolon – imaging findings. Clin Radiol 1998;53(12):875-1.

32. Obaro RO, Lata A. Journey through the abdominal underpass: the subperitoneal pathway of disease spread revisited. Can Assoc Radiol J 1995;46(5): 353-62.

33. Mastromatteo JF, Mindell HJ, Mastromatteo MF, Magnant MB, Sturtevant NV, Shuman WP. Communications of the pelvic extraperitoneal spaces and their relation to the abdominal extraperitoneal spaces: helical CT cadaver study with pelvic extraperitoneal injections. Radiology 1997;202(2):523-30.

34. Oliphant M, Berne AS, Meyers MA. The subserous thoracoabdominal continuum: embryologic basis and diagnostic imaging of disease spread. Abdom Imag 1999;24(3):211-9.

Chapter **4**

Overview of respiratory and EENT systems

The aim of this chapter is to review the general and relational anatomy of the respiratory and EENT systems, and discuss physiology in terms of its applicability to osteopathic practice and osteopathic models of intervention. The chapter includes an overview of the salivary glands which, although part of the gastrointestinal system, are included here as many of the techniques and considerations used for various ear, eye, nose and throat structures can be applied to salivary gland examination and treatment.

This chapter includes a basic anatomical overview of the respiratory system and an introduction to the examination and treatment techniques that can be used. It gives an indication of the integration between the somatic and visceral systems, and of reflex relationships, which builds upon information in previous chapters. Patient management is discussed together with the other body systems in Chapter 9 on patient management. All case management discussions are included in that integrated patient management chapter as it is important in osteopathy to remember that treating patients with respiratory and EENT problems does not involve work to the lungs and pharynx alone.

INTRODUCTION

Osteopathy has a lot to offer people with respiratory problems. Helping children and adults cope with the effects of asthma and other chronic respiratory disorders, including hyperventilation syndrome, centres around understanding how the chest wall, respiratory muscles and reflex relationships interact to compromise respiratory function. These disorders also impact on general musculoskeletal system efficiency and many biomechanical problems can trace their roots to restrictions and tensions within the respiratory system and associated tissues. The chest is an area often prone to trauma and strain; in various sports, in road traffic impacts, and as a result of poor posture (rounded shoulders, leaning forwards to the computer screen and so on) at work.

SURFACE ANATOMY

Knowledge of the surface anatomy of the lungs and pleura and related structures helps palpation and interpretation of findings on examination of the musculoskeletal system, as they relate to respiratory function. If the osteopath examines the flexibility of the ribcage in particular ways, a distinction can be made between tensions and restrictions in movement of the musculoskeletal components of the ribcage, such as the costotransverse articulations or the manubriosternal articulation, and visceral mobility such as the ease of slide in the costodiaphragmatic pleural recess or between the lobes of the lung along the oblique fissure, for example. The location of the palpating hand and its direction of movement will determine which underlying structure is being assessed: visceral or musculoskeletal.

The lung fields spread over a large portion of the torso and most of the interpretation of respiratory function is done in the first instance through evaluating the compliance, flexibility and elasticity of the ribcage and intercostal muscles. If one examines the ribcage above the anatomical height of the thoracic diaphragm, one can be more certain that the underlying tissues are those of the lungs and pleura. If the lower portion of the ribcage below the level of the diaphragm is examined, then the underlying tissues include many other visceral structures than just lung or pleura.

POINTS TO REMEMBER

The anatomical height of the diaphragm is approximately the D8–9 vertebral body level. This approximates to the level of a line drawn between the inferior angles of the scapulae, which bisects the tip of the D7 vertebral spinous process.

- Palpation above this height will assess the bulk of the respiratory system
- Palpation below this height will also assess subdiaphragmatic organs such as the liver, kidneys, spleen and stomach.
- The costodiaphragmatic recess is found between ribs 10 and 12, bilaterally, and overlaps the surface projection of the renal fascia.

Table 4.1 shows musculoskeletal landmarks for the respiratory tract. The locations of respiratory landmarks are reasonably consistent and they can be used to guide contact points for various palpatory, examination and treatment techniques.

Table 4.1   Musculoskeletal landmarks for the respiratory system

Respiratory structure	Musculoskeletal landmark	Comments
Suspensory ligament of the pleural dome	Just above clavicle, 1/3 of way from sternoclavicular to acromioclavicular joint	Links lung and mediastinal mechanics to the cervical spine
Costovertebral ligament		Links lungs to thoracic inlet mechanics
Sibson's fascia		Links lungs to thoracic inlet mechanics
Oblique fissure		
Horizontal fissure on the right	From midaxillary line, anteriorly along rib 4	
Bifurcation of the trachea		
Height of the diaphragm in neutral respiration	D8–9 vertebral body height (inferior angles of scapulae)	The abdominal cavity is in fact very 'thoracic' and the subdiaphragmatic organs are much higher than many remember
Costodiaphragmatic recess	Between the 10th and 12th thoracic vertebrae	Restrictions here bind the posterior wall of the diaphragm, indirectly reduce renal mobility and can impact on dorsolumbar spinal mechanics
Costomediastinal recess	Costal cartilages 2–6, either side of the sternum (slight deviation to the anterior ends of ribs 4–6, on the left)	Mediastinal recess restrictions bind the mobility of the costal cartilages and can impact on anything from respiratory function and lung volume to internal thoracic artery and vein circulation (and hence mediastinal and mammary function, for example)

LIGAMENTS AND SUPPORTS

EYES

The eyeball is surrounded by a fascial sheath which is fused anteriorly to the sclera and posteriorly to the sheath of the optic nerve. The extrinsic muscles of the eye link into this fascial sheath and take fascial extensions to their bony insertions (where made). The lateral rectus joins to the zygomatic arch and the medial rectus joins to the lacrimal bone. These fascial extensions are called the lateral and medial check ligaments, respectively. The suspensory ligament of the eyeball is a thickening of the fascia of the inferior rectus. Surrounding the orbit and its fascial sheath as a whole is an orbital septum, linking the eye to the rim of the bony orbit. The lacrimal nerves and vessels pierce this, as do the superior orbital vessels and nerve. The orbital septum, medial and lateral check ligaments all attach either side to the medial and lateral palpebral ligaments, which connect to a tubercle on the zygomatic bone (laterally, just inside the orbit and to the upper part of the

lacrimal crest and the frontal process of the maxilla, medially). The lacrimal gland sits on the superior orbital septum. The lacrimal sac ultimately drains into the inferior meatus of the nasal cavity, via the nasolacrimal duct.

The dural/meningeal attachments with the optic nerve, and the fact that the eyes are literally an extension of the brain, make contact with them (fingers gently resting on the orbits via closed eyelids) an excellent way of evaluating and treating complex dural and reciprocal tension membrane torsion patterns. It is often easier to feel dural torsion through the eyes than it is through contact with the bony cranium. Orofacial and cranial restrictions are therefore critically important for eye function.

The main movements of the eye are:

- medial and lateral, and superior and inferior movements from muscular action
- general three-dimensional mobility within the orbit
- global eye movement, which depends on optic nerve elasticity and dural/membranous elasticity within the cranium.

UPPER RESPIRATORY TRACT AND MIDDLE EAR

The oronasopharyngeal tonsils are embedded in the pharyngeal tissues and the base of the tongue. The pharyngeal tissues and muscles are linked to various cranial structures, such as the basiocciput via the pharyngobasilar fascia. The superior constrictor attaches to the pterygomandibular raphe (linking the medial pterygoid plate to the mylohyoid line on the mandible); the middle constrictor attaches to the hyoid cartilage and lower part of the stylohyoid ligament; the inferior constrictor attaches to the thyroid cartilage, the cricoid, and is continuous with the upper fibres of the oesophagus.

The eustachian tube connects the middle ear and the nasopharynx. Its lateral third is a bony canal in the petrous portion of the temporal bone. Its medial two-thirds are cartilaginous and lie between the petrous temporal and the greater wing of the sphenoid. The cartilage is a folded-over plate, secured joined on its underneath by fibrous tissue. Its lateral end inserts onto bone and the medial end projects through the muscles of the nasopharynx. The tensor veli palatini is attached to the anterolateral portion of the cartilaginous tube, linking it to the soft palate, and the salpingopharyngeus links it to the superior constrictor muscle.

These attachments make the cranial structures, throat, sternoclavicular, temporomandibular and cervical fascial mechanics all important for effective upper respiratory function.

The main movements of the upper respiratory tract are:

- generalized stretch of the upper pharynx with global head and jaw movements
- the throat should be generally elastic and supple to accommodate mandible, shoulder girdle and cervical movements
- stretching and bending of the eustachian tube with palate mobility, temporomandibular joint and cranial bone movements.

LOWER RESPIRATORY TRACT

There are a number of connective tissue structures which are called 'ligaments' that support or attach to the lungs, to help 'anchor' them. These ligaments are mostly pleural reflections or remnants of embryological tissues, which can contain various vessels and/or nerves. The pericardial and pleural 'sacs' all arise from the same structure as the peritoneal 'sac', namely the intraembryonic coelum. This is a horseshoe-shaped hollow structure which makes the serous membranes of the body cavities, into which all the organs invaginate (pushing inwards, dragging folds and layers of serous membrane with them, to become enveloped), thereby eventually forming the many ligaments and mesenteries that support the organs and form conduits for their vascular and nerve supply. This is indicated in Figure 4.1.

Figure 4.2 shows the general pleural, pericardial, mediastinal and other fascial relationships that blend within the thorax in the adult. The heart has descended from the throat area, dragging a 'stocking' of cervical fascia with it, so that the heart is enveloped in a tube of fascia that extends from the cranial base to the central tendon of the diaphragm. The heart is then 'pushed' into the top of the horseshoe-shaped coelum, forming the pericardial layers. The two lungs, which arise from the foregut (the developing oesophagus), 'push' into the rest of the top of the coelum, forming the pleural layers. As a result, the pleural and pericardial layers remain united at the level of the hilum of the lungs and the posterior wall of the heart, where the great vessels enter and leave.

The parietal pleura lines the inside of the ribcage (and so connects all of the ribs). Embryologically, the ribs grow into the sides of the chest, stabilizing the somatic and pleural structures of the body wall at that level. The pleura also covers the two domes of the diaphragm inferiorly and various thoracic inlet structures (such as Sibson's fascia and the underneath of the scalenes) superiorly (see Fig. 4.2). Medially it is reflected alongside the pericardium. The visceral pleura covers the external surface of the lungs and invaginates in between the various lobes of the lungs. There are also two parietal pleural recesses, where the parietal pleura is reflected upon itself, creating 'pockets' so that the lungs can expand into them during inspiration. These are shown in Figures 4.3 and 4.4.

The parietal and visceral pleural layers meet together at the hilum of the lung, where they are also attached to the back of the pericardium and other mediastinal fascial structures. A section of this 'gathering up' of the pleural layers gives an inferior 'extension' which passes towards the diaphragm.

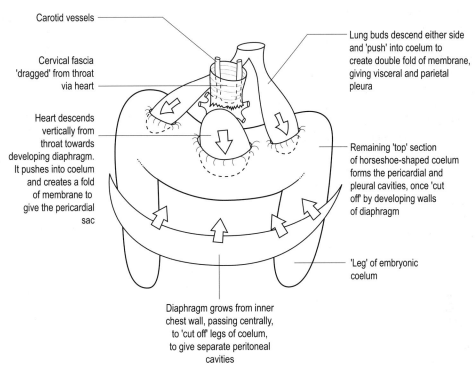

Carotid vessels

Cervical fascia 'dragged' from throat via heart

Heart descends vertically from throat towards developing diaphragm. It pushes into coelum and creates a fold of membrane to give the pericardial sac

Lung buds descend either side and 'push' into coelum to create double fold of membrane, giving visceral and parietal pleura

Remaining 'top' section of horseshoe-shaped coelum forms the pericardial and pleural cavities, once 'cut off' by developing walls of diaphragm

'Leg' of embryonic coelum

Diaphragm grows from inner chest wall, passing centrally, to 'cut off' legs of coelum, to give separate peritoneal cavities

Figure 4.1   Intraembryonic coelum and development of pleural and pericardial cavities.

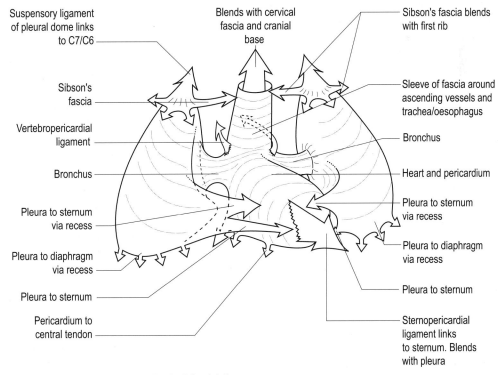

Suspensory ligament of pleural dome links to C7/C6

Sibson's fascia

Vertebropericardial ligament

Bronchus

Pleura to sternum via recess

Pleura to diaphragm via recess

Pleura to sternum

Pericardium to central tendon

Blends with cervical fascia and cranial base

Sibson's fascia blends with first rib

Sleeve of fascia around ascending vessels and trachea/oesophagus

Bronchus

Heart and pericardium

Pleura to sternum via recess

Pleura to diaphragm via recess

Pleura to sternum

Sternopericardial ligament links to sternum. Blends with pleura

Figure 4.2   Generalized pleural and mediastinal fascial ligaments.

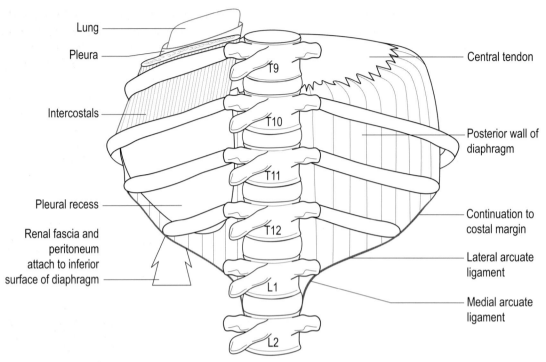

Figure 4.3 Costodiaphragmatic recess.

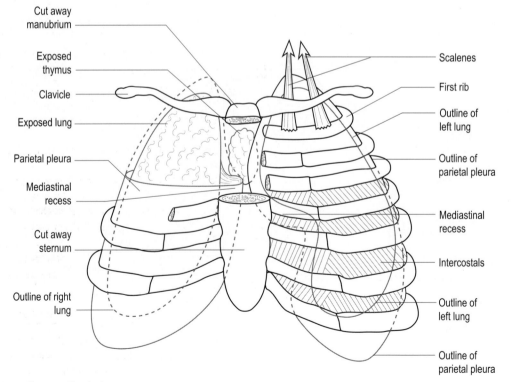

Figure 4.4 Costomediastinal recesses.

This is called the pulmonary ligament and it is effectively a part of the 'mesentery' for the pulmonary vessels, which extends from the hilum of the lung inferiorly. The lower border of the pleural membrane that wraps around the pulmonary vessels extends towards the diaphragm, and this lower free edge/border specifically is referred to as the pulmonary ligament. Some authors consider it might be better labelled as the 'mesopneumonium' to reflect this general arrangement.[1]

Between the two hilar areas of the lungs, the parietal pleural layers have a midline communication called the bronchopulmonary ligament or membrane. This passes between the upper parts of the two pulmonary ligaments and inferior to the bronchi. It blends anteriorly with the posterior pericardial structures. This structure is effectively examined and treated as part of the posterior pericardium. It is not often referred to in standard anatomy texts. It is shown in Figure 4.5.

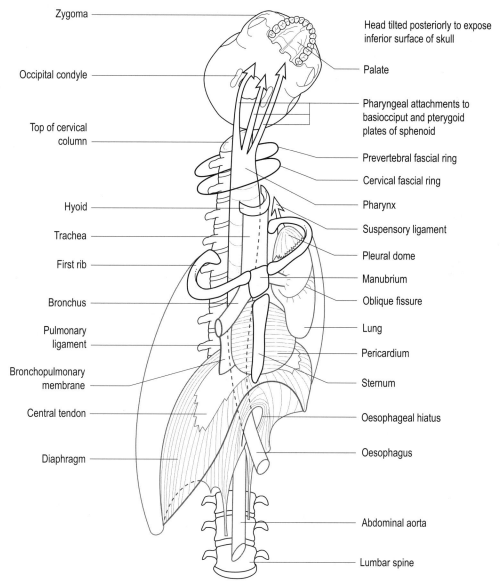

Figure 4.5   Other pleural relations and cervical connections.

Other fascial structures connected with the parietal pleura include the suspensory ligament of the pleural dome (see Fig. 4.5) and links with pre-vertebral and cervical fascial systems. They also include the vertebropericardial ligament, which passes from the anterior upper dorsal spine area, either side of the oesophagus, to insert onto the posterosuperior part of the pericardium and bronchi. These have all been discussed in Chapter 3 and are shown in Figure 4.2.

The main movements of the lungs are:

- torsional movements along the walls of the bronchi should be elastic and not interfere with normal bronchial compliance and stretch
- the trachea should be able to slide superiorly and inferiorly with neck extension and flexion respectively
- the lungs should slide anteriorly into the costomediastinal recesses ('medial rotation'), and inferiorly into the costodiaphragmatic recesses on inspiration
- the lobes of the lungs should slide over each other to accommodate general respiratory

movements and global torso and thoracic cage motion.

MOTILITY

Please refer to the appendix for illustrations of the motility patterns for the respiratory system. The motility can be affected by tensions in any of the ligaments described above, by smooth muscle tension, and tissue irritation within the organs themselves, or indirectly from somatic relations which are biomechanically affected or irritated.

Many of the techniques described at the end of this chapter can be used as palpating contacts to evaluate and treat the motility of the organ concerned.

REFLEX RELATIONSHIPS

Table 4.2 shows the reflex relationships for the respiratory system and the ear, eye, nose and throat structures.

Table 4.2 Reflex relationships for the respiratory and EENT systems

Organ	Anatomical name	Somatic level/relationship
Eyes		
Sympathetic – spinal cord	T1–4	T1–4, and ribs 1–4
Sympathetic – paravertebral chain ganglia	Superior cervical ganglion to the sphenopterygoid (pterygopalatine) ganglion, located in the pterygopalatine fossa. It is attached to the maxillary nerve. Sympathetic fibres in this ganglion form the plexus around the internal carotid artery (deep petrosal nerve) via the pterygoid canal	Upper cervical spine
Sympathetic – plexus	Via the internal carotid plexus	Cervical fascia
Parasympathetic	Sphenopterygoid ganglion, receiving fibres from facial nerve (greater petrosal nerve)	
Ears/eustachian tube		
Sympathetic – spinal cord	T1–4	T1–4, and ribs 1–4
Sympathetic – paravertebral chain ganglia	Superior cervical ganglion to the sphenopterygoid ganglion in the pterygopalatine fossa	Upper cervical spine
Sympathetic – plexus	Via the internal carotid	Cervical fascia
Parasympathetic	Sphenopterygoid ganglion, receiving fibres from facial nerve (greater petrosal nerve)	

Table 4.2 Reflex relationships for the respiratory and EENT systems—cont'd

Organ	Anatomical name	Somatic level/relationship
Nasopharynx/sinuses		
Sympathetic – spinal cord	T1–4	T1–4, and ribs 1–4
Sympathetic – paravertebral chain ganglia	Superior cervical ganglion to the sphenopterygoid ganglion in the pterygopalatine fossa	Upper cervical spine
Sympathetic – plexus	Via the internal carotid	Cervical fascia
Parasympathetic	Sphenopterygoid ganglion, receiving fibres from facial nerve (greater petrosal nerve)	
Oropharyngeal glands (adenoids and tonsils)		
Sympathetic – spinal cord	T1–4	T1–4, and ribs 1–4
Sympathetic – paravertebral chain ganglia	Superior cervical ganglion to the sphenopterygoid ganglion in the pterygopalatine fossa	Upper cervical spine
Sympathetic – plexus	Via the internal carotid	Cervical fascia
Parasympathetic	Sphenopterygoid ganglion, receiving fibres from facial nerve (greater petrosal nerve)	
Salivary glands (parotid, sublingual, submandibular)		
Sympathetic – spinal cord	T1–4	T1–4, ribs 1–5
Sympathetic – paravertebral chain ganglia	Otic ganglion to the parotid gland	TMJ function
	Submandibular ganglion to the sublingual and submandibular glands	TMJ and tongue function
Sympathetic – plexus		
Parasympathetic – parotid	Glossopharyngeal nerve, running through the petrous temporal bone and joining with the otic ganglion (on the tensor veli palatini muscle) and then passing with auriculotemporal nerve to the parotid gland	Temporomandibular joint (TMJ) and related soft tissues
Parasympathetic – submandibular and sublingual	Via submandibular ganglion	
Trachea		
Sympathetic – spinal cord	T1–6	T1–6
Sympathetic – paravertebral chain ganglia	Direct fibres to the trachea	Ribs 1–6
Sympathetic – plexus		
Parasympathetic	Vagus	Upper cervical spine
Bronchi		
Sympathetic – spinal cord	T1–6	T1–6
Sympathetic – paravertebral chain ganglia	Direct fibres to the bronchi	Ribs 1–6
Sympathetic – plexus	Posterior pulmonary plexus	Mediastinal fascia
Parasympathetic	Vagus	Upper cervical spine
Lungs and visceral pleura		
Sympathetic – spinal cord	T1–6	T1–6
Sympathetic – paravertebral chain ganglia	Direct fibres to the tissues	Ribs 1–6
Sympathetic – plexus	Posterior (larger) and anterior (smaller) pulmonary plexus	Mediastinal fascia
Parasympathetic	Vagus	Upper cervical spine

VEINS, ARTERIES AND LYMPHATICS

Table 4.3 shows the major blood and lymph vessels of the respiratory and EENT systems. The visceral ligaments and fascial conduits that contain the blood vessels are important to consider, as work on those structures will help influence venous drainage, blood flow (as ligamentous torsion may affect the arteries/arterioles, and the sympathetic nerves that course along their length) and lymphatic drainage, all of which are important for organ health. The somatic relations also

Table 4.3   Blood and lymph vessels

Organ	Anatomical name	Cervical, mediastinal or pleural ligament or fascial relation	Somatic relation, where applicable
Eyes			
Veins	Ophthalmic vein, and to cavernous sinus, pterygoid plexus and anterior facial vein		Bones of orbit
Arteries	Ophthalmic artery		Bones of orbit
Lymphatics	Facial nodes, parotid and submandibular nodes, to deep cervical nodes	RIGHT THORACIC DUCT	Upper cervical spine, sternocleidomastoid (upper portion) to region of hyoid and cricoid, 1st rib right
Ears/eustachian tube			
Veins	Communication between the intracranial venous sinuses and the extracranial pterygoid plexus		Upper neck, cranial and face mechanics
Arteries	Branches of the posterior auricular, maxillary and internal carotid arteries		Upper neck, cranial and face mechanics
Lymphatics	Eustachian tube drains into retropharyngeal glands, and the tympanic membrane drains into posterior auricular and parotid lymph glands, to deep cervical nodes	RIGHT THORACIC DUCT	Upper cervical spine, sternocleidomastoid (upper portion) to region of hyoid and cricoid, 1st rib right. TMJ
Nasopharynx/sinuses			
Veins	Corresponding with arteries (note the nasal veins can communicate with the frontal lobe via the cribriform plate)		Nasal bone mechanics
Arteries	Branches of the ophthalmic, maxillary and facial arteries		Nasal bone mechanics
Lymphatics	All the sinuses drain inferiorly, except the maxillary, which drains superiorly. Link with retropharyngeal glands, glands either side of hyoid, and into upper deep cervical nodes	RIGHT THORACIC DUCT	Throat, cervical fascia and upper cervical spine mechanics, 1st rib right
Oropharyngeal glands			
Veins	Internal jugular and facial veins		Upper neck and face mechanics
Arteries	Tonsillar artery from the facial artery; branches of the maxillary and lingual		Upper neck and face mechanics
Lymphatics	Retropharyngeal nodes, deep cervical nodes	RIGHT THORACIC DUCT	Upper cervical spine, sternocleidomastoid (upper portion) to region of hyoid and cricoid, 1st rib right

Table 4.3   Blood and lymph vessels—cont'd

Organ	Anatomical name	Cervical, mediastinal or pleural ligament or fascial relation	Somatic relation, where applicable
Salivary glands			
Veins	Internal jugular and facial veins		Submandibular and jaw/hyoid mechanics
Arteries	Tonsillar artery from the facial artery; branches of the maxillary and lingual		Submandibular and jaw/hyoid mechanics
Lymphatics	Parotid, submandibular, to deep cervical	RIGHT THORACIC DUCT	General cervical spine, sternocleidomastoid (upper portion) to region of hyoid and cricoid, 1st rib right
Trachea			
Veins	Inferior thyroid vein		Thoracic inlet mechanics
Arteries	Inferior thyroid artery		Thoracic inlet mechanics
Lymphatics	Tracheobronchial and mediastinal nodes	LEFT THORACIC DUCT	Cervical fascia and thoracic inlet, mechanics of the throat and upper ribcage
Bronchi			
Veins	Pulmonary vein, bronchial veins to the azygos system		Thoracic inlet and upper chest mechanics
Arteries	Pulmonary artery, bronchial arteries from thoracic aorta		Thoracic inlet and upper chest mechanics
Lymphatics	Nodes around hilum of lung	LEFT THORACIC DUCT	Mediastinal fascia and thoracic inlet
Lungs			
Veins	Pulmonary vein		Mediastinal mechanics
Arteries	Pulmonary artery		Mediastinal mechanics
Lymphatics	Nodes around hilum of lung	LEFT THORACIC DUCT	Mediastinal fascia and thoracic inlet

indicate where the musculoskeletal system may be engaged to aid fluid movement in the structures concerned.

SOMATIC AND VISCERAL INTERACTIONS

GENERAL CHEST MECHANICS

Although it commences prior to birth, ossification of the sternum is not complete until around 25 years of age. Thus childhood respiratory problems could have a long-lasting impact on sternal structure and hence biomechanics of not only the ribcage and shoulder girdle but also the respiratory system itself. The need for effective sternal movement in respiratory function is discussed below.

LOCAL THORACIC MECHANICS

There are many interesting ribcage–costal margin, sternum and spinal–vertebral motion patterns that determine how the thorax functions as a complete unit. These smaller movements of the ribs and associated cartilages will relate directly to many pleural and pericardial restrictions, and will be interdependent with respiratory system and general mediastinal function.

Rib mechanics

Rib movements are traditionally discussed in terms of inspiration and expiration, with pump handle and bucket handle motions (and the consequent rotations about a horizontal axis of the posterior aspect of the rib) being described. All the ribs should move in concert and there remains some ongoing debate as to which movement (inspiration or expiration) is performed by which intercostal muscles. Osteopaths were historically taught about individual rib 'lesions', where the term 'lesion' describes a restriction in mobility either in 'inspiration' or 'expiration'. The concept would imply individual movement, independent of adjacent ribs. In practice, generalized restrictions through the ribcage are more common, as all the ribs move together, linked by the parietal pleura.

The pleural layer is like a large sheet of tissue into which the ribs are embedded (embryologically, the ribs grow out to stiffen the parietal pleural sheets and body wall). The ribs are thus stabilized and are 'at the mercy' of tensions and irritations that act on the pleural sheet. Many respiratory diseases lead to stiffening and inelasticity (lack of compliance) in the pleural layers, and hence the ribcage. These tensions can persist for a long time after resolution of any chest infection or irritating foci, and can therefore contribute to long-standing somatic biomechanical problems (and vice versa). Other pleural restrictions will be discussed later, which again can influence certain areas of the ribcage more than others.

The above-mentioned pump handle and bucket handle motions involve rotatory movements at the costovertebral and costotransverse articulations. These rotations will also cause the anterior end of the rib to move superiorly or inferiorly, and hence create a hinge effect at the costochondral and chondrosternal articulations. This in turn leads to shearing movements of the sternum in relation to the ribs such that, on initial inspiration, the sternum appears to move inferiorly with respect to the anterior end of the ribs (as the 'slack' in the chondral articulations is taken up). Once this slack is taken up, then the ribs and sternum move in concert, and both move superiorly through the rest of the inspiration, with a similar relationship occurring during expiration.[2] This is shown in Figure 4.6. These sheer forces are important for pleural compliance and the mobilization of the costomediastinal pleural recesses. It is very important to ensure that, if appropriate thoracic cage volume changes are going to occur uniformly, anterior chest mobility is unrestricted.

Rib influences on vertebral motion

The function and stability of the dorsal vertebral articulations depend very much on balanced rib movement.[3,4] Many scoliosis studies have looked at how the vertebral stacking stability of the thoracic spine is literally dependent upon two ribs pushing equally on the vertebra, with the forces acting along the transverse processes onto the interarticular pillar and onto the facet angles on the vertebral bodies. The rib pair has to have a dynamic equilibrium and equal pressure acting on both sides of the vertebra to stabilize the thoracic spine in between (also indicated in Fig. 4.6). If tension or pressure differs from one lateral component to the other, the vertebra will eventually twist and rotate. If a flexible rod (the spine) is twisted, it sidebends and scoliotic patterns start to emerge. Clinically confined areas of scoliosis can arise from pleural and rib restrictions that result in localized unilateral chest wall stiffening, which affects the above-mentioned rib–vertebra relationship.

Hence in scoliosis (and very probably in most general thoracic restriction patterns) it is the movements of the ribs that dictate the vertebral alignment, rather than the other way around. Once the thoracic cage starts to distort, the 3D shape of the internal thoracic cavity changes, which will have an effect on thoracic organ function.[5,6] It is very interesting to consider that in a patient with compromised respiratory function, it is not the inspiration/expiration movements of the ribcage that are always the most important to preserve, but the rotational movements. Maintenance of rotation is more efficient than inspiration/expiration movements at preserving lung function test values. These concepts also fit together with theories of sliding surfaces in thoracic organ movement, which will be discussed later.

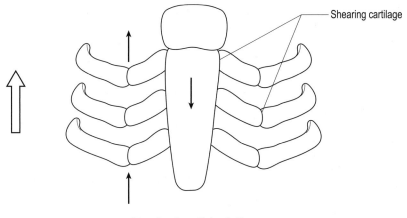

Sternal motion with inspiration

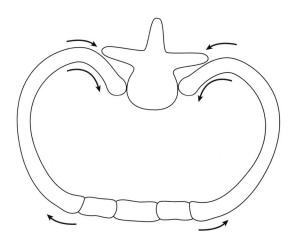

Rib head motion with thorax rotation

Figure 4.6 Sternal and cartilage movements with respiration and rib movement with rotation.

INTERNAL MECHANICS OF THE THORAX

When thoracic cage movements as a whole are considered, movement dynamics depend upon more than rib articulations. Three-dimensional movement of the thoracic and visceral/mediastinal structures depends upon a series of sliding surfaces which are created by the pleura and the pericardium.

Sliding surfaces

Figure 4.7 shows a cross-section of the chest at around D4 showing the ribs either side, the vertebral body posteriorly, a lung either side and the heart in the middle. The heart and lungs are wrapped in their serous membranes (visceral pleura and pericardium) and the inside walls of the ribcage are also lined by serous membranes (parietal pleura). When torso movement as a whole is considered (compared to just motion within the dorsal spine), the axis about which the torso rotates is located within the thorax itself (dorsal spine axis of rotation, as defined by the plane of the vertebral facets, is located outside the thorax, anterior to the sternum). Interestingly, this fulcrum (axis of rotation) is at the posterior wall of the heart at its superior–posterior border, which is just in

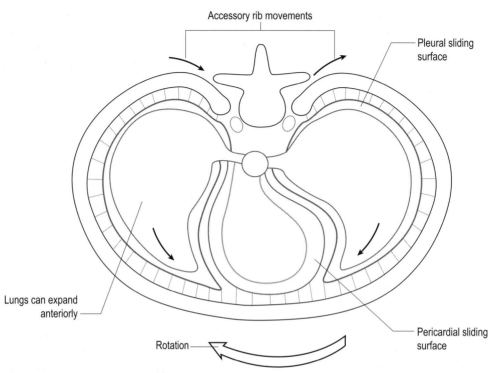

Figure 4.7 Sliding surfaces from pleural and pericardial layers.

front of D3–4. This point represents the least mobile part of the thoracic cage and visceral contents. It is very relevant that the static point of the thorax is at the back wall of the heart, which needs to be stabilized in order to function properly.

During torso movement and especially during any sort of rotation, the external thorax should 'slide around' the internal structures, without unduly impacting on organ function. The parietal pleura is intimately attached to the internal face of the ribs and as the ribcage moves, then the parietal pleura slips over the visceral pleura, enabling the lungs to move somewhat independently of the ribs. Also, as the fibrous pericardium is attached to the internal aspect of the sternum (and the internal thoracic muscle), each time the sternum is moved, the pericardium is dynamically engaged. Effectively, anterior chest motion will torsion the heart (via surrounding soft tissues) such that it is necessary to have good sliding of the pericardium and its fluid to allow the heart to move independently of the pericardium.

Although during respiration there is a negative pressure created such that the movement of the ribs and parietal pleura will cause the lung (and visceral pleura) to expand outwards, the lung must still be able to slide and expand anteriorly and inferiorly, into the recesses of the pleural sacs. It is interesting to note that although the external ribcage effectively expands outwards and externally rotates, as it does so the sliding of the lungs into the recesses is in a different direction. The lungs and ribcage are moving in nearly opposing directions in some parts. Figures 4.3 and 4.4 show the pleural recesses, enabling lung movement posteroinferiorly (inferior expansion) and anteromedially ('internal rotation') during inspiration.

It is therefore very necessary to maintain global and three-dimensional movement dynamics in the ribcage, thoracic muscles and serous membranes, in order to have efficient somatic as well as visceral function. Ribcage restriction can limit movement in these recesses, which can impact on the viscosity of the pleural fluid at this level and reduce overall lung expansion and tidal volume. Similarly, inflammation as a consequence of respiratory dysfunction can lead to adhesion and limited movement within the recesses, which will bind the mobility of the overlying ribs.

Rib motion associated with the sliding surfaces concept

As a corollary to the pattern of thoracic cage rotatory motion and the sliding surface concept, individual rib mechanics need to be reconsidered as they have an additional axis of motion as a result (in addition to those described earlier). When the whole thorax moves in rotation there is an anterior–posterior sliding of the rib heads which is a very necessary passive, accessory movement. This is indicated in Figure 4.7.

With rotation to the right, for example, the head of the rib on the left will move anteriorly and the one on the right will move posteriorly. The ribs act like cog wheels that are engaging a third cog wheel – the vertebra. There is actually an A–P shifting of the rib heads along the arm of the transverse process and side of the vertebral body, and this is a very good movement to try to preserve for any biomechanical or visceral functions within the thorax. The movement itself is quite small and represents a taking up of the slack in the articular tissues, rather than a gross range of motion; however, although the motion is small it is very significant. It has an important function for the articulation of the paravertebral chain ganglia (thereby maintaining effective vascular drainage for the sympathetic chain), and aiding optimal function and neural processing.

Other sliding surfaces

There are other sliding surfaces within the thorax that are also determined by the way in which the visceral pleura wraps around the lobes of the lungs. So, not only is there sliding motion around the outside of the lung, there is sliding between the lobes of the lung as well. Figure 4.8 shows the fissures of the lung, illustrating the lobar sliding dynamics created by the visceral pleural layers.

Any movement restriction between the fissures of the lung can affect the local pleural fluid flow, which can become 'stickier' over the area of the affected fissure. If this occurs, the parietal pleura in contact with the area of the fissure will also become restricted, and ultimately this will limit movements of the associated rib and vertebral complexes. Restrictions in the oblique fissure (for example, from some inflammatory change or fibrosis subsequent to an infection or irritation) lead to a restriction of the ribs overlying that oblique fissure, namely ribs 3–6. Note that the oblique fissure starts at around rib 3 posteriorly, is next to ribs 4–5 in the midaxillary line and is next to ribs 6–7 at its anterior end. Both oblique fissures (left and right) follow approximately the same course along the ribcage. The horizontal fissure is only found on the right and passes from the midaxillary line along rib 4, anteriorly. If there is a horizontal fissure problem or a middle lobe restriction on the right that binds up rib 4 on that side, it will affect the mobility of the midsection of the ribcage at that level.

To manage this sort of problem, it is possible to get hold of the ribcage in such a way that motion passes through into the thoracic cavity itself and creates an impetus for mobilizing the lungs themselves. Lobar articulation can be performed, as can sliding tests for all the mediastinal, pleural and pericardial layers. Lung tissue compliance can also be evaluated through a careful contact with the chest wall. These techniques are discussed later.

The thoracic inlet

The influence of lung and mediastinal mechanics on the thoracic inlet has already been introduced in a previous chapter. Lobar articular problems and compliance restrictions within the body of the lung can be quite influential in cervicobrachial mechanics and the dynamics of the thoracic inlet. When these latter become affected then the sympathetic chain ganglia in the neck can become quite irritated and the lymphatics for the whole body (via the right and left lymphatic trunk links to the venous system at the point) can become compromised. Hence lung and thoracic inlet function is key to management concerns for many (if not all) other visceral system functioning.

Whiplash and other chest impact traumas (such as through various sports, for example) can often lead to internal chest injury or dysfunction, which can be meaningful to cervicodorsal mechanics. There are many complex traumatic forces that occur in whiplash, which can have wide-ranging effects. During a whiplash (or similar trauma),

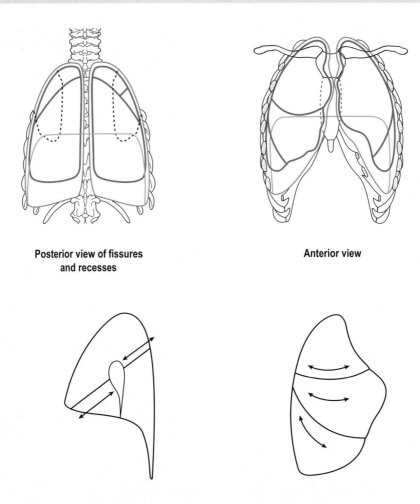

**Posterior view of fissures
and recesses**

Anterior view

Side view of oblique and horizontal fissures

Figure 4.8   *Fissures and other sliding surfaces.*

oscillation forces are created, leading to a momen-
tum-induced movement within the organs and
mediastinal tissues.[7] The organs are quite fluid,
heavy structures attached into the body cavities at
a couple of places, and chest traumas and
whiplash often create contrary motion to the
somatic structures as a result of this momentum.
This dramatically strains many tissues, including
the suspensory ligament of the pleural dome, giving
a very complex strain at the level of the lower cervical spine. This can subsequently conflict with
the hypermobility strains that commonly occur at
C4–5 as a result of the same injury process.

Recognizing the pleural and lung component
can suggest another avenue of management when
someone presents with an acute neck problem
post whiplash. The neck-mediastinal indicator
test described in Chapter 3 will help differentiate
the level of influence of the internal thoracic
structures.

Other considerations of thoracic mobility: changes over time

From all the above discussions, a three-dimensional
picture of the thoracic cage and visceral biomechanics within the thorax should emerge. However,
it is important to remember that certain aspects of
chest movement or dynamics alter over time (with
growth and aging).

In the infant, the chest wall is very soft and compliant and it is the lung which actually controls the action of the chest wall.[8] Through childhood and in adulthood, the opposite occurs: the chest wall helps to control lung function. So, infants have a floppy chest wall and diaphragm that initially cannot cope well with the changing pressures within the chest during respiration. In this situation, inhomogenous movements within the chest and ordinary changes of motion within the lungs can cause strain within the respiratory muscles, and can sometimes cause muscle fatigue and distress.[9] After 1–2 years of life, the chest wall stiffens and the respiratory function improves.[10] Other changes to the chest include the way in which the chest stiffens over the years and the anteroposterior diameter diminishes during puberty. This can impact on cardiac function[11] as well as respiratory function.

Osteopathic management of respiratory function in children therefore requires subtlety as very small changes in chest wall mechanics could have a very large effect upon respiratory function. Overall biomechanical balance (from head to toe) is necessary for effective respiratory function through life, as if a child adopts a slightly poor postural balance or torsion pattern, this will have an ongoing (underlying) impact on respiratory function. Other aspects of management for respiratory function will be discussed in Chapter 9.

EENT FUNCTION

Whilst reviewing respiratory function, it is important not to overlook the impact of the nose, sinuses, pharynx and other throat structures on a person's overall respiratory balance and function.

SOMATIC AND VISCERAL INTERACTIONS

Oronasal–pharyngeal function

There are many complex soft tissue, bony and cartilaginous movements that occur in sucking, eating, swallowing, nasal and chest breathing and speech, all of which need to be coordinated and unhindered for effective orofacial development,[12] for respiratory function[13] and for auditory and language skills[14] to develop optimally. Even dentition and the temporomandibular joint can be influenced

by these adverse mechanics,[15] and many cases requiring orthodontic intervention may be helped osteopathically by addressing mechanical imbalance in the orofacial head, chest and general body dynamics.

Having an oral breathing pattern leads to many anatomical adaptations. Craniomorphological changes (such as 'adenoid face') can result from mouth breathing and upper respiratory obstruction[16] and these can also lead to general somatic biomechanical and postural compensation and balance.[17,18] Changes to the nasopharynx from adenotonsilar hyperplasia can also lead to sleep apnoea and failure to thrive.[19] Tongue movements are also very important in the overall dynamics of the orofacial-pharyngeal complex.[20]

Swallowing, for example, has many complex movements. It is initiated by tongue pressure on the hard palate (from intrinsic muscle contraction and actions of the styloglossus muscles); the floor of the mouth is raised by contraction of the mylohyoid muscles which elevate the hyoid bone; the palatoglossal folds are brought together; the pharyngeal constrictors initiate a wave of motion; the soft palate approximates to the posterior pharynx; the soft palate is raised by the levator veli palatini and kept taut by the tensor veli palatini. The larynx is lifted by the stylopharyngeus, palatopharyngeus and salpingopharyngeus, and the distal oesophagus will dilate.

Speech, swallowing and head movements will all affect upper pharyngeal soft tissue dynamics, which can also affect eustachian tube movements and therefore middle ear function. The middle ear is part of a functional system consisting of the nasopharynx and eustachian tube (anteriorly) and the mastoid air cells (posteriorly). There is only one muscle that opens the eustachian tube, the tensor veli palatini. This action helps maintain airflow into and out of the middle ear. The eustachian tube also helps protect the ear from strong sound pressures and invasion by nasopharyngeal secretions.

The anatomical relationships of the oropharyngeal complex suggest that (1) the levator veli palatini opens the eustachian tube by isotonic contraction that results in displacement of the medial tubal cartilage and the tubal membrane, and (2) the tensor veli palatini opens the tube directly by traction on the lateral tubal membrane and indirectly by rotation of the medial tubal cartilage by means of traction on the lateral tubal cartilage.[21]

The craniofacial and oropharyngeal dynamics and anatomical orientations change dramatically from birth to adulthood. Promoting balanced and supple soft tissue dynamics from infanthood to adolescence will help to ensure appropriate development of these regions and limit the aetiology of and effects of EENT disorders. One very interesting dynamic for osteopaths involved in paediatrics is the role that factors such as sucking, breast feeding and pacifier ('dummy') use play in orofacial and nasopharyngeal development.[22,23]

Sinus function

Sinus function can also be affected by mechanical tensions through the head and neck region. The physiology and function of the sinuses have been the subject of much debate and multiple theories of function exist. These include the functions of warming/humidification of air, assisting in regulation of intranasal pressure and serum gas pressures, contributing to immune defence, increasing mucosal surface area, lightening the skull, giving resonance to the voice, absorbing shock and contributing to facial growth. Because of the sinuses' copious mucus production, they contribute heavily to the immune defence and air filtration performed by the nose. The thickened superficial layer of nasal mucus serves to trap bacteria and particulate matter in a substance rich with immune cells, antibodies and antibacterial proteins. Unless obstructed by disease or anatomical variance, the sinuses move mucus through their cavities and out of their ostia toward the nasal cavity.

The nose and sinuses prepare the air for the lower respiratory tract and condition it for pulmonary gas exchange. The nose requires the integration of many autonomic neural reflexes for this task, influencing the function of the nasal blood vessels and glands, and some consider that non-eosinophilic non-allergic rhinitis may in fact be a disease of autonomic imbalance.[24] Without effective nose and sinus function, other respiratory function could be compromised. Sinusitis and asthma often coexist in patients, where the asthma may be worsened by sinus disease through reflex neural irritation and interference with the nasal functions of heating, humidification and filtration.

Asthma can also be worsened by allergic rhinitis and gastro-oesophageal reflex disease.[25]

It is difficult to overestimate the range of functional interrelationships between orofacial structures, respiratory function, throat mechanics, including the hyoid and associated muscles, jaw and tongue mechanics, overall posture, and head and neck mechanics and cervical fascial tension and torsion.[26,27] Coupled with the movement dynamics are the influence of the neuroendocrine immune system and the functioning of the autonomics and lymphatic tissues in relation to the above-mentioned types of disorders and pathologies.

The sympathetic supply to the head and neck arises from the upper dorsal segments of the spinal cord and passes through the thoracic inlet region and the cervical region, forming the inferior, middle and superior cervical ganglia, which can be affected by cervicodorsal, upper chest, shoulder girdle, TMJ and throat mechanics, as well as restrictions in the upper cervical spine and cranium. Whenever there is a problem in this region (such as allergic rhinitis, tonsillitis, mouth breathing or something similar), the mechanics of the head and neck alter but this in itself sets up a negative cycle as these very restrictions will adversely impact on the autonomics and lymphatic tissues involved in homeostatic and physiological function of the affected tissues. It is often necessary to work not only locally but also through the chest and shoulder girdle, and then through the rest of the body to reduce the overall biomechanical disturbances that culminate in altered local tissue distress, congestion and dysfunction. Many of the autonomic reflexes and upper airway functions are mediated by the sphenopterygoid ganglion, situated in the upper nasopharynx (as shown in Figure 4.9). Tensions in and around this ganglion can adversely affect its function.

Eye function

Osteopaths have long been interested in eye mobilization and drainage and release of orbital musculature, to ease eye strain and other ocular conditions. Eye massage or mobilization is not a new concept, nor is it confined to osteopathic circles. Chinese acupuncture has advocated the

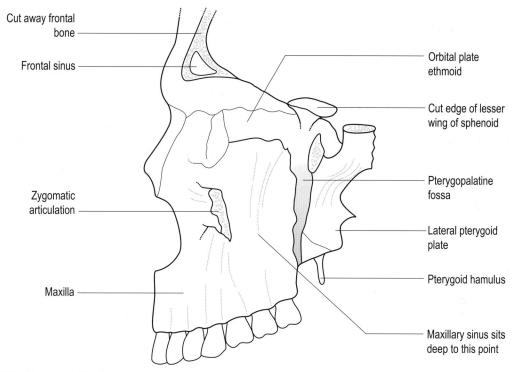

Figure 4.9   Pterygopalatine fossa.

use of eye massage and acupressure around the eye for various problems of myopia and vision disturbances due to close visual work.[28] Stereoscopic eye exercises are also thought to have a beneficial effect on visual acuity.[29] Local massage to the eye region may have a role to play in a general management plan for nasolacrimal duct obstruction[30] and for dry eye syndrome/chronic eye irritation.[31] However, significant (heavy) or prolonged eye rubbing (over years) may irritate the optic nerve, cornea and eye in general, and be detrimental to eye function and trigger such things as migraine.[32] Also, some very old-fashioned techniques included the lifting or levering of the eye out of the orbit (restrained only by the elasticity of the optic nerve). This has fallen out of favour and indeed, if performed, may result in optic neuropathy.[33] That said, gentle periorbital mobilization of the eye within the orbit does not appear to be contraindicated and empirically seems to help in several eye conditions, through improving drainage, relieving tension on ocular muscles, relieving dural and fascial tensions around the optic nerve

and easing sympathetic nervous irritation to the eye.

As the eye is a major sensory organ, it is linked to the major proprioceptive and balance systems of the body. As such, any eye disorder will lead to significant postural and movement pattern disorders. Indeed, a person may need to adapt all their actions when eye disorders are present and many musculoskeletal torsion, tension and restriction patterns may be maintained purely on a reflex basis as a result. Behavioural optometrists work with local eye movement coordination (vision training) to help redress these imbalances, which makes it a very useful corollary to osteopathic work which can focus on the whole-body reflex disturbances in posture, movement behaviours and somatoemotional expressions that accompany vision disturbances.

Although it is not possible to discuss all the above relations in detail, nor to outline the complex cranial movement dynamics that accompany disorders in this region, it should be noted that mobilization and release of these many tissues and movement dynamics are essential for ear, eye, sinus, upper respiratory tract, dental, auditory and speech function. Some techniques to achieve this are discussed below.

EXAMINATION AND TREATMENT OF THE RESPIRATORY AND EENT SYSTEMS

It is possible to illustrate only a small number of the myriad osteopathic techniques available for the examination and treatment of the EENT and respiratory systems.

Some tests for the pleura and lungs will also test heart structures and relations. Other mediastinal and sternal/thoracic cage tests that relate to the heart are also included in the chapter on the vascular, endocrine and lymphatic systems.

TECHNIQUES FOR THE COSTOVERTEBRAL ARTICULATIONS AND THE DIAPHRAGM

In any EENT or respiratory disorder, the impact of the rib head movement of the paravertebral sympathetic chain, and therefore autonomic neural reflexes, cannot be overestimated. For this reason, work to improve the anteroposterior mobility of the rib heads against the vertebral body will help normalize sympathetic function. Figure 4.10 shows one technique for achieving this. The practitioner

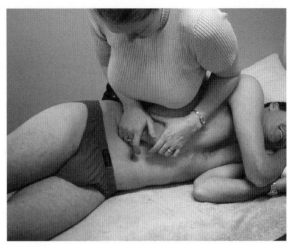

Figure 4.11 Diaphragmatic mobilization and stretch.

is stabilizing the ribcage with one forearm, and contacting onto the rib angles. The other hand (using either a thumb or finger contact, as is comfortable) can 'hold back' on the spinous process(es) of the associated vertebra, creating a strong local stretch to the costovertebral articulations. General compression with the forearm resting on the chest wall of the patient will improve the focus of the technique.

Another very useful technique for any respiratory and head/neck problem is a release of the thoracic diaphragm muscle, shown in Figure 4.11. The practitioner is stabilizing the lateral ribcage with their abdomen, and contacting the diaphragm subcostally. With plenty of skin slack under the costal margin between the two palpating hands, a contact is taken onto the diaphragm and ribcage. Now, a slight separating movement is made to stretch adjacent ribs 'caudally and cephalically', to help increase the ability of the domes of the diaphragm to expand laterally. This is one direction of stretch that is often forgotten. The stretch on the diaphragm is aided by a slight compression onto the lateral chest, to help the hands 'splay' the costal margin without too much finger pressure being applied.

TECHNIQUES TO MOBILIZE THE PARIETAL PLEURA

General pleural restrictions can be relieved by working through the ribcage and creating shearing

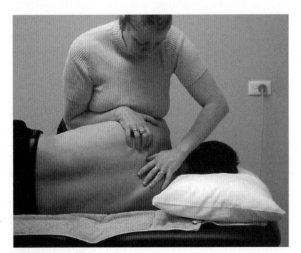

Figure 4.10 Rib articulations to move rib head in AP direction.

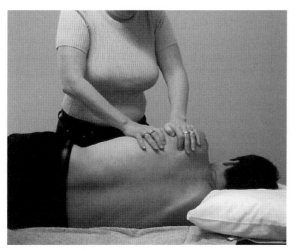

Figure 4.12   Sidelying mobilization of pleura.

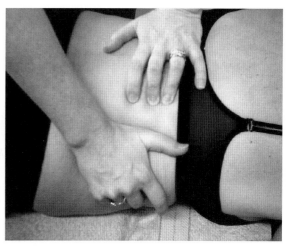

Figure 4.13   Pleural recess testing.

and stretching movement to adjacent ribs (ensuring sufficient skin slack is present between contacts, prior to commencing). Figure 4.12 shows a sidelying contact for mobilization of the parietal pleura. The hands can be moved up or down the ribcage, and can come slightly anterior or posterior to the position shown. In this way, the whole parietal sheet can be evaluated and treated. Functional or fascial unwinding techniques are also useful, as are recoil techniques (used with a tissue barrier found during a shearing/rib-pleural test, for example). These sorts of general mobilizations to the ribs, pleura and diaphragm make a good precursor to other more specific tests and treatments.

TECHNIQUES TO MOBILIZE THE PLEURAL RECESSES

As discussed before, the pleural recesses are important, as restriction there can limit overall lung expansion and impact on many rib/vertebral movement patterns. There are costodiaphragmatic as well as costomediastinal tests. Costodiaphragmatic tests can be done in a number of positions, and a contact similar to that shown in Figure 4.15 can be made, although in this latter case, more inferiorly to cover the lower ribs over the underlying fissure. Alternatively, the test can also be made with the patient lying prone, so as to contact the posterior surface of ribs 10–12 (but not covering the vertebral structures) to access the underlying pleural recess. The contact can be bilateral, to test both

recesses together, or unilateral. The ribs should be gently moved around in several directions, with the practitioner focusing down to the pleural layer and visualizing the sliding of the two adjacent layers of parietal pleura over each other. This is shown in Figure 4.13. This technique can also be used to explore the posterior diaphragm, the arcuates of the diaphragm, the kidneys and adrenals, the spleen on the left and the liver on the right (especially the right triangular ligament).

Figure 4.14 shows a mobilization of the costomediastinal recesses, which is very similar to a global release for the sternum and costal cartilages. The practitioner should remember to 'follow' the

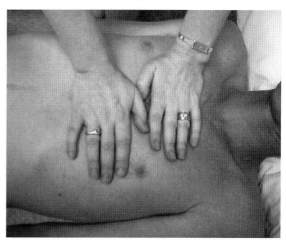

Figure 4.14   Sternal sliding and costomediastinal testing.

curvature of the chest wall, in whatever section is being evaluated, as inducing shearing or torsional movements without doing so in an arcing manner will create movement that passes into the chest and so bypasses the pleural layers (reducing the effectiveness of the technique at that level). This is true for all sections of the thoracic cage and chest.

In this contact, the aim is not to perform cardiac massage but to gently mobilize the anterior chest tissues such that only the ribs and underlying pleura are engaged. This requires some practice to 'descend' through the layers, without creating too much compression. The hands can move to the right or left, up and down or in oblique/torsional directions, to create a number of shearing movements, to test the fibres of the pleura in multiple directions. This is necessary as the pleura should be globally elastic and compliant and may be restricted in only a few directions, depending on the traumas and irritations it has been exposed to.

When testing in different directions, it is important to consider the diagnostic impact of 'push–pull tensions'. This means that if the hands move the sternum or ribs to the right and there is a movement block or tissue barrier, the tension could be on the right ribcage (where the hands 'push' against a tissue block) or it could be on the left, where the hands feel a 'pull' or tethering sensation. This can guide the practitioner towards a more specific location for further testing, to isolate the most significant area of restriction (rather than work on myriad 'compensatory' patterns). It should not be forgotten that the rib and pleural restrictions can indicate underlying organ problems and therefore the surface anatomy of heart, lungs, kidneys, spleen and liver must be remembered in order to accurately describe tensions once located.

The orientation of the costomediastinal recesses is shown in Figure 4.4 and this should be remembered when placing the hands for the above technique, as the surface anatomy changes from right to left.

This technique is also used for evaluating the sternopericardial ligament which passes between the pericardium and the inside of the lower sternum and transversus thoracis muscle. Note: there is a superior band to the sternopericardial ligament, which passes from the pericardium to the area of the manubrium and upper sternum. This can be

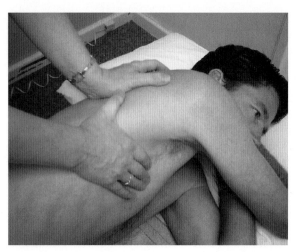

Figure 4.15 Mobilizing oblique fissure and lobes of lung.

evaluated by moving the chest contacts slightly superiorly.

Having explored general pleural tensions, the fissures of the lungs can be evaluated. Figure 4.15 shows a basic contact for the midsection of the oblique fissure. The aim is to place a hand either side of the expected position of the fissure. In the midaxillary line on either side, the oblique fissure is found at the level of the fourth and fifth ribs. The cephalad hand needs to partly cover the scapula in order to be superior enough to stabilize ribs 3 and 4. The lower hand then stabilizes ribs 5 and 6. All of the palm and fingers are used, to avoid gripping with the finger tips, which can be painful. The ribs are gently sheared or moved in opposing directions to create some degree of slide that passes into the fissure. Despite the presence of the ribs, these should still be flexible enough for the practitioner to 'feel' through and into the fissure. If the fissure is free, there will be a sensation of more 'give' along its line. If it is restricted, there will be a blocked sensation. The other parts of the fissure can be evaluated in the same way, if the practitioner moves their hand either posteriorly, to lie either side of ribs 3 and 4 near the angles of the ribs, to test the first third of the fissure, or anteriorly, either side of ribs 6 and 7 near the midclavicular line, to test the last third of the fissure.

The hand can also be moved up and down the chest, feeling into different parts of the lung tissue, depending on location. In this sidelying position, the middle and lower lobes on the right and the lower lobe on the left can be best felt. There are other contacts which suit the upper lobes more in a sidelying position.

If the hand contact as shown in figure Figure 4.15 is adapted slightly, the middle lobe of the right lung can be assessed. The cephalad hand continues to contact the lower scapula on the chest wall, to stabilize the ribs above rib 4. The caudal hand moves slightly anteriorly so that the palm of the hand is just anterior to the midaxillary line and the index finger is at rib 4. If the palm and index finger rock towards the sternum and back again, the middle lobe is moved and the horizontal fissure is articulated. In women this will mean some contact that is effectively over the lateral-inferior breast. With explanation as to the aim of the technique, this should not be a particularly sensitive contact, as the breast itself is not being treated. If necessary, the fingers can be used to contact the middle lobe, rather than the palm of the hand. This will reduce the contact on the breast area but make it more awkward for the practitioner to ensure effective mobilization onto the lung tissue.

When testing the lung tissue as opposed to the fissures, remember that testing should be carried out in multiple directions, as the pattern of contracture, spasm, torsion or tension found will depend on the individual. Treatment can be direct stretch, vibration, rhythmic mobilization or fascial/functional indirect 'unwinding' techniques.

A global release of the upper lobe and shoulder girdle (scapulothoracic joint) is sometimes useful. Figure 4.16 illustrates one method of achieving this. The posterior hand contacts the scapula, the practitioner's abdomen can stabilize the posterior ribcage and elbow, and the anterior hand contacts the upper ribs (with the palm). The fingers of the anterior hand are not part of the active technique and are just gently resting over the thoracic inlet area, without exerting pressure. In effect, the two hands are cupping the upper lobe, which is situated above rib 4 (front and back). The two hands move in concert, stretching or engaging the lung tissue via the ribcage. The scapula contact utilizes some compression so as to move the underlying ribs. If desired, the anterior hand can stabilize the ribs and the posterior hand can mobilize the scapula. This releases the scapulothoracic tissues, which are

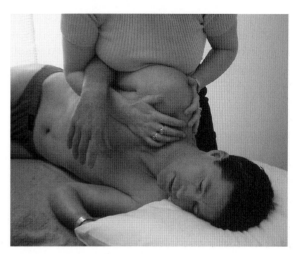

Figure 4.16   Generalized release of upper lobe and shoulder girdle.

often compromised in chronic breathing disorders. Mobilizing the scapula and upper lobe of the lung in these ways can help free up the thoracic inlet and clavicle quite effectively, improving drainage and neural reflexes operating from triggers within the thoracic spine and from the upper dorsal and rib articulations.

This contact can be adapted to release the subclavius muscle, which stabilizes the medial third of the clavicle onto the first rib and is affected in many respiratory and shoulder girdle problems. In this situation, the anterior hand is moved to the medial end of the clavicle and the index finger and thumb gentle contact around the medial end of the clavicle. The index finger makes the deeper contact, to be placed next to the belly of subclavius, just underneath the clavicle. The thumb rests over the top surface of the clavicle but care is taken not to compress the neurovascular structures of the thoracic inlet.

This contact can also be adapted to release the axillary fascia and lymph nodes, which can be useful in many chest conditions and cervicobrachial and upper limb problems. This time, the basic placement of the hands will be the same but the thumbs are now moved to be within the axillary space. The thumb of the anterior hand is now underneath the pectoral tissue and the thumb of the posterior hand is now underneath the latissimus dorsi and the posterior rotator cuff. It is necessary that both contacts are high up into the axillary space, to release the fascia at this level. This type of release is beneficial in cases such as adhesive capsulitis, after breast surgery and shoulder surgery, and in many respiratory problems, as the axilla is often compromised with long-term accessory respiratory muscle use.

TECHNIQUES TO MOBILIZE THE LOBES OF THE LUNGS AND THE LUNG TISSUE DIRECTLY

The upper lobe of the lung can also be evaluated in a sitting position, which is shown in Figure 4.17. The posterior hand uses the thenar eminence for this technique, and it is placed such that the superior angle of the scapula is nestled right into the centre of the palm. This should bring the thenar eminence medial to the border of the scapula but just lateral to the transverse processes. This is important, as the vertebra should be avoided to ensure a good contact with the lung. The rest of the fingers can gently lie over the top of the trapezius fibres. The fingers should not be held rigidly. The anterior hand is placed so that the palm and thenar eminence are covering the first three ribs. It is important to keep the anterior contact *below* the clavicle. Any contact on the clavicle will not only be uncomfortable, it will block the effect of the technique onto the lung tissue. Where the anterior arm passes over the patient's

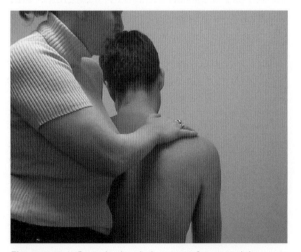

Figure 4.17   Posterior hand placement for upper lobe techniques.

shoulder, some additional support to the patient can be provided, by gently compressing the overlying arm against the shoulder girdle. The heel of the anterior hand should be lateral to the sternum, and be around the level of the chondrocostal articulations. Again, the fingers of the anterior hand should be relaxed and can rest over the pectoral tissues and anterior shoulder.

There are several options to test out the lung in this position. One is to use a local 'listening' approach; another is to feel for general fascial and connective tissue tensions within the lung tissue itself. Often in asthmatic cases and post whiplash or chest injury situations, there is quite a lot of sensitization to the lung tissue and this can be palpated quite effectively with a global upper lobe contact. Seatbelt injuries, for example, often involve the upper lobe of the lung. The contact can be used to unwind and balance through the tissues, easing torsions and so reducing spasms, irritability and sensitization.

Another approach is to mobilize directly into the lung tissue, which is useful when there is chronic congestion or stiffening of the lung in problems such as chronic bronchitis, or from scarring after rib injury, for example. Here the contact is the same but a vibratory or rhythmic pendular movement can be made. If performing a vibratory technique, the practitioner starts with some compression between the two hands, to descend past the ribs and pass into the lung tissue. The posterior hand compresses in an inferior and slightly anterior direction, and the anterior hand compresses in a superior and slightly posterior direction. Maintaining this compression, the two hands then vibrate quite quickly. The amplitude of this movement is quite small and should not rock the patient backwards and forwards at their hips, for example. The patient should be somewhat resting against the practitioner, so that they are not holding themselves up in any way. In effect, the practitioner uses the compression between their two hands to slightly support the weight of the patient. In this way, any subsequent movements of the practitioner's hands will pass immediately into the chest, and supporting the weight of the patient helps to create depth within the technique.

A variation of this technique is to perform a rhythmic pendular movement instead of a vibration.

The pendular movement can be quite slow and gentle, and can be very useful as a basic mobilization or to induce balance and desensitization within the tissues. It can also be useful for fluid-balancing techniques. The practitioner takes the same basic contact as already described, and shown in Figure 4.17. The compression between the two hands is still made, to pass deep to the ribs. Now, whilst maintaining a degree of mutual compression, the two hands move in a slightly aphasic rhythm, as though they were gently batting a tennis ball between the two palms. First the posterior hand pushes forwards and downwards, and the anterior hand waits for the tissues to 'bulge'. The anterior hand allows the tissues to 'bulge' or 'swell' and then it 'gathers them up' and gently pushes them back to the posterior hand (in a superior and slightly posterior direction). So, first one hand induces a wave of motion and then the other, in an equal and opposite direction. The tissues of the lung are gently reflected to and fro between the two hands. The wave of motion should pass evenly through the lung and pleural tissues, and any restriction is felt by the wave not reflecting through as it should, or being 'bounced' back. Effectively, this is a bit like a manual ultrasound technique and is both an evaluation and a treatment.

All of the lung fields can be mobilized in this way; the hand contacts are moved up and down the chest accordingly. Figure 4.18 shows the

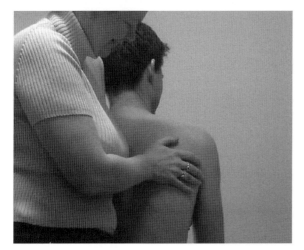

Figure 4.18 Posterior hand placement for lower lobe (above diaphragm level).

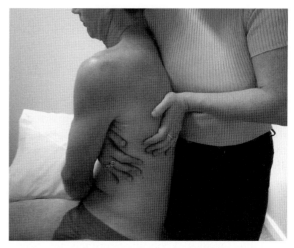

Figure 4.19 Sitting global lower lobe release.

posterior placement for the lower lobe (in this technique only that section which is above the level of the diaphragm is being tested/treated). The posterior hand should remain above the inferior angle of the scapula to ensure that the lower lobe above the level of the diaphragm is being evaluated. The anterior hand is placed quite laterally, so that the palm is just lateral to the midclavicular line and is at the level of the seventh and eighth ribs. This ensures that it contacts the anterior margin of the lower lobe of the lung (this anterior contact is shown in Figure 4.19).

If the hands contact the chest below the level of the diaphragm, then the movement can pass through other organs such as the spleen or liver, as well as the sliver of lower lobe that passes down between the posterior diaphragm and the lower ribcage. The direction for mobilizing the lower lobe is slightly more oblique, compared to the direction for testing the upper lobe. The upper lobe is tested with the compression/movement occurring from back to front (from posterosuperiorly to anteroinferiorly). The lower lobe is tested with the compression/movement occurring from posterosupero-medial to anteroinfero-lateral, as indicated in Figure 4.19. Again, it should be remembered that the practitioner takes part of the weight of the patient, supports the patient's lumbar region with a small pillow if necessary, and does not use enough movement to rock the patient to and fro on their hips.

TECHNIQUES FOR THE STELLATE GANGLION, COSTOVERTEBRO–PLEURAL LIGAMENT AND SIBSON'S FASCIA

Having globally released the lobes of the lung, more specific tests can be considered for the thoracic inlet and suspensory ligament of the pleural dome. There are many techniques for this region that can stretch the scalenes, the brachial plexus, the upper fibres of trapezius, the cervical erector spinae and so on. All of these can be adapted to help mobilize tissues within the thoracic inlet. As with all techniques, it is necessary to have a thorough and three-dimensional appreciation of the anatomy in order to develop any number of individual techniques. A couple of contacts are shown below, to help begin releasing tissues in the thoracic inlet region.

Figure 4.20 shows a sidelying technique which uses leverage from the shoulder girdle to ease tissue tensions from the clavicle and upper ribs, across the thoracic inlet, whilst the other hand contacts into the scalenes, suspensory ligament of the pleural dome or whatever tissue is being explored. In this technique, the thumb is used as a direct contact and care should be taken not to use too much pressure and to avoid sensitive vascular structures. The technique shown places the thumb quite low down, near the transverse processes of C6 and C7, to mobilize the suspensory ligament via the scalenes and other musculofascial tissue that runs from this point down to the pleural

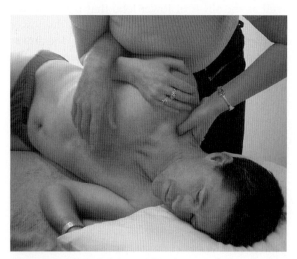

Figure 4.20 Thoracic inlet mobilization.

dome level. The ligament is covered by the scalenes, so it is not possible to contact it directly.

Palpating close to the posterior arch of the first rib, as near to the head of the rib as possible (tucked deep to the fibres of trapezius), the practitioner can release the posterior thoracic inlet fascia, the posterior part of Sibson's fascia and the pleural dome and the costovertebro-pleural ligament. In this region (on top of the pleural dome and near the head of the first rib) is the stellate or inferior cervical ganglion. This is an important structure for all head and many thoracic structures, as the upper four dorsal spinal cord segments send the majority of their fibres upwards through this ganglion, to pass then to some throat and mediastinal structures or upwards to the middle and superior cervical ganglia. Functional or unwinding release through this region of the posterior thoracic inlet will directly affect the stellate ganglion, and help balance autonomic neural reflexes and function for many head, neck, throat and mediastinal structures. Inhibition can also be applied, via a direct stretch to the surrounding tissues, to ensure good neural circulation and drainage.

TECHNIQUES FOR THE SUSPENSORY LIGAMENT OF THE PLEURAL DOME, CERVICAL FASCIA, VAGUS AND PHRENIC NERVES

The suspensory ligament and other thoracic inlet structures can also be evaluated in a supine position, as shown in Figure 4.21. Here, the posterior cervical column is supported with one hand, which can induce cervical rotation or lateral flexion, or anterior-posterior translation, if required. The other hand will contact the anterior cervical region. The suspensory ligament is found deep to the anterior scalene muscle, just inferior to the sternal head of the sternocleidomastoid (SCM). The palpating fingers may also have to feel through some of the outer fibres of the clavicular head of the SCM.

To test the ligament, there are several options. One is to 'listen' to the fascial pulls created as the patient breathes in. If there are any mediastinal or lung restrictions, the tissues between the thoracic diaphragm and the palpating contact will be less elastic than normal. As the patient inspires, the

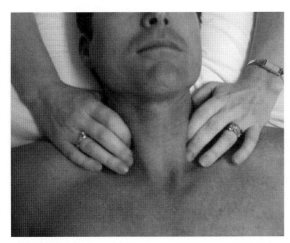

Figure 4.21   Palpation of suspensory ligament and other neck fascias.

diaphragm descends and the slack in the mediastinal and lung tissues is taken up. This quickly engages the suspensory ligament of the pleural dome and the cervical fascia, when there is a problem. The practitioner will feel the cervical fascia being 'drawn inferiorly' as the patient breathes in. Normally, with no tissue restriction present, it is only at the end of a deep inbreath that some inferior movement of the fascia may be felt. With a restriction, this dragging comes on almost immediately. The posterior hand around the neck can gently tilt the cervical column into one direction or another, to ensure that the cervical fascia is not too tautly tensioned in advance of the technique. If desired, both hands can palpate on the cervical fascia, so that the test can be performed bilaterally (which makes comparison easier). To release the cervical fascia, direct stretches or functional/indirect unwinding can be utilized. The posterior hand contact is very useful when functionally releasing or balancing the cervical fascias and suspensory ligament, as it can induce motion so that the most optimal direction for treatment can be created between the two hands.

The phrenic nerve is relatively easily treated in the cervical region. It overlies the lower part of the anterior scalene muscle, lateral to the carotid sheath and vessels, and inferior to the SCM. Balancing of the cervical fascia overlying the scalenes can help to reduce irritation within the phrenic nerve. The tissues can also be 'inhibited' by using very slight pressure onto the nerve. It is

very important not to cause compression onto the carotid sheath, which lies just medial to this contact. However, bearing this in mind, with very careful contact the carotid sheath can be 'listened' to and in so doing, it may be possible to influence the vagus nerve (which runs within it).

TECHNIQUES FOR THE MEDIASTINAL PLEURAL ARTICULATIONS

The mediastinal pleural articulations (or sliding surfaces) ensure mobility between the lungs and the heart/pericardium. These sliding surfaces are illustrated in Figure 4.7. In these techniques, one hand is using the sternum to stabilize the heart and pericardium, and the other uses the ribcage to contact the lung (usually the lower lobe). When contacting the heart and the left lower lobe, the heart/sternal contact should be from the midline of the sternum to the left midclavicular line.

Figure 4.22 shows a supine contact, with the practitioner at the head of the patient. The anterior hand is placed over the left lateral sternum as described. The posterior hand contacts the lower lobe, by ensuring that it is slightly posterior to the midaxillary line, and the inferior angle of the scapula is placed in the centre of the palm. This will keep the bulk of the contact above the level of the diaphragm. The anterior hand will make a small supination-pronation movement about an axis just deep to the left costal cartilages. This will effectively rotate the heart and pericardium around

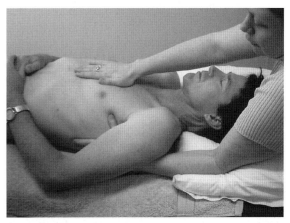

Figure 4.22   Balancing the left lower lobe in relation to heart.

its own axis, and begin to create some movement within the mediastinal sliding surfaces. The posterior hand will make an arcing movement with the side of the chest wall, in a direction that is slightly more curved than the periphery of the ribcage. The thumb and thenar eminence will first move towards the ceiling, and then the ulnar border of the hand and fifth finger will scoop towards the spine, and will end up lifting against the angles of the ribs, to create an arc that will move the lower lobe of the lung around the heart. During the actual technique, the hands can move at the same time or one can stabilize whilst the other mobilizes. If the hands are moved at the same time, the sternal hand supinates (to the patient's left) whilst the posterior hand curves the chest wall up and around (towards the ceiling).

This type of contact makes an excellent starting point to evaluate the pulmonary vessels, and structures of the hilum of the lungs, which pass from the lungs to the heart. Many of the mediastinal lymph nodes are located along the bronchi, around the hilum of the lung, and posterior to the heart, so releases in this region are very useful for lymphatic drainage and immune function within the chest. Remember that the still point for active movement within the thoracic cage as a whole is just posterosuperior to the heart, meaning this is the least mobile part of the chest. So, any tissue tension at this point will negatively impact on function and any technique that approaches this mediastinal balance should be of value.

Figure 4.23 shows a contact onto the right side of the chest to explore the sliding surfaces between the heart and the right lung.

TECHNIQUES FOR THE BRONCHI AND PULMONARY VESSELS

The tests introduced for the sliding surfaces between the heart and the lung will also test/treat the bronchi and pulmonary vessels as the contacts are stabilizing the heart and the lung, between which the vessels and bronchi pass (see Figs 4.22 and 4.23). Contacts that palpate just through the lobes themselves are also clearly relevant to the function of the bronchi and pulmonary vessels.

Figure 4.24 shows a bilateral posterolateral contact of the lower lobes of the lungs, to evaluate

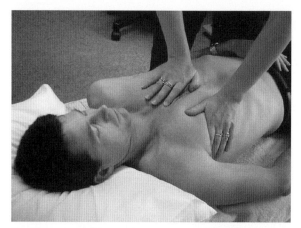

Figure 4.23   Mediastinal/heart and right lung sliding surfaces.

the lungs and the bronchi. The hands are placed with the palms contacting the inferior angles of the scapulae, just posterior to the midaxillary lines. The left hand should be very slightly higher than the right, as the left bronchus has a slightly more oblique (less vertical) orientation than the right, due to the placement of the heart. This contact is particularly good for functional/fascial unwinding releases along the bronchi and between the two lower lobes. It is also a very good contact for working with the motility of the lungs. Often the bronchi exhibit a spiral torsion running along their length. They also often feel contracted along their length. Feeling into these patterns and

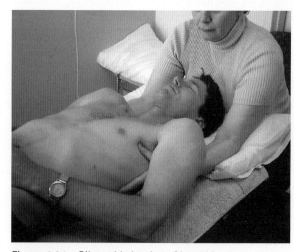

Figure 4.24   Bilateral balancing of bronchi.

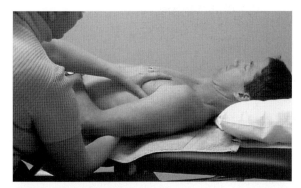

Figure 4.25 Alternative lower lobe contact.

allowing lateral expansion can be very effective in restoring normal bronchial compliance.

Figure 4.25 shows the same contact but performed unilaterally, with the practitioner at the patient's side. The sidelying technique shown in Figure 4.16 illustrated an upper lobe contact, which can be used to evaluate the bronchioles that relate to the upper lobe. These are oriented fairly vertically and the practitioner feels for spiral torsions operating in this vertical alignment.

Figure 4.26 shows a technique for the tissues that link the two hilums of the lungs, the posterior wall of the heart, and the fascia running upwards to the posterior pharynx/cervical region, to that attaching to the posterior section of the central tendon of the diaphragm. This layer of tissue is called the bronchopulmonary ligament and work

in this region helps to balance the whole of the posterior mediastinum and the visceral core-link of fascia to the cranial base. The practitioner has one hand placed under the ribs/spine at the level of the middorsal spine. The other hand is placed over the sternum and engages the pericardium and through to the posterior wall of the heart. The posterior hand contacts through the dorsal spine and into the posterior mediastinum, to engage the posterior wall of the heart 'from behind'. The two hands reach a point of balanced equilibrium, where the bronchopulmonary membrane (just behind the posterior wall of the heart) can be worked on.

This technique makes a good contact to release the cardiac and pulmonary autonomic plexi that are found in and around the pericardium and posterior mediastinal tissues.

TECHNIQUES FOR THE THROAT, CERVICAL FASCIA, LARYNX AND PHARYNX

These techniques help to release the structures relevant to EENT function.

Figure 4.27 shows a contact for the anterior throat. This technique can access the thyroid, the infrahyoid tissues and middle cervical fascia and the trachea and beginning of the oesophagus. It can balance these tissues with the sternum and anterior chest and mediastinal tissues. The cephalic hand contacts the sides of the thyroid and/or

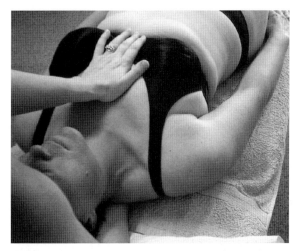

Figure 4.26 Bronchopulmonary ligament and posterior cardiac contact.

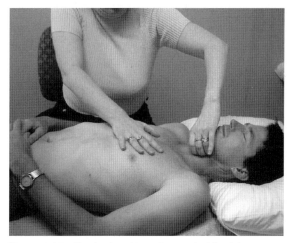

Figure 4.27 Tracheal and anterior cervical fascial tests.

hyoid cartilages, just so that the posterior soft tissue (the trachea) is being engaged as part of the contact. It is important not to compress the anterior throat or to press near or on the carotid sheath. The caudal hand contacts the sternum and manubrium, to engage the infrahyoid soft tissues and the cervical fascia. It can also feel down through the layers of the chest, to contact with the pericardium or the bifurcation of the trachea. Depending on the depth of the contact at the chest, various different tissues can be evaluated when combined with movement from the cephalic hand, engaging the tissues from 'above down'. A functional unwinding or balancing technique is useful between these two contacts, as is a slight traction/vertical stretching, to slightly ease the trachea towards the mandible. This will subtly elongate the trachea and can be used as a soft tissue stretch to diffuse irritation within the trachea. Stretch of the infrahyoid muscles is also useful and can help improve hyoid mobility, which is necessary for tongue function, as well as throat drainage and upper mediastinal balance (as well as linking into the cranial base).

Figure 4.28 shows a contact to release the tongue, submandibular tissues and glands, and the upper anterior throat. One hand stabilizes the head, whilst the other contacts just on the medial (inside) border of the mandible. From here, the fingers can gently release (using inhibition, direct soft tissue or unwinding/balancing techniques) the base of the tongue, the suprahyoid tissues and the larynx.

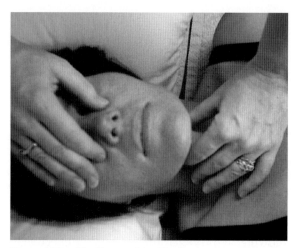

Figure 4.29   Maxillary and hyoid release.

The fingers can be eased medially to apply a gentle compression on the base of the tongue, taking care not to press too firmly onto the hyoid. This type of release is very useful for any EENT congestion and middle ear/eustachian tube problems, for example.

Figure 4.29 shows a contact which is moving up into the nasopharynx. The caudal hand is contacting the hyoid and the cephalic hand is contacting over the two maxillae. This contact is designed to use the maxillary contact as a 'handle' into the pterygoid plates of the sphenoid and the palatine bones, to engage the pharyngeal tissues. The hyoid engages the constrictors from below and the maxillary contact engages them from above. An inferior stretch to the hyoid can be given, a maxillary spreading technique and a superior traction can be applied, and a general unwinding and balancing between the two contacts can also be given.

There are myriad techniques that can be applied to the face which could also be of value to the management of EENT problems. There are also many intraoral techniques for the palate, the pterygoids, the vomer and so on that usually need addressing in chronic EENT problems, which should not be overlooked.

TECHNIQUES FOR SINUS DRAINAGE AND FOR FACIAL AND OTHER CRANIAL BONE ARTICULATION

A key point to release the face and its articulation with the cranium is to mobilize the ethmoid, and

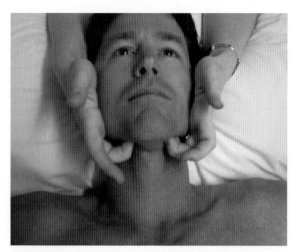

Figure 4.28   Tongue and submandibular release.

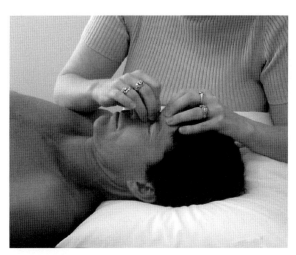

Figure 4.30   Ethmoid release.

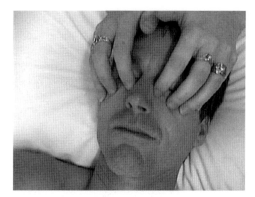

Figure 4.31   Sinus release.

create some movement in and around its relations. In Figure 4.30 one hand is contacting the frontal bone either side of the bridge of the nose, just inside the medial upper orbit. The other hand contacts the bridge of the nose directly, to engage the nasal bones. Now, a gentle but definite traction can be applied, to separate the two contacts and to give some space to the underlying ethmoid articulations. A rhythmic gapping technique is used. Note: the actual range of movement is minimal (less than a millimetre) but this is a direct articulatory technique, not a functional unwinding. Of course, the indirect type of technique can also be very usefully applied but in cases of chronic congestion and long-standing irritation of the sphenopalatine ganglion, the gapping technique is very effective.

Figure 4.31 shows a technique for spreading the zygomas and the maxillae (depending on exact contact) to help decongest the sinuses. A rhythmic pumping or gapping technique is useful. Also, a vibratory technique where the finger tips are gently but definitely 'drummed' against the facial contacts can help to loosen the maxillary sinuses and ease drainage. This vibratory technique can also be applied over the frontal area, to help with the frontal, ethmoid and sphenoid sinuses.

TECHNIQUES FOR THE EYE

As mentioned before, eye mobilization techniques can be useful if applied carefully. Figure 4.32 shows

a contact with one eye, where the finger tip is being gently applied to the outside of the eye, within the rim of the orbit. The eye is gently compressed in a rhythmic pumping manner (that utilizes a very small amplitude and a slow rhythm). The contact can be moved around the eye, testing all its quadrants. The eye should be freely mobile within the orbit and should also feel equally soft and relaxed all around, in all quadrants. Supraorbital nerve inhibition or unwinding can be applied at the supraorbital notch, and lacrimal mobilization can be applied in the medial upper quadrant of the eye. As mentioned before, the eyes make a very good window into the dura and meninges and if the index, middle and third fingers are gently placed over the closed eyelids, they can gently hold onto the eye and evaluate its torsion, and that of the optic nerve and cranial membranes.

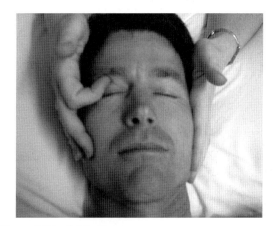

Figure 4.32   Orbit release.

Often, as a result of tissue tension and different torsion patterns, the eyes feel as though they are being dragged into very different directions and this can lead to fatigue and irritation within the eye muscles, thereby compromising vision and accommodation. A functional unwinding or balancing applied directly to the eye can help with many eye problems, many cases of migraine and headache, and many other situations where dural and meningeal release is required.

References

1. Mirilas P, Siatitsas Y, Skandalakis JE. Benign anatomical mistakes: inferior pulmonary ligament. Am Surg 2002;68(10):922-6.
2. De Troyer A, Wilson TA. Sternum dependence of rib displacement during breathing. J Appl Physiol 1993;75:334-40.
3. Oda I, Abumi K, Lu D, Shono Y, Kaneda K. Biomechanical role of the posterior elements, costovertebral joints, and rib cage in the stability of the thoracic spine. Spine 1996;21(12):1423-9.
4. Pal GP. Mechanism of production of scoliosis. A hypothesis. Spine 1991;16:288-92.
5. Culham EG, Jimenez HA, King CE. Thoracic kyphosis, rib mobility, and lung volumes in normal women and women with osteoporosis. Spine 1994;19:1250-5.
6. Upadhyay SS, Mullaji AB, Luk KD, Leong JC. Relation of spinal and thoracic cage deformities and their flexibilities with altered pulmonary functions in adolescent idiopathic scoliosis. Spine 1995; 20:2415-20.
7. Fung YC, Yen RT, Tao ZL, Liu SQ. A hypothesis on the mechanism of trauma of lung tissue subjected to impact load. J Biomech Eng 1988; 110(1):50-6.
8. Papastamelos C, Panitch HB, England SE, Allen JL. Developmental changes in chest wall compliance in infancy and early childhood. J Appl Physiol 1995;78(1):179-84.
9. Gaultier C. Respiratory muscle function in infants. Eur Respir J 1995;8(1):150-3.
10. Grivas TB, Burwell RG, Purdue M, Webb JK, Moulton A. A segmental analysis of thoracic shape in chest radiographs of children. Changes related to spinal level, age, sex, side and significance for lung growth and scoliosis. J Anat 1991; 178:21-38.
11. Mishiro Y, Oki T, Iuchi A, et al. Echocardiographic characteristics and causal mechanism of physiologic mitral regurgitation in young normal subjects. Clin Cardiol 1997;20(10):850-5.
12. Faria PT, De Oliveira Ruellas AC, Matsumoto MA, Anselmo-Lima WT, Pereira FC. Dentofacial morphology of mouth breathing children. Braz Dent J 2002;13(2):129-32.
13. Cottle MH. A consideration of nasal, pulmonary and cardio-vascular interdependance and nasal-pulmonary function studies. Rhinology 1980;18(2):67-81.
14. Tasko SM, McClean MD. Variations in articulatory movement with changes in speech task. J Speech Lang Hear Res 2004;47(1):85-100.
15. Hruska RJ Jr. Influences of dysfunctional respiratory mechanics on orofacial pain. Dent Clin North Am 1997;41:211-27.
16. Principato JJ. Upper airway obstruction and cranio-facial morphology. Otolaryngol Head Neck Surg 1991;104(6):881-90.
17. Tourne LP. Growth of the pharynx and its physio-logic implications. Am J Orthod Dentofacial Orthop 1991;99(2):129-39.
18. Zafar H. Integrated jaw and neck function in man. Studies of mandibular and head-neck movements during jaw opening-closing tasks. Swed Dent J 2000;143(Suppl):1-41.
19. Darrow DH, Siemens C. Indications for tonsillectomy and adenoidectomy. Laryngoscope 2002;112(8 Pt 2 Suppl 100):6-10.
20. Carlson CR, Sherman JJ, Studts JL, Bertrand PM. The effects of tongue position on mandibular muscle activity. J Orofac Pain 1997;11(4):291-7.
21. Huang MH, Lee ST, Rajendran K. A fresh cadaveric study of the paratubal muscles: implications for eustachian tube function in cleft palate. Plast Reconstr Surg 1997;100(4):833-42.
22. Viggiano D, Fasano D, Monaco G, Strohmenger L. Breast feeding, bottle feeding, and non-nutritive sucking; effects on occlusion in deciduous dentition. Arch Dis Child 2004;89(12):1121-3.
23. Carreiro J. An osteopathic approach to children. Edinburgh: Churchill Livingstone; 2003.
24. Jones AS. Autonomic reflexes and non-allergic rhinitis. Allergy 1997;52(36 Suppl):14-19.
25. Virant FS. Sinusitis and asthma: associated airway diseases. Curr Allergy Asthma Rep 2001;1(3):277-81.
26. Takahashi S, Ono T, Ishiwata Y, Kuroda T. Breathing modes, body positions, and suprahyoid muscle activity. J Orthod 2002;29(4):307-13; discussion 279.

27. Behlfelt K, Linder-Aronson S, Neander P. Posture of the head, the hyoid bone, and the tongue in children with and without enlarged tonsils. Eur J Orthod 1990;12(4):458-67.

28. Ostberg O, Horie Y, Feng Y. On the merits of ancient Chinese eye acupressure practices. Appl Ergon 1992;23(5):343-8.

29. Lasky DI, Lasky AM. Stereoscopic eye exercises and visual acuity. Percept Mot Skills 1990;71(3 Pt 1):1055-8.

30. Ciftci F, Akman A, Sonmez M, Unal M, Gungor A, Yaylali V. Systematic, combined treatment approach to nasolacrimal duct obstruction in different age groups. Eur J Ophthalmol 2000;10(4): 324-9.

31. Gilbard JP. Dry eye, blepharitis and chronic eye irritation: divide and conquer. J Ophthalmic Nurs Technol 1999;18(3):109-5.

32. Jacome DE. Migraine triggered by rubbing the eyes. Headache 1998;38(1):50-2.

33. Borruat FX, Kawasaki A. Optic nerve massaging: an extremely rare cause of self-inflicted blindness. Am J Ophthalmol 2005;139(4):715-16.

Chapter 5

Overview of gastrointestinal system

i Note: details for the overview of the pancreas are also included in Chapter 8. Details for the salivary glands are included in Chapter 4.

This chapter includes a basic anatomical overview for the gastrointestinal system, and an introduction to the examination and treatment techniques that can be used. It gives an indication of the integration between the somatic and visceral systems, and of reflex relationships, which builds upon information in previous chapters. Patient management is discussed, together with the other body systems, in Chapter 9. All case management discussions are included in Chapter 9 as it is important in osteopathy to remember that treating patients with gastrointestinal tract problems does not only involve work to the gut tube.

SURFACE ANATOMY

The gastrointestinal tract (GIT) has a very large surface area and there are many musculoskeletal landmarks indicating the general location of various parts of the GIT. As a result of the large amount of movement in embryological formation, there is commonly some variability in landmarks, for example of the appendix, the position of the greater curvature of the stomach or the length of the sigmoid colon.

Thus, it is better to identify GIT structures using palpation in general geographical locations, rather than relying on tape measures and 'average' positions. The illustration **Figure A1** in the appendix shows anterior, posterior and lateral views of the body, indicating which GIT structures are generally related to which skeletal structure. This gives a guide for the palpating hand. It should be noted that when dealing with infants and babies, the relative size and location of the GIT organs do alter somewhat (for example, the liver is relatively a much larger organ in the infant).

As the GIT is soft to palpation (especially when healthy), exact location of structures through the abdominal wall or other body parts can be difficult and requires skill. That said, some parts (and other adjacent organs) are more easily identifiable than others and form good palpation localizing points.

Table 5.1 shows a breakdown of musculoskeletal landmarks for the GIT. This table should be read in conjunction with the surface anatomy illustrations in the appendix.

LIGAMENTS AND SUPPORTS

The 'ligaments' of the GIT are formed by remnants of the dorsal and ventral mesenteries during embryological rotation and migration of the gut tube. The gut tube invaginates into the intraembryonic coelum, a hollow, horseshoe-shaped structure that forms the pleural, pericardial and peritoneal cavities. Figure 5.1 illustrates the development of the peritoneal cavity, and consequently some of the visceral 'ligaments' and mesenteries that support the gut tube and form conduits for its blood vessels, nerves and lymphatics.

OESOPHAGUS

Within the throat and thorax, the oesophagus is first attached to the cranial base via the pharyngeal tubercle, and then the pharyngeal constrictor attachments to the pterygoid plates of the sphenoid, and the hyoid and thyroid cartilages. It is then attached along the posterior surface of the trachea, then the posterior wall of the heart (and the bronchopulmonary ligament, discussed in Chapter 4), before passing through the diaphragmatic hiatus.

The phreno-oesophageal ligament attaches the oesophagus to the diaphragm, at the level of the diaphragmatic hiatus. The ligament divides into a prominent upper leaf and an ill-defined lower leaf before inserting into the wall of the oesophagus.[1]

The oesophageal hiatus of the diaphragm is a spiral 'figure of eight' arrangement of the fibres of the crurae. The ligament of Treitz (described below) is a suspensory ligament for the last part of the duodenum. It appears clinically that the ligament of Treitz, through its crural attachments, links the oesophageal hiatus to the terminal part of the duodenum, thereby creating a sort of mechanical 'sphincter link' between the oesophagus/cardiac sphincter and the duodenojejunal junction. This may be relevant in cases of reflux and hiatus hernia.

As the oesophagus enters the abdominal cavity, it also becomes enclosed by the lesser omentum, which is discussed below. The oesophageal ligaments and relations are shown in Figure 5.2.

The main movements of the oesophagus are as follows.

- Stretch and general mobilization in pharynx area following cranial base, tongue, hyoid and thyroid movements
- Slight longitudinal slide against the posterior trachea and posterior heart
- Up-and-down slide through the diaphragmatic hiatus
- Straightening and re-curving of the J-shaped cardiac section of the oesophagus as it enters the stomach

STOMACH

There are several ligaments and peritoneal structures that support the stomach, as shown in Figure 5.4. From the pictures showing the embryological formation of the peritoneal ligaments, it can be seen that many of the stomach ligaments are essentially part of one extended structure. The different parts of it have different names and in fact, the nomenclature can be as complex as desired, separately labelling many small segments. However, this level of detail does not help practically. It is more important to have a global picture of the overall arrangement and orientation of the ligamentous structures, so that when it comes to techniques, the required subtlety can be achieved

Table 5.1   Musculoskeletal landmarks for the gastrointestinal tract

GIT structure	Musculoskeletal landmark	Comments
Dome of diaphragm	Although the right dome is slightly higher, in general the upper reach of the diaphragm is adjacent to the 8–9th dorsal vertebrae	The 8–9th vertebral level approximates to a line drawn between the two inferior angles of the scapulae, which in turn bisects the tip of the spinous process of the 7th dorsal vertebra
Cardiac sphincter	To the left of the midline, posterior to the midaxillary line and medial to the posterior equivalent to the midclavicular line	The oesophageal hiatus is related to the suspensory ligament of the duodenum (ligament of Treitz), therefore functionally linking the duodenojejunal junction and the cardiac sphincter
Pylorus	L1–2 on right, lateral to midline on the right, but still deep to the rectus abdominis muscle	A line drawn between the two tips of the 9th costal cartilages also bisects the L1–2 vertebral body level and is called the transpyloric line
Duodenum	The C-shaped curve of the duodenum sits to the right of the first 3 lumbar vertebrae	The descending and transverse parts are immobile, being retroperitoneal. The other parts are intraperitoneal and less influenced by lumbar Ispinal mechanics
Sphincter of Oddi	To the right of the midline, approximately lateral to the 2nd lumbar vertebral body	Approximately the same height as the duodenojejunal junction but more medially situated
DJ junction (duodenojejunal junction)	To the left of the midline, usually around the L2–3 vertebral level.	The DJ junction is slightly lower and slightly more lateral than the pylorus is on the right. The DJ junction is near the border of the rectus muscle, whereas the pylorus is covered by it
Ileocaecal valve	On a line between the umbilicus and the anterior superior iliac spine on the right	The valve is usually found between half and two-thirds of the way from the umbilicus to the ASIS along this line
Caecum	Superior to the ASIS on the right	As the caecum can swell depending on contents, its exact size will vary. However, it shouldn't be found lower than the ASIS
Ascending and descending colons	Lateral to the midclavicular line bilaterally (and anteriorly to the midaxillary lines)	The ascending and descending colons are relatively easy to palpate and are fixed in position, so are consistently locatable on top of either kidney and psoas muscles
Sigmoid colon	Inferior to the ASIS on the left	The sigmoid will be found nestled into the left iliac fossa and can run along the pubis, and also cross the midline, before turning and passing posteriorly, towards the rectum
Left lobe of the liver	Near the midclavicular line on the left, at the 6–7th intercostal space	The left-sided position of the tip of the left lobe of the liver is variable, and in some people is quite close to the midline
Falciform ligament	This is found in the medial notch on the anterior inferior border of the liver	This is usually slightly behind the right insertion of the rectus muscle
Gall bladder	This is found in the lateral notch on the anterior inferior border of the liver	This is usually slightly lateral to the border of the rectus muscle insertion to the right costal margin
Appendix	This is highly variable in position but is most commonly found in the right iliac fossa or along the lower half of the ascending colon	There is no set landmark for the appendix and pain on palpation in the iliac fossa can be related to a number of conditions, such as ovarian pathology, for example

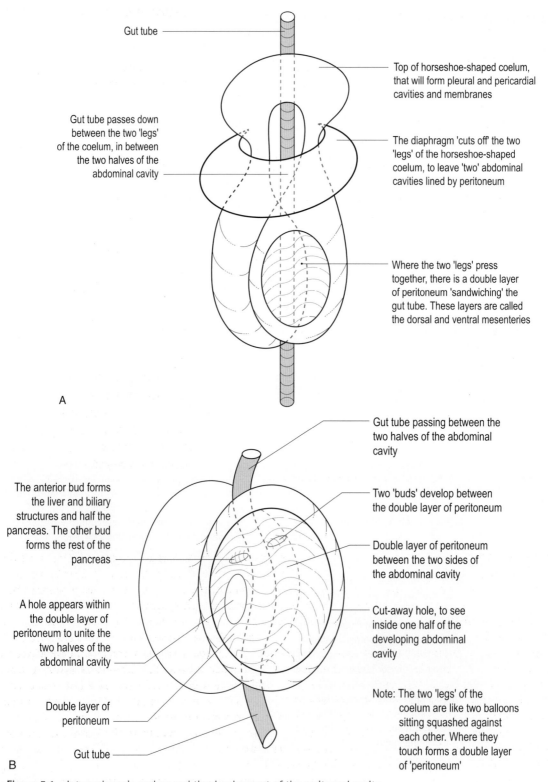

Figure 5.1   Intraembryonic coelum and the development of the peritoneal cavity.

Continued

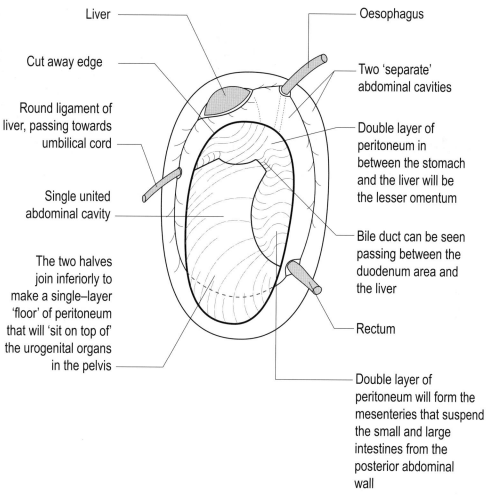

Liver

Cut away edge

Round ligament of
liver, passing towards
umbilical cord

Single united
abdominal cavity

The two halves
join inferiorly to
make a single–layer
'floor' of peritoneum
that will 'sit on top of'
the urogenital organs
in the pelvis

Oesophagus

Two 'separate'
abdominal cavities

Double layer of
peritoneum in
between the stomach
and the liver will be
the lesser omentum

Bile duct can be seen
passing between the
duodenum area and
the liver

Rectum

Double layer of
peritoneum will form the
mesenteries that suspend
the small and large
intestines from the
posterior abdominal
wall

C

Figure 5.1   Cont'd

by ensuring all of them are properly visualized to guide the palpating hand.

In basic terms, the two main supports are the greater and lesser omentum. These link the stomach to the diaphragm, spleen and kidney, and to the liver and gall bladder/bile duct. The lesser omentum contains the oesophagus at one end and the bile duct, portal vein and various nerves and lymph vessels at the other. It is continuous with the coronary and falciform ligaments of the liver. The greater omentum contains the spleen in its top left 'corner' between the stomach and the diaphragm, and effectively gives rise to the gastrophrenic, gastrosplenic, gastrocolic and gastrolienal ligaments where it merges with the diaphragm, spleen, colonic flexure and kidney, respectively. It then

hangs inferiorly from the greater omentum and can influence the position and mobility of the bulk of the lower segments of the stomach when the greater omentum 'migrates' around or becomes adhesed.

This ligamentous relationship ensures that the stomach swings like a hammock under the liver and diaphragm. The alignment for the stomach suspensory mechanism is 'equal and opposite' in orientation to that of the liver, giving 'opposing' movements (see Fig. 5.4).

The main movements of the stomach are as follows.

■ A pendular swinging motion underneath the liver and diaphragm.

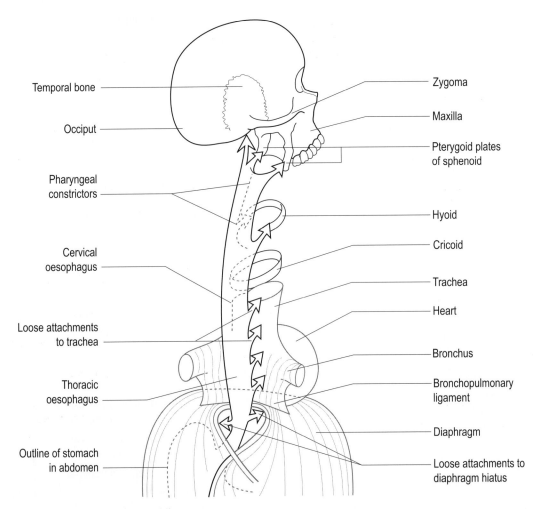

Temporal bone

Occiput

Pharyngeal constrictors

Cervical oesophagus

Loose attachments to trachea

Thoracic oesophagus

Outline of stomach in abdomen

Zygoma

Maxilla

Pterygoid plates of sphenoid

Hyoid

Cricoid

Trachea

Heart

Bronchus

Bronchopulmonary ligament

Diaphragm

Loose attachments to diaphragm hiatus

Figure 5.2 Oesophageal relations and ligaments.

- A hinging motion where the mobile pylorus and first part of the duodenum (duodenal cap) meets the immobile descending part of the duodenum. This hinging motion aids in the functions of the pyloric sphincter and gives a particular motion to the right lateral edge of the lesser omentum, rather like a curtain being swished aside a little. This mobilization of the free edge of the lesser omentum is important for those structures embedded within it, namely the bile duct, portal vein and various arteries.
- The lesser curvature of the stomach is more constant in its anatomical position between subjects compared to the greater curvature, which can be anywhere from umbilical level

to the pubis. Hence, the articulations of the greater curvature of the stomach (and consequently the greater omentum) are variable in description, depending on where the curvature is located in that individual.
- The transverse colon is always attached to the underneath of the greater omentum, at the border of the greater curvature of the stomach, and so the movements of the transverse colon and stomach are linked.

DUODENUM

The duodenum has some interesting peritoneal and fascial relations. It is also the point at which embryological rotation of the gut was initiated

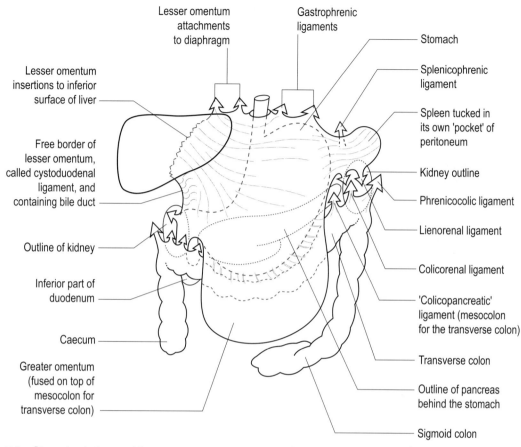

Lesser omentum attachments to diaphragm

Gastrophrenic ligaments

Stomach

Splenicophrenic ligament

Lesser omentum insertions to inferior surface of liver

Spleen tucked in its own 'pocket' of peritoneum

Free border of lesser omentum, called cystoduodenal ligament, and containing bile duct

Kidney outline

Phrenicocolic ligament

Lienorenal ligament

Outline of kidney

Colicorenal ligament

Inferior part of duodenum

'Colicopancreatic' ligament (mesocolon for the transverse colon)

Caecum

Transverse colon

Greater omentum (fused on top of mesocolon for transverse colon)

Outline of pancreas behind the stomach

Sigmoid colon

Figure 5.3   Stomach relations and ligaments.

(in order to bring the two halves of the embryonic pancreas together). Hence, any alteration in mobility at this level will affect the whole impetus and vitality of the gut tube. The duodenum is a retroperitoneal organ 'by default'; initially it was covered on both sides by the peritoneum. As it rotated, it swept back and dragged the pancreas and bile duct so that when all three structures met the posterior abdominal wall, the peritoneum in between disappeared and the bile duct became trapped behind the descending part of the duodenum/head of the pancreas and the posterior abdominal wall, attaching to the renal fascia, psoas, arcuate ligament of the right side of the diaphragm and indirectly from these to the upper lumbar spine on the right, and the cysterna chyli, for example. Specifically, the descending and transverse sections of the duodenum are retroperitoneal and the first

and fourth parts are still intraperitoneal. This gives the duodenum two 'hinges' at either end.

Both the bile duct and the pancreatic duct enter into the medial side of the descending part of the duodenum and these ducts are surrounded by the sphincter of Oddi, which influences the flow of pancreatic enzymes and bile into the small intestine. Duodenal tension at the sphincter of Oddi can therefore influence pancreatic function, as well as gall bladder function. The last part of the duodenum is not separated from the jejunum by a defined sphincter. However, the suspensory ligament of the duodenum ('ligament of Treitz') forms a spiralling, twisting hinge motion at the junction between the duodenum and jejunum, thereby conferring some degree of sphincteric action to this section of the gut tube.[2] The duodenum and its relations and fascial attachments are outlined in Figure 5.5.

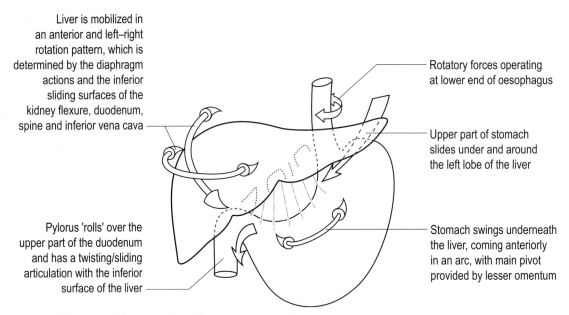

Liver is mobilized in an anterior and left–right rotation pattern, which is determined by the diaphragm actions and the inferior sliding surfaces of the kidney flexure, duodenum, spine and inferior vena cava

Rotatory forces operating at lower end of oesophagus

Upper part of stomach slides under and around the left lobe of the liver

Pylorus 'rolls' over the upper part of the duodenum and has a twisting/sliding articulation with the inferior surface of the liver

Stomach swings underneath the liver, coming anteriorly in an arc, with main pivot provided by lesser omentum

Figure 5.4   Alignment of the stomach and liver suspensory mechanisms.

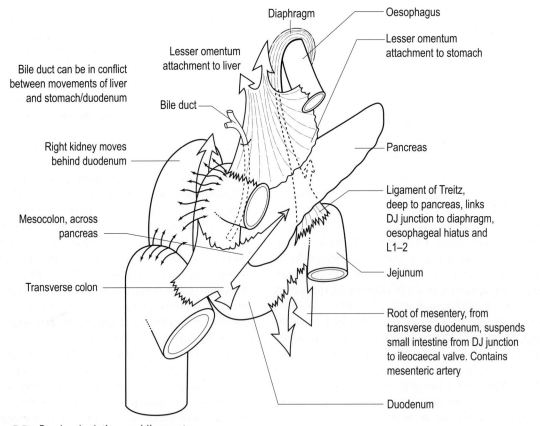

Diaphragm

Oesophagus

Lesser omentum attachment to liver

Lesser omentum attachment to stomach

Bile duct can be in conflict between movements of liver and stomach/duodenum

Bile duct

Pancreas

Right kidney moves behind duodenum

Ligament of Treitz, deep to pancreas, links DJ junction to diaphragm, oesophageal hiatus and L1–2

Mesocolon, across pancreas

Jejunum

Transverse colon

Root of mesentery, from transverse duodenum, suspends small intestine from DJ junction to ileocaecal valve. Contains mesenteric artery

Duodenum

Figure 5.5   Duodenal relations and ligaments.

The main movements of the duodenum are as follows.

- A hinging/swinging motion where the first part of the duodenum and the pylorus articulate against the immobile descending part of the duodenum.
- An elastic suppleness is required in the descending and transverse sections, to accommodate the motions of the lumbar spine and posterior abdominal wall.
- The descending section of the duodenum is influenced by the renal fascia posteriorly and the mesentery for the transverse colon anteriorly, which attaches to the anterior surface of the duodenum, just above the level of the sphincter of Oddi.
- A hinging/swinging motion of the last part of the duodenum, against the immobile transverse section, with the swinging influenced by the superior suspension provided by the ligament of Treitz to the posterior abdominal wall.
- Where the duodenum 'turns a corner' between the descending and transverse sections, this angle must be elastic and supple so as not to interfere with the transit of food, and duodenal peristaltic action.
- The transverse section of the duodenum is influenced by the 'root of the mesentery for the small intestine' (the jejunum and ileum), which attaches to the anterior surface of the transverse section of the duodenum.

LIVER, GALL BLADDER AND BILE DUCT

The peritoneal attachments of the liver are extensive and serve to hold the liver in a 'bag' suspended from the underneath surface of the diaphragm and anterior abdominal wall, and from which other organs are suspended. The weight of the liver is mostly taken by the relatively negative pressure acting across the diaphragm from the thoracic cavity. As can be seen from Figure 5.4, the attachments of the liver are continuous with those of the stomach and they contain the remnants of the umbilical vein (which eventually forms the ligamentum teres/round ligament of the liver) enclosed in the free border of the falciform ligament.

The ligaments which suspend the liver superiorly are the left and right triangular ligaments, the coronary ligaments and the falciform. These ligaments are continuous structures and labelling them as 'separate' structures misleads the reader about their interconnectedness. Indeed, there is ongoing debate about how these peritoneal structures should be labelled, with some authors suggesting the terms 'left triangular peritoneal attachment' of the liver and 'coronary peritoneal attachment' instead of 'left triangular ligament' and 'coronary ligament', for example.[3] Either way, the nomenclature is less important than the fact that the liver is globally suspended under the diaphragm, and any movements made affect all the 'ligaments' to some degree. The liver is also suspended by vascular pedicles, which limit the amount of possible movement. The hepatic veins pass from the posterior aspect of the liver to the inferior vena cava, anchoring the liver fairly firmly in place. This leads to much less movement than would be possible from the ligamentous attachments alone. The liver is also wrapped around the side and front of the lower dorsal spine, and this curvature lends a degree of immobility to the liver if surrounding tissues and the spine are tense and tight. The liver is essentially wedged under the right lobe of the diaphragm and against the lower dorsal spine. It is encompassed by the ribs, and has a slight rocking and rolling motion which is heavily influenced by the actions of the diaphragm.

The lesser omentum, which is also a continuation of the posterior coronary ligament, has been described above with the stomach. The falciform, which is an extension of the anterior coronary ligament, passes from the anterior surface of the liver and initially attaches to the inside of the diaphragm. Its upper part attaches to the superior part of the inside of the right rectus abdominis muscle, and its lower part to the linea alba, finally finishing at the level of the umbilicus. The falciform ligament is joined by the ligamentum teres, which is the obliterated umbilical vein. This runs in the free border of the falciform and connects the undersurface of the liver to the umbilicus. The right triangular ligament is continuous with the peritoneum that sweeps over the whole underside of the diaphragm and, as such, is continuous with the peritoneum that covers the hepatic flexure of the colon and the renal fascia over the right kidney.

As a result, some authors consider that the liver is attached to the colon via the hepatocolic ligament, and the kidney via the hepatorenal ligament. This relationship is sometimes absent and depends on whether the right triangular ligament extends inferiorly enough to enable a small section of peritoneum to pass in between the liver and the kidney or adrenal area or the hepatic flexure of the colon (the hepatocolic being far less frequently present). This does not mean that the hepatic flexure of the colon and the kidney are not mechanically related to the liver in all cases. Both, in fact, can block liver movement (posteroinferiorly) when they are tense and irritated and, of course, if the liver is restricted or tense this can influence these organs, as they are nestled directly underneath the posteroinferior surface of the liver (the liver has indentations in its underside for the flexure, the kidney and the angle of the duodenum).

The term 'hepatoduodenal' refers to the section of the lesser omentum that passes between the liver and the duodenum, and the hepatogastric ligament is the section of the lesser omentum between the liver and stomach. These relationships are illustrated in Figure 5.6.

The gall bladder is attached by a fibrous sling to the underneath of the liver, and the peritoneum that sweeps over the liver also wraps the gall bladder in its own separate fold. The bile duct, as stated before, is situated in the right-hand edge/free border of the lesser omentum, and this edge is often referred to as the hepatoduodenal ligament.

The main movements of the liver and gall bladder are as follows.

- When viewed from the front, the liver swings backwards and forwards in an arc that follows the curve of the right dome of the diaphragm.

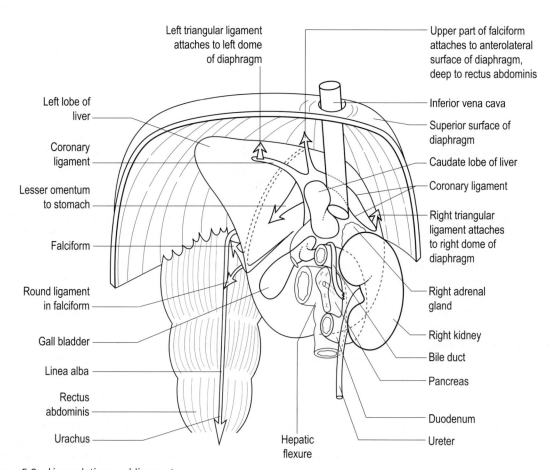

Figure 5.6   Liver relations and ligaments.

This means that the anterior inferior border rises superiorly and then drops inferiorly, whilst the posterior surface drops inferiorly and then rises superiorly as the liver rotates back again.

- This movement can be blocked at the back by stiffness or restriction in the hepatic flexure of the colon, the right kidney or the angle of the duodenum.
- The liver also moves in such a way that it can swing around the front of the spine and back again. When viewed from the front, this means that the right side of the liver moves anteriorly with the left lobe acting as a pivot.
- The liver can also drop to the right and rise up again. In other words, the right lobe of the liver can sink slightly inferiorly, resulting in the left lobe moving more to the midline, towards the right. This dropping motion is usually said to pivot around the falciform ligament attachments.
- All these movements are rocking, rotatory movements which follow the curves of the underside of the diaphragm and the front to the lower dorsal spine.
- The gall bladder does not move much against the underneath of the diaphragm and is hard to identify separately. However, it should be elastic and supple against the underneath of the liver. It generally moves with the liver.

SMALL INTESTINE

The rest of the small intestine, the jejunum and ileum are attached and supported by the 'root of the mesentery of the small intestine', which is usually known just as the root of the mesentery. The root of the mesentery commences at the ligament of Treitz and ends at the level of the ileocaecal valve. It traverses the transverse section of the duodenum and therefore indirectly attaches to the front of the third lumbar vertebra (thereby linking the spine with the mechanics of the small intestine).

The ileocaecal valve is an interesting structure. It is not a proper sphincter but definitely acts as a gateway between the small and large intestines. The valve is formed by an invagination of the ileum into the caecum, as though the ileum pokes into

the caecum slightly, creating two 'lips' or flaps. These can effectively open or close, depending on the contractile activities of the caecum, the peristaltic waves of the terminal ileum, and tension or torsion in the root of the mesentery/adjacent peritoneum.

Interestingly, the caecum is rather like the stomach, in that the peristaltic waves in the caecum are quite 'ruminatory' – like those in the stomach, they churn the food into all sorts of directions, mixing it thoroughly. The ileum is to the caecum as the oesophagus is to the stomach, therefore gastro-oesophageal reflux (and all its attendant problems) is mirrored by an incompetent ileocaecal valve, giving a type of ileocaecal reflux which has accompanying pain, discomfort and irritation to the digestive tissues and therefore function in the affected area. One way in which this reflux causes irritation is to allow bacterial flora from the colon to colonize the small intestine, which is normally sterile of those organisms. This creates a lot of irritation and disturbance to local digestive function. Mechanical factors maintained by the caecum or terminal ileum and the external anatomy of the surrounding peritoneum contribute to competence at the ileocaecal valve/junction.[4]

The root of the mesentery is attached to the renal fascia either side, and to the fascia over the lumbar spine structures such as the aorta, inferior vena cava, autonomic plexi and ganglia and various nerves of the lumbar plexus. It allows the long length of the small intestine to be 'gathered together' and attached across a relatively small section of the posterior abdominal wall. The mesentery allows the gut to 'cascade' down towards the pelvic bowl, and the whole mesentery can be 'flapped' backwards and forwards or turned over like a page in a book. This, of course, does not happen in real life; normally the mesentery simply hangs freely downwards and this freedom allows the peristaltic waves to pass unhindered.

The coils of the small intestine are free to wriggle about and are quite sinuous in mobility. The coils will ride around alongside and in between each other, and will wriggle and slither over and between the tops of the pelvic organs such as the rectum, uterus (where present) and bladder. As the small intestine itself is very soft and long, it is not possible to physically palpate each and every centimetre in turn along the full length of the jejunum and ileum. The small intestine coils are treated as one organ en masse (rather like a heavy brocade curtain hanging from the mesentery) and the mesentery itself is treated as a separate organ, which is much more easily felt, examined and treated.

The root of the mesentery contains the superior mesenteric artery and vein, and various lymphatic vessels and nerves. It effectively controls the nutrition to the gut tube and the initial drainage of absorbed products back to the rest of the body's systems. Any tension in the root of the mesentery will affect vascular function to the gut tube, and blood and lymph drainage from it. As mentioned previously, there are also many tension receptors within the mesentery, helping the central nervous system to monitor food transit, and torsion within the gut and mesentery. Therefore any tension, irritation and contraction or immobility within the mesentery will affect the body both mechanically and reflexly.

The relations of the root of the mesentery are shown in Figure 5.7.

The main movements of the small intestine are as follows.

- Individual wriggling and sinuous movements that cannot be individually palpated but can be observed on real-time MRI studies.
- Global general articulation between the lower aspects of the coils of the small intestine and the pelvic organs such as the top of the bladder, the sigmoid, the rectum and the top of the broad ligament and uterus, where present.
- A generalized subtle swinging from side to side as the coils of the intestine hang and 'waft' below the root of the mesentery.
- The coils of the small intestine should not be adhesed onto the pelvic organs or structures, and it should be possible to 'scoop'

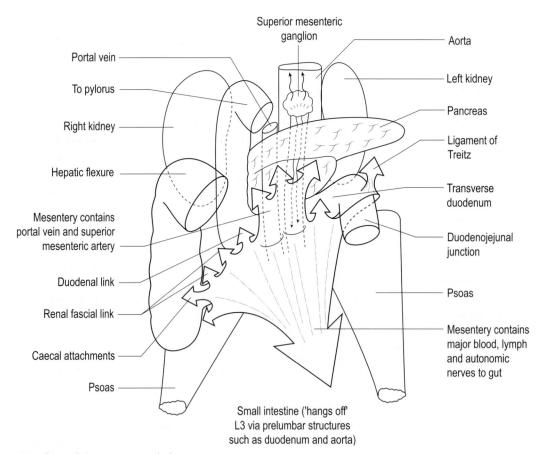

Figure 5.7   Root of the mesentery relations.

them up out of the pelvic bowl towards the head. The root of the mesentery should be relatively soft and pliable, and the global mass of the small intestine should not be tense, hard or particularly resistant to global mobilization.

LARGE INTESTINE

The colon has extensive peritoneal attachments and reflections, which are indicated in Figure 5.8. From Figure 5.4, it can be seen that the colon is wrapped in large sheets of peritoneum that then get 'flattened' against the posterior abdominal wall, 'trapping' various sections (the ascending and descending colon and the rectum) against the posterior abdominal wall. The flattened peritoneal layers adhere to the posterior abdominal wall and in this position become labelled as Toldt's fascia.

This gives three fixed sections of the colon, the ascending and descending colons and the rectum, and three mobile sections, the caecum, the transverse colon and the sigmoid colon. Of these, the caecum is the least mobile. The ascending colon is attached to the renal fascia and the iliopsoas muscle posteriorly and inferiorly, and medially

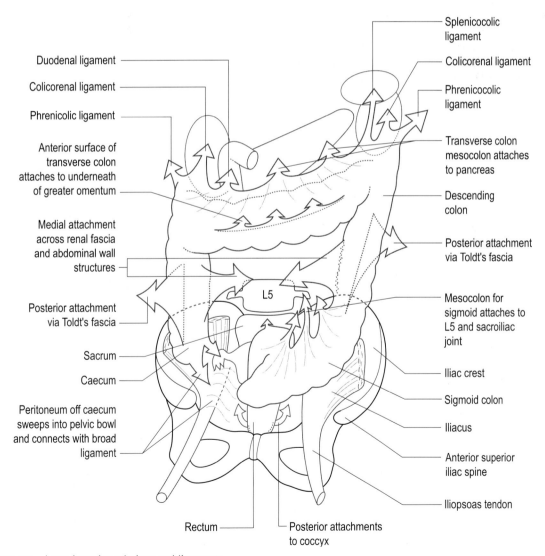

Figure 5.8 Large intestine relations and ligaments.

the peritoneum sweeps off the colon into the paracolic gutter and over the descending part of the duodenum. Superiorly, the peritoneum sweeps up onto the diaphragm, sometimes passing up onto the back of the liver or to the gall bladder (cystoduodenal ligament, spreading mainly between the gall bladder and duodenum when present). The descending colon is similarly attached posteriorly to the renal fascia and the iliopsoas muscle inferiorly. Superiorly, the peritoneum sweeps off onto the diaphragm and also to the spleen. Medially, the peritoneum passes into the left paracolic gutter and then onto the pancreas and terminal part of the duodenum. The rectum is attached posteriorly to the sacrum, and the anal sphincter is attached via the anococcygeal raphe to the coccyx posteriorly and the perineal body anteriorly.

The sigmoid is suspended by the mesocolon for the sigmoid, which is reflected on the posterior abdominal wall in an inverted V-shape. The apex of this V lies around the left lumbosacral joint, and one side of the V passes in front of the left sacroiliac joint to the iliac fossa, and the other passes from the lumbosacral region to the front of the sacrum, to meet the rectal attachments. The mesocolon for the transverse (colon) attaches to (but can be separated from) the undersurface of the greater omentum just below the greater curvature of the stomach. Its reflection on the posterior abdominal wall forms a line along the length of the pancreas; effectively, the transverse colon hangs off the pancreas. The mesocolon for the transverse starts at the hepatic flexure and finishes at the splenic flexure, where it terminates in the phrenicocolic ligament. As it passes from side to side, it also hangs off the right and left renal fascia, where exposed.

The phrenicocolic ligament acts somewhat like the ligament of Treitz does for the terminal part of the duodenum. It provides a superior suspensory mechanism and can help the splenic flexure form a sort of 'spiralling gateway' to the descending colon.[2] The phrenicocolic ligament on the right is much less commonly referred to in standard anatomy texts, but the peritoneum that sweeps from the top of the hepatic flexure onto the undersurface of the diaphragm is considered by osteopaths to have similar suspensory effects to the splenic phrenicocolic ligament. Hence the right phrenicocolic ligament is often referred to in relevant osteopathic texts.[5]

The main movements of the large intestine are as follows.

- The ascending and descending colons must remain elastic and flexible along their fixed length. They should be able to be rolled slightly from side to side, and not resist some degree of twisting or torsion along their lengths.
- The hepatic and splenic flexures act like hinges and either end of the transverse colon should swing slightly from side to side, against the fixed sections of the ascending or descending colons.
- The hepatic flexure can be compressed from above by the liver.
- The splenic flexure is less affected by the spleen but does have a reciprocal relationship with it.
- The caecum should swing slightly from side to side on its very short mesentery, and it should be possible to 'scoop' it out of the right iliac fossa slightly.
- The sigmoid colon should swing reasonably well from side to side as it has a longer mesentery than the caecum; it should articulate over the pubis and bladder (and usually the uterus as well, when present) and it should be possible to 'scoop' it out of the left iliac fossa and pelvic bowl.
- The transverse colon is quite mobile where it hangs down between the two flexures. As it is attached to the greater curvature of the stomach, these two organs are mechanically linked. However, as the position of the greater curvature and the transverse can be very variable, it is only specifically examined at the level of the two flexures. The rest of the transverse is considered as part of the general abdominal visceral mass, and is treated as part of a global technique (like the mass of the coils of the jejunum and ileum).

MOTILITY

Please refer to the appendix for illustrations of the motility patterns for the gastrointestinal tract. The motility can be affected by tensions in any of the ligaments described above; by smooth muscle tension, and tissue irritation within the organs themselves; or indirectly from somatic relations which are biomechanically affected or irritated.

> Many of the techniques described at the end of this chapter can be used as palpating contacts to evaluate the motility of the organ concerned.

REFLEX RELATIONSHIPS

Table 5.2 shows reflex relationships for the gastrointestinal tract. The somatic level or relationship indicates those parts of the musculoskeletal system that can be worked on to influence the

neural tissues related to that section of the gut. Note: these should be examined, and treated only if found to be mechanically disturbed in some way. Work to these areas when they are not expressing any sort of somatic dysfunction will not influence neural activity.

VEINS, ARTERIES AND LYMPHATICS

Table 5.3 shows the major blood and lymph vessels for the gastrointestinal tract. It is important to consider the visceral ligaments and fascial conduits that contain the blood vessels, as work on

Table 5.2   Reflex relationships for the gastrointestinal system

Organ	Anatomical name	Somatic level/relationship
Oesophagus		
Sympathetic – spinal cord	Upper oesophagus served via the recurrent laryngeal nerve from the cervical ganglia; lower two-thirds by direct fibres	T1–6
Sympathetic – paravertebral chain ganglia	Mostly direct fibres in thoracic region	Ribs 1–7
Sympathetic – plexus	NA	
Parasympathetic	Vagus	Upper cervical spine (left>right)
Stomach		
Sympathetic – spinal cord	T5–9	T5–9 (L)
Sympathetic – paravertebral chain ganglia	Greater splanchnics	Ribs 6–10
Sympathetic – plexus	Coeliac plexus	Anterior to T12–L1
Parasympathetic	Vagus (left and right gastric nerves). The left vagus serves the greater curvature and the right vagus serves the lesser curvature	Upper cervical spine (left>right)
Duodenum		
Sympathetic – spinal cord	T5–9	T5–9 bilaterally
Sympathetic – paravertebral chain ganglia	Greater splanchnics	Ribs 6–10
Sympathetic – plexus	Coeliac plexus	Anterior to T12–L1
Parasympathetic	Right and left vagus	Upper cervical spine (left>right)
Pancreas		
Sympathetic – spinal cord	(T5–9, but especially T7)	T5–9
Sympathetic – paravertebral chain ganglia	Greater splanchnics	Ribs 5–9
Sympathetic – plexus	Coeliac	Dorsolumbar spine
Parasympathetic	Left vagus	Upper cervical spine (left>right)

Continued

Table 5.2 Reflex relationships for the gastrointestinal system—cont'd

Organ	Anatomical name	Somatic level/relationship
Liver		
Sympathetic – spinal cord	T5–9, but especially T5	T5–9
Sympathetic – paravertebral chain ganglia	Greater splanchnics	Ribs 5–9 (right>left)
Sympathetic – plexus	Hepatic plexus, which is an extension of the coeliac plexus (around coeliac trunk)	Dorsolumbar junction
Parasympathetic	Anterior gastric (branch of right vagus) goes to hepatic plexus. Travels in lesser omentum	Upper cervical spine (left>right)
Gall bladder and bile duct		
Sympathetic – spinal cord	Around T7–9 but especially T6	T7–9
Sympathetic – paravertebral chain ganglia	Greater splanchnics	Ribs 6–9 (right>left)
Sympathetic – plexus	From the coeliac plexus	Dorsolumbar spine
Parasympathetic	Right and left vagus, joining in with coeliac plexus	Upper cervical spine (left>right)
Small intestine		
Sympathetic – spinal cord	T9–10	T9–10
Sympathetic – paravertebral chain ganglia	Lesser splanchnics	Ribs 9–11
Sympathetic – plexus	Superior mesenteric	Upper lumbar spine
Parasympathetic	Right vagus	Upper cervical spine (left>right)
Large intestine		
Sympathetic – spinal cord	T10–L2	T10–L2
Sympathetic – paravertebral chain ganglia	Least splanchnics, lumbar splanchnics	Ribs 10–12
Sympathetic – plexus	Superior mesenteric plexus for ascending colon and inferior mesenteric for descending colon	Mid and upper lumbar spine, and psoas muscles
Parasympathetic	Right vagus to the left colic flexure, and then the pelvic parasympathetics from S2–4	Upper cervical spine (left>right), then sacrum, sacroiliacs and coccyx
Rectum		
Sympathetic – spinal cord	L1–2	L1–2
Sympathetic – paravertebral chain ganglia	Lumbar splanchnics	Psoas muscles
Sympathetic – plexus	Superior hypogastric	Prevertebral fascia
Parasympathetic	Pelvic parasympathetics (pelvic splanchnics) from S2–4	Sacrum, sacroiliacs and coccyx

those structures will influence venous drainage, blood flow (as ligamentous torsion may affect the arteries/arterioles and the sympathetic nerves that course along their length) and lymphatic drainage, all of which are important for organ health. The somatic relations also indicate where the musculoskeletal system may be engaged to aid fluid movement in the structures concerned.

CIRCULATORY ISSUES

As with all tissue, vascular supply and drainage is very important for gut function. Although the gut is a large organ and has many blood vessels serving it, they essentially all originate from three main trunks or stems, which arise from the blood supply to the developing gut in the embryo. The embryological foregut is served by the coeliac

Table 5.3   Blood and lymph vessels

Organ	Anatomical name	Mesenteric or peritoneal ligament relation, where applicable	Somatic relation, where applicable
Oesophagus			
Veins	Azygos system of veins and the portal system (linking systemic and portal venous systems)	Lesser omentum	Prevertebral fascia
Arteries	Lower oesophagus supplied by the coeliac and left gastric arteries and the abdominal aorta	Lesser omentum, or direct	Median arcuate ligament of diaphragm (for aorta) and oesophageal hiatus
	The upper oesophagus is supplied by by the inferior thyroid artery and the descending thoracic aorta	Cervical fascia	Sternum is important for upper oesophagus
Lymphatics	Posterior mediastinal nodes draining to the thoracic duct	Thoracic trunk and dorsal prevertebral fascia	Prevertebral fascia and the anterior longitudinal ligament
Stomach			
Veins	Hepatic and portal veins	The splenic and superior mesenteric veins unite behind the neck of the pancreas, in the root of the small intestine	The upper lumbar spine mechanics are important for movement in this section of the root of the mesentery
Arteries	Coeliac trunk and branches. The left and right gastric run along the lesser curvature	Lesser omentum	Diaphragmatic, subcostal and upper gastrointestinal tract mechanics
	The right and left gastroepiploic run along the greater curvature (the left coming from the splenic artery, the right from the gastrohepatic artery)	Greater omentum and gastrosplenic ligament	Diaphragmatic, subcostal and upper gastrointestinal tract mechanics
Lymphatics	The fundus and upper half of the left stomach drain to the gastroomental nodes, then to the splenic nodes, and then to the coeliac nodes	Greater omentum and gastrosplenic ligament	Diaphragmatic, subcostal and upper gastrointestinal tract mechanics
	The lower part of the left stomach nodes along the greater curvature and pylorus, and then to the coeliac nodes	Greater omentum and lesser omentum	Diaphragmatic, subcostal and upper gastrointestinal tract mechanics
	The right part of the stomach	Lesser omentum (many ulcers and inflammatory problems in the stomach are sited along the lesser curvature)	Diaphragmatic, subcostal and upper gastrointestinal tract mechanics
Duodenum			
Veins	Pancreaticoduodenal veins join the superior mesenteric and the splenic to form the portal vein	Lesser omentum	Diaphragmatic, subcostal and upper gastrointestinal tract mechanics

Continued

Table 5.3   Blood and lymph vessels—cont'd

Organ	Anatomical name	Mesenteric or peritoneal ligament relation, where applicable	Somatic relation, where applicable
Arteries	From foregut and midgut arteries: the upper duodenum is supplied by the gastroduodenal and the superior pancreaticoduodenal (from the coeliac trunk) and the lower part by the inferior pancreaticoduodenal, from the superior mesenteric artery	Lesser omentum and posterior abdominal wall fascias	Diaphragmatic, subcostal and upper gastrointestinal tract mechanics
Lymphatics	Nodes between the head of the pancreas and the duodenum, passing to pre-aortic nodes near the superior mesenteric artery	Lesser omentum and posterior abdominal wall fascias	Dorsolumbar junction
Pancreas			
Veins	Pancreaticoduodenal veins, draining to the portal vein	Posterior abdominal wall, root of mesentery and mesocolon for the transverse colon	Upper gastrointestinal tract visceral dynamics are important
Arteries	To the head: the superior and inferior pancreaticoduodenal arteries; to the neck, body and tail: the splenic artery	Posterior abdominal wall, root of mesentery and mesocolon for the transverse colon	Upper gastrointestinal tract visceral dynamics are important
Lymphatics	Pancreatic nodes, and superior mesenteric nodes	Posterior abdominal wall, root of mesentery and mesocolon for the transverse colon	Upper lumbar spine
Liver			
Veins	Hepatic veins, going to inferior vena cava	No ligament: form vascular pedicle for liver	Spine and inferior vena cava are 'wrapped' up by the right lobe of the liver, with the hepatic veins being very short
Arteries	Hepatic artery, which comes from the common hepatic artery, which is a branch of the coeliac trunk	Lesser omentum, to porta hepatis	Upper lumbar and subdiaphragmatic mechanics are important
	'Portal vein' – included on the arterial side, as flow is towards the liver	Lesser omentum, to porta hepatis	Upper lumbar spine, where portal vein emerges from root of mesentery (attached to lumbar region) and goes to lesser omentum
Lymphatics	Diaphragmatic surface of liver drains through diaphragm and goes into thoracic duct	Subdiaphragmatic tissues and arcuate ligaments of diaphragm	Diaphragm, and associated articulations are important
	Deep lymphatics go to nodes near diaphragm or near aorta and coeliac trunk	Subdiaphragmatic tissues and arcuate ligaments of diaphragm	Lower dorsal articulations are important
Gall bladder			
Veins	Pass directly into the liver and the portal vein	Lesser omentum	Lower ribcage and diaphragm mechanics are important

Continued

Table 5.3 Blood and lymph vessels—cont'd

Organ	Anatomical name	Mesenteric or peritoneal ligament relation, where applicable	Somatic relation, where applicable
Arteries	From the cystic artery, coming from the right hepatic artery	Liver ligaments and peritoneal relations	Lower ribcage and diaphragm mechanics are important
Lymphatics	Hepatic nodes, near the porta hepatis	Subdiaphragmatic tissues and arcuate ligaments of diaphragm	Lower dorsal articulations are important
Bile duct			
Veins	Pass directly into the liver and the portal vein	Hepatoduodenal ligament	Lower ribcage and diaphragm mechanics are important
Arteries	Cystic artery, from the right hepatic artery	Hepatoduodenal ligament	Lesser omentum and liver/subcostal mechanics are important
Lymphatics	Hepatic nodes	Subdiaphragmatic tissues and arcuate ligaments of diaphragm	Lesser omentum and liver/subcostal mechanics are important
Small intestine			
Veins	Superior mesenteric vein	Mesocolon, Toldt's fascia, and root of mesentery	Right and left paracolic gutters
Arteries	Superior mesenteric artery and its branches (jejunal, ileal, pancreaticoduodenal)	Mesocolon, Toldt's fascia, and root of mesentery	Right and left paracolic gutters
Lymphatics	Mesenteric nodes		Mid lumbar spine
Large intestine			
Veins	Superior mesenteric vein, to the left colic (splenic) flexure, and the inferior mesenteric below	Mesocolon, Toldt's fascia, and root of mesentery	Right and left paracolic gutters
Arteries	Superior mesenteric artery branches (caecal, middle colic and right colic), to the left colic flexure, and the inferior mesenteric below	Mesocolon, Toldt's fascia, and root of mesentery	Right and left paracolic gutters
Lymphatics	Mesenteric nodes	Posterior abdominal wall fascias	Posterior abdominal wall fascias
Rectum			
Veins	Superior rectal vein, to the inferior mesenteric vein, the middle rectal vein to the internal iliac vein and the inferior rectal vein via the internal pudendal vein	Pelvic fascia	Sacrum and ischiorectal fossa
Arteries	Superior rectal artery, middle rectal artery and inferior rectal artery	Pelvic fascia	Sacrum and ischiorectal fossa
Lymphatics	Nodes near the inferior mesenteric artery, and the internal iliac nodes	Pelvic fascia	Pelvic fascia and pelvic floor mechanics are important

artery, the midgut by the superior mesenteric artery and the hindgut by the inferior mesenteric artery. All the blood vessels to the gut pass through the remnants of the dorsal and ventral mesenteries and as such, become 'plastered' against the posterior abdominal wall, 'trapped' between various visceral or somatic structures or pass through peritoneal mesenteries to reach their target organ. Hence, global peritoneal elasticity and suppleness are very important for circulatory issues. Chapter 8 considers circulatory issues in more depth.

The root of the mesentery is vitally important for the superior mesenteric artery, as is Toldt's fascia for the inferior mesenteric arteries, and the dorsolumbar junction and the median arcuate ligament for the coeliac trunk. This latter can also be accessed from the front by passing 'through' the lesser omentum in the midline epigastric region. Figure 5.9 shows the main arteries to the gut.

Figure 5.10 shows the main venous and lymphatic vessels of the abdomen.

SOMATIC AND VISCERAL INTERACTIONS

The abdominal cavity, and therefore the gastrointestinal tract, are influenced by whole-body biomechanical disturbances, as discussed earlier when posture and visceral support were reviewed. Unlike the thorax, there are fewer specific viscerosomatic mechanical relationships that are important for

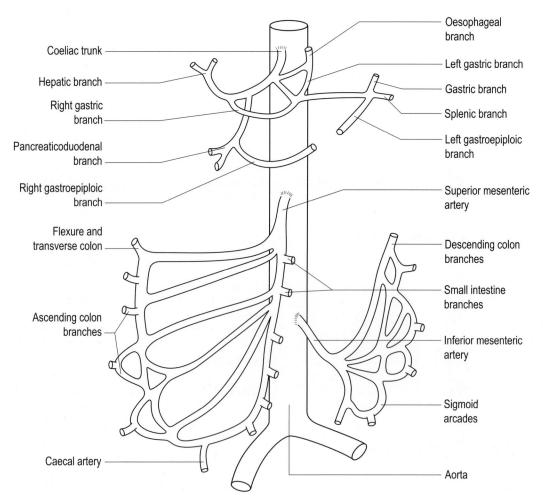

Figure 5.9   Coeliac and mesenteric branches.

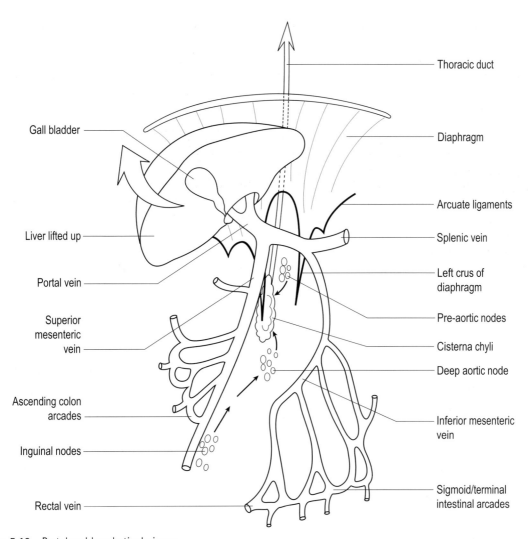

Gall bladder

Liver lifted up

Portal vein

Superior
mesenteric
vein

Ascending colon
arcades

Inguinal nodes

Rectal vein

Thoracic duct

Diaphragm

Arcuate ligaments

Splenic vein

Left crus of
diaphragm

Pre-aortic nodes

Cisterna chyli

Deep aortic node

Inferior mesenteric
vein

Sigmoid/terminal
intestinal arcades

Figure 5.10   Portal and lymphatic drainage.

visceral function, beyond general visceral support, the general moving of the diaphragms and
the integration of the spinal column and the posterior abdominal wall. Generalized peritoneal
'bag' concepts, which are strongly relevant, were
also introduced previously (see Chapter 3).

EXAMINATION AND TREATMENT OF THE GASTROINTESTINAL TRACT

GENERAL PERITONEAL TECHNIQUES

These were introduced in Chapter 3.

TECHNIQUES FOR THE GREATER OMENTUM

The greater omentum is a unique organ, having
many functions, including immune functions,
friction buffering, healing and wound repair, and
other biochemical attributes.[6] It is a very mobile
structure and moves around the abdomen (using
chemoattraction), searching for irritated, infected
or otherwise compromised tissues. The omentum
can then isolate the area by forming adhesions all
around – so 'glueing' itself over the affected part.
It can then promote healing, detach itself and
move on to another area.

As a result of all this movement, adhesion formation and resorption, the greater omentum may be found stretched or 'tucked' into varied sites or around various organs, depending on the individual. It is usually found hanging between the anterior abdominal wall and the mass of the small intestines, as shown in Figure 5.11.

Figure 5.12 shows a general anterior abdominal contact, where the practitioner will feel 'through' the anterior abdominal wall, through the parietal peritoneum and into the peritoneal cavity, just deep to the peritoneum. The greater omentum is the first structure that is felt as the contact passes into the abdominal cavity. Listening and unwinding techniques are best applied. There can be confusion when palpating the greater omentum, as it is very soft and can easily be overlooked. It is necessary to descend 'through the layers' very carefully or else the omentum may be missed. The greater omentum passes from the greater curvature of the stomach and hangs down over the transverse colon, where it is attached to the mesocolon. This makes a good landmark; if the flexures of the colon are identified and followed medially, then the transverse colon can be identified, which gives a landmark for the upper sections of the greater omentum. If the omentum is adhesed, then gentle traction and stretching techniques can be applied, as can recoil techniques.

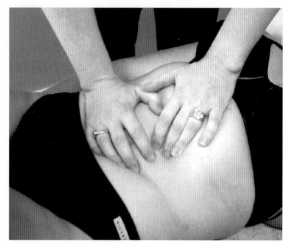

Figure 5.12 Greater omentum contact.

TECHNIQUES FOR THE COLON

The most accessible places to palpate the colon are the ascending and descending colons, which are fixed either side of the abdomen, lateral to the midclavicular lines, to the renal fascia and iliopsoas, by Toldt's fascia. These sections of the colon palpate a little like rubbery tubes, and they can easily be mobilized by a number of techniques.

Figure 5.13 shows a general technique for mobilizing the ascending colon, which involves a

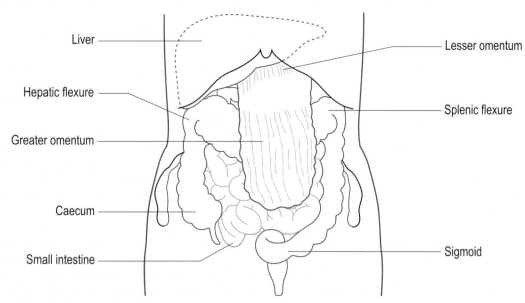

Figure 5.11 Greater omentum

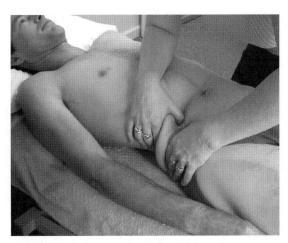

Figure 5.13   Ascending colon.

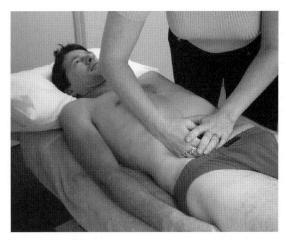

Figure 5.14   Caecum.

torsioning movement applied along the length of the tube. The thumbs do not pass any more medially than the midclavicular line and are palpating into the paracolic gutter. The fingers are wrapping gently around the lateral abdomen, thereby covering the bulk of the ascending colon. The fingers can feel into the soft space between the lower ribs and the iliac crest. If further leverage is required, then the ulnar borders of the hand or palm can contact onto these bony parts and twist the lateral trunk and the colon all together. The actual range of motion involved is small and the fingers can freely palpate and monitor any tension within the gut tube. The colon can also be stretched longitudinally; inhibition can be used, as can functional or indirect unwinding techniques. The contact can also be applied on the left, for the descending colon. Note that this has a slightly narrower diameter and is sometimes partly covered by coils of the small intestine, which should be moved aside before commencing the technique (by applying some lateral-to-medial scooping movements, for example). This technique can also combine a non-specific release of the renal fascia and quadratus lumborum with that of the colon.

A number of visceral restrictions are often found at the ileocaecal valve and caecum. These are commonly associated with right sacroiliac joint problems. Figure 5.14 shows a general contact to scoop the caecum away from or out of the right iliac fossa. Note that the caecum is usually found on or above the level of the anterior superior iliac spine (ASIS) on the right (whereas the sigmoid is found

at the ASIS or lower on the left). This technique relies on gaining sufficient skin slack, before attempting to cup around the inferior border of the caecum (or sigmoid, if applied to the left iliac fossa). The skin is slightly eased towards the hip area and when the fingers reach the inferior margin of the fossa, near the inguinal canal, they can now gently start to ease downwards (towards the table) in order to pass deep to the colon. Now, maintaining this depth and the skin slack gathered at the beginning, the fingers/hands can gently raise or scoop the caecum away from the hip area and out of the iliac fossa. One hand can palpate and one hand can cover over this and be the motor or active hand, if required. The patient's knee can be raised and, if desired, the practitioner can perform the technique with one hand, whilst the other supports the patient's knee, using it as a lever to gently move the hip and pelvis, to aid the technique within the iliac fossa. The caecum is more mobile than the ascending or descending colons but not as mobile as the sigmoid. This technique applied on the left for the sigmoid requires the hands to cup along the superior pubic arch, as the sigmoid usually reaches as low as the pubis and often crosses the midline to the right, before turning back to form the rectum.

Figure 5.15 shows a sidelying contact for the ascending colon. This is useful when a combined release with the posterior abdominal wall muscles and the lumbar spine is required. It is also useful as articulation and treatment to the dorsal and lumbar regions can be given, followed by visceral

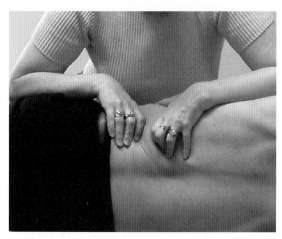

Figure 5.15 Sidelying colon.

work to the colon, without having to move the patient. The practitioner's cephalad hand can reinforce a contact with the lower ribs and work on the superior attachments of Toldt's fascia and indirectly stretch the phrenicocolic ligament. The caudal hand can either ease away the pelvis, for more indirect stretch, or 'hold back' on the lower part of the colon, for added focus. Remember that the colon is no more posterior than the midaxillary line and any contact onto the mass of the lumbar erector spinae will have moved off the colon.

Figure 5.16 shows a contact for the hepatic flexure, where the practitioner is attempting to gain access to the inside angle of the colon. The medial

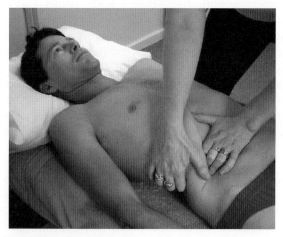

Figure 5.16 Hepatic flexure.

border of the ascending colon can be located (by rolling from lateral to medial over the ascending colon 'tube') and once the medial border is found, the practitioner can feel in the sulcus (paracolic gutter) immediately medial to the colon. If the practitioner 'walks' up the sulcus (remaining lateral to the descending part of the duodenum) and gently eases away any other intestinal mass that lies superficially in this region, they will arrive in the angle between the ascending colon and the transverse colon. With the hand in the position shown, the practitioner's palm and fingers will be covering the beginning of the transverse colon and the pylorus. The other hand is shown supporting the lower right ribcage, with a fairly lateral contact. This is to create some tissue slack in the subcostal region, to enable sufficient depth for the practitioner to palpate into the inside angle of the hepatic flexure. If the practitioner now moves the abdominal hand medially in a small arc (slightly scooping towards the left chest) the transverse colon will be slightly swung away from the ascending colon. There is no need to stabilize the ascending colon, as it is firmly attached along its length by Toldt's fascia. This swinging/scooping motion will open out the hepatic flexure from the inside, and allow relaxation and mobilization of this section of the gut tube.

The angles are frequently irritated because of their mechanical arrangement (mobile area next to a fixed area). In the case of the hepatic flexure, pressure and irritation from the liver can compromise colonic function and using this technique, the hand contacting the ribcage can combine an indirect mobilization of the liver (via the ribcage) as part of the technique if desired.

This basic type of contact, with a few modifications, can also be used to release the phrenicocolic ligament, which suspends the hepatic flexure to the underneath of the diaphragm. Firstly, the lateral border of the ascending colon is followed until the costal margin is reached. The aim now is to cup over the top of the hepatic flexure, and not the inside of the angle. Using the rib contact, sufficient slack should be created to ease underneath the costal margin, between the liver and the top of the hepatic flexure. Once this has been achieved (sometimes with the aid of a little gentle rocking of the rib contact, to coax tissue relaxation in the region), the abdominal hand can be rotated to face inferiorly. If the practitioner applies a caudal stretch from this point, the tissues superior to the hepatic flexure will be engaged, including the phrenicocolic ligament.

It is important to remember with these two techniques that if the practitioner has the basic point of contact medial to the midclavicular line, then the duodenal/pyloric angle will be worked on, either as a hinge using the first technique or a stretch to the hepatoduodenal ligament using the second technique.

The hinge technique described above for the hepatic flexure can be used for the splenic, but it is not possible to reach right into the inside of the angle between the descending colon and the transverse colon, as this is too deeply located under the ribcage. The principles of the technique are the same, however. The practitioner 'walks' up the medial border of the descending colon, as far as possible, and then scoops medially the intestines and tissues located under the palm, at this point. The transverse colon will be included in this mass and so an indirect opening of the splenic flexure will be created. The ribcage contact can be used to mobilize the flexure via the ribs, which will increase the efficacy of the technique. Work can be applied to the flexures of the colon using the sitting position which is sometimes more effective for the splenic flexure.

The splenic flexure effectively hangs off the inside of ribs 8–10 and the hepatic flexure hangs off the inside of ribs 10 and 11. The mechanics of these ribs can be affected, creating spinal restrictions in the lower dorsal spine as a result of mechanical links to the colon. This gives a mechanical link to the spine that is slightly higher than the neural reflex one (for the large intestine as a whole, which links to the T10–L2 region).

Figure 5.17 shows part of the contact for the sitting release of the splenic flexure. This posterior contact is the same for techniques that also release the stomach and the spleen. The anterior contact for this series of techniques is shown in Figure 5.25. That image shows the release of the stomach but the release of the splenic flexure is similar. The posterior arm passes around the back of the lower ribcage. The spleen and splenic flexure are found approximately at ribs 8–10, lateral to the rib angles and posterior to the midaxillary line. The practitioner is using the posterior arm to support the patient.

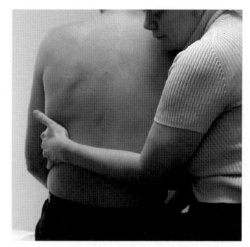

Figure 5.17 Posterior hand and forearm contact for stomach, spleen and splenic flexure.

It is best to have the patient slightly leaning against the practitioner, so that a global movement and support of the trunk can be achieved using slight practitioner body movements and adjustments with the rib contact. Moving the patient in a side-to-side direction will begin to create some slack in the subcostal region and the anterior hand contact can now be commenced. The anterior hand will contact under the left costal margin. For the splenic flexure, the palpating part of the contact should be lateral to the midclavicular line. The palm can lie flat against the rest of the abdomen, which usually makes things more comfortable for the patient and allows the practitioner to gently move the general visceral mass laterally, to help create slack for the palpating part of the hand (usually the fingers). With the fingers under the costal margin, it is important to remember that they must be kept relaxed at all times, as digital tension will be uncomfortable and block the technique. With the basic contact in place, the patient can be gently moved from side to side, and as the patient is moved towards the practitioner, the abdominal hand will emphasize an 'opening' out of the splenic flexure, by cupping the intestines medially. Sometimes applying a slight inferior drag to the subcostal tissues will engage the transverse colon nearer the flexure and improve the technique. The patient can be moved slightly into rotation, sideshifting, a little compression or traction, depending on the individual tissue barriers noted. These accessory

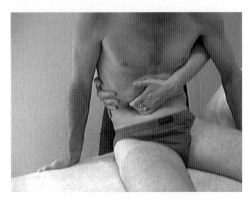

Figure 5.18 Anterior hand contact for hepatic flexure.

movements are best created using the posterior arm contact on the ribcage (which is why a broad, solid contact here is required). Figure 5.18 shows the anterior hand contact for this technique when applied on the right, for the hepatic flexure.

Figure 5.19 shows a contact for the terminal root of the mesentery and the ileocaecal valve area of the ascending colon. Although the ileocaecal valve is not a true sphincter, the arrangement of tissues at this point creates a sphincter-like action, and regulation of food transit between the small and large intestines is a very important function for the ileocaecal valve. The valve is actually created by a small invagination of the ileum into the caecum (like beginning to turn the sleeve of a jacket inside out at the level of the shoulder. Where the sleeve is slightly pulled inwards, this creates a

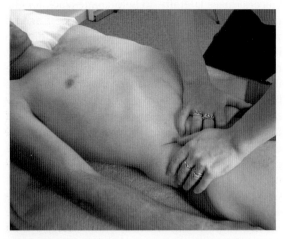

Figure 5.19 Terminal root of mesentery and ileocaecal valve.

fold of sleeve that protrudes inside the jacket). The turned-in sections of ileum can lie flat against each other, rather like a pair of lips, and can be referred to as being 'opened' or 'closed'. Tensions in the caecum, ileum or fascia attaching to these sections of the gut can create torsion and dysfunction at the level of the valve. The lower part of Toldt's fascia binds the caecum to the iliopsoas in the iliac fossa and the terminal part of the root of the mesentery for the small intestine attaches the terminal ileum to the renal fascia, psoas and anterior lumbar spine structures, in the right iliac region.

Parietal peritoneal extensions that sweep off the caecum laterally, inferiorly and medially can also create tension in the ileocaecal valve area. Inferior-medial extensions of the peritoneum that sweeps off the caecum will pass into the lateral pelvic bowl. Here they can blend with the broad ligament (especially the posterior layer) and with the ovarian ligaments. Scarring from appendix operations can interfere with the uterine and ovarian ligaments and tissues, and adhesions from ovarian or fallopian tube problems can pass superolaterally towards the lower caecum peritoneal attachments, creating tension at the ileocaecal valve, for example.

To relax tissue in the ileocaecal area, the practitioner can palpate with one hand onto the viscera and use the other onto the iliac crest, to create tissue slack and also to utilize pelvic movements to aid the technique indirectly. The abdominal hand cups over the organs of the lower abdomen and gently eases them towards the right iliac fossa, to create slack. Once slack is created (taking care not to push the palm of the hand onto the front of the lumbar spine), the palpating fingers can ease into the abdomen, to create a contact close to the posterior abdominal wall, at the level of the root of the mesentery and the iliopsoas muscle. Maintaining this contact and depth, the palpating hand can then very gently stretch the tissue towards the patient's left costal margin, thereby stretching the terminal ileum, the ileocaecal valve and the supporting peritoneum/fascia. The exact direction of stretch or mobilization can vary, depending on the exact pattern of tensions in any given patient. The hand resting on the iliac crest can do several things. It can act as a basic stabilizer, it can move the iliac crest medially, to aid slack in the technique, and it can be moved laterally again, once the abdominal contact is correct, to create stretch from lateral to medial. This is particularly useful if the abdominal contact is a little tender, as the practitioner can keep the abdominal contact still whilst moving the pelvis and still create sufficient mobilization onto the ileocaecal tissues to be effective. This contact also makes a very good general 'functional' or indirect unwinding release for this area of the intestines and body wall. It can also be used as a starting point for a recoil technique to chronic fibrosed scar tissue, for example.

There is no equivalent valve between the sigmoid and the descending colon, so this technique cannot be exactly replicated on the left side. However, the basic contact makes an effective way of accessing the mesocolon for the sigmoid, which hangs the sigmoid off the left iliopsoas muscle, the left sacroiliac joint and the left lumbosacral region. Any restrictions in the right or left sacroiliac joint, hip or psoas may be eased by working on the sigmoid mesocolon or ileocaecal valve tissue as just described, when indicated (by the presence of local tissue restrictions and irritations).

Another approach for the caecum or sigmoid is to use a sidelying contact to 'scoop' them out of the iliac fossae. This is shown in Figure 5.20. The practitioner ensures that the patient is placed towards the rear of the table, so that the practitioner can use their body/torso as a stabilizer to the posterior lumbopelvic region of the patient. To place the abdominal contact, the practitioner first rotates the patient's pelvis slightly backwards, to reveal the right ASIS. The practitioner places the ulnar border of their hand next to the ASIS, so that the hand can slide gently between the inner wall

of the ilium and the caecum as the patient is gently rolled forwards again. The patient's abdominal wall should relax and the caecum should 'fall forwards' into the practitioner's hand. It is very important for the practitioner to utilize a lot of supination of the wrist and hand, to ensure that the ulnar border of the hand and fingers cups up enough (and with enough depth) to engage the tissues posterior to the caecum. If necessary, the practitioner can remove their other hand from the lateral pelvis and use it to support the abdominal hand, to maintain this depth of contact. The direction of pressure of the ulnar border of the hand is posterosuperiorly, towards the practitioner's umbilicus. If the other hand is left on the pelvis, this can create general pelvic movements (sideshift, compression, rotation and so on) to help mobilize the tissues and create movement, whilst the abdominal hand makes very small movements or changes in direction to subtly release the tissues. It is important to remember that the amount of movement available is usually only a few millimetres.

This can be a very comfortable technique for the patient, as their pelvis and lower abdomen can be gently rocked to and fro, and kept in motion, whilst the abdominal tissues are gently released. The technique can also be applied for the sigmoid but the abdominal contact must be lower, towards the superior pubic arch, in order to effectively scoop under the sigmoid to lift it out of the left iliac fossa.

TECHNIQUES FOR THE LIVER AND GALL BLADDER

There are many ways of releasing the liver and gall bladder and here it is possible only to discuss the most commonly applied techniques. As with all techniques, once the practitioner is familiar with the anatomy, many variations become possible and the reader should think of the techniques described as a starting point for their visceral exploration, not as the limits of it. Although the following are 'active' or direct techniques, all the contacts shown can be used for fascial, functional or other indirect explorations and treatments. Indeed, in many cases these more subtle techniques are often the first port of call and the stronger, more direct techniques are applied later, once the tissues are partly released and less irritated.

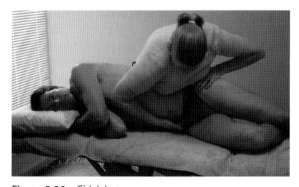

Figure 5.20   Sidelying caecum.

Care should be taken when using some of the liver and general subcostal techniques, as ulceration of the upper gastrointestinal tract can render the tissues very weak. Fibrotic change from cirrhosis of the liver and other biliary conditions, for example, may create oesophageal varices and portal venous congestion, which again are weak and easily damaged further. Vigorous subcostal techniques are contraindicated in circumstances such as these, and the practitioner should be careful to be guided by tissue reaction and patient history, and only to apply subtle and gentle contacts to gradually release the tissues rather than using strong, direct techniques in the first instance.

As indicated previously, the liver swings underneath the diaphragm in several different axes and all its supportive ligaments are connected. It is not possible to move the liver so that only one part of the suspensory mechanism is engaged; all sections will be somewhat engaged in all techniques. However, the techniques here are described as working on particular ligaments to illustrate the contacts that best focus the movement on particular sections of the suspensory mechanism. As discussed in Chapter 4, many subcostal tensions are relevant for the respiratory system, heart and mediastinum, so many of these subcostal and liver techniques may be utilized when there is respiratory distress or dysfunction.

Figure 5.21 shows a basic subcostal, sitting liver contact. For any sitting subcostal technique, the position and orientation of the practitioner's arms and torso are very important. If the practitioner is working under the right costal margin, they must stand slightly to the patient's left and support the

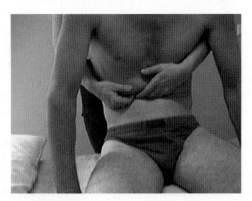

Figure 5.21   General liver technique.

left side of the patient's ribcage. If they are working on the left subcostal region, they must shift position so that they are contacting and supporting the right ribcage, lateral to the spinal column. Next, the practitioner's shoulders must remain relaxed and lowered at all times. Most cases of error with subcostal visceral release occur when the practitioner tenses the shoulder and raises the arms, so that the fingers grip the costal margin and the practitioner lifts too strongly under the diaphragm with fingers that are far too rigid. Another error is that the practitioner often tries to perform the technique using the finger tips of the index and middle fingers. These are usually 'poked' directly under the ribs, pointing towards the patient's lumbar spine, and this creates much pain and discomfort for the patient. In Figure 5.21, the practitioner is shown using the ulnar border of the hand and the sides of the middle to little fingers as the palpating part. The index fingers do not participate in the active technique at all and are just gently resting without poking.

If the patient is relatively small compared to the practitioner, then one hand should be used rather than two (the 'spare' hand can support the other hand, by contacting on the back of the hand). Another essential point is that the anterior ribs should not be compressed and the costal margin should not be gripped. To avoid this, the forearms of the practitioner must be supinated, allowing the wrists to roll outwards, and for the most lateral hand to drape more inferiorly than the midline hand. This is to avoid contact with the costal margin that, of course, slopes inferiorly as it passes laterally. The subcostal depth is created by allowing the forearms and wrists to roll into supination, which means the ulnar border is gently raised under the ribcage without irritation. Another useful tip is to utilize the contacts of the practitioner's arms and body with the lateral and posterior ribcage to gently guide the torso of the patient into different positions such as flexion, extension, sideshifting and rotation. In this way, the patient can be 'moved around' the subcostal contact, allowing it to remain relatively still and therefore even more relaxed and comfortable for the patient.

So, with the above points in mind, the liver is usually first explored by taking a subcostal contact slightly to the right of midline, in the sitting position, as shown in Figure 5.21. Just under the costal margin, the inferior border of the liver can be located. The practitioner's finger/hand contact is oriented towards the practitioner's umbilicus, not towards their pelvis (which would mean they are contacting directly posteriorly towards the patient's kidneys). This is a technique that can be used for the kidneys and ureters, for example, but in this instance, to affect the liver, the contact and movement must be oriented posterosuperiorly. The next point to remember is that the inferior surface of the liver slopes posterosuperiorly, so that as the practitioner feels a little more deeply, the hands must move more superiorly in order to remain in contact with the undersurface of the liver. In practice, most liver techniques are done by remaining in contact with the inferior border, just inside the costal margin, so there is no need to palpate any deeper than this in most instances.

Once the basic contact is made, the practitioner can gently lift the liver, which will tip it upwards and backwards, under the right dome of the diaphragm. Having applied a little lift (and only a millimetre or so of movement may be available), the liver must be allowed to fully relax down again, before attempting to re-lift it. It is most uncomfortable if the liver is continually pressed upwards, without being allowed to return to its neutral position in between motions.

Moving the liver in a superior direction and letting it rebound inferiorly will emphasize movement and elasticity in the coronary ligaments. As the liver is lifted, the practitioner must feel for additional tissue resistance in a number of different planes to properly interpret liver restriction: if the liver does not move superiorly or does not return inferiorly to neutral very easily, then several tissues may be at fault. Poor superior movement when the tissue tension is felt as a drag to the inferior border may mean that falciform ligament tension is involved (from an umbilical problem, for example). Poor superior movement in midrange may implicate the anterior and posterior sections of the coronary ligament. Poor superior movement that feels as though the liver is being blocked at the back as it tries to rotate under the right dome of the diaphragm can suggest a problem with its vascular pedicle (hepatic veins) or with the kidney/adrenal or hepatic flexure of the colon, as the liver has to press against these when it rolls

under the diaphragm. In this instance the muscular tube of the gut may be tight or the kidney may be restricted in movement. If the liver does not return inferiorly very easily, then it may be tethered by renal fascial problems (where there is an indirect peritoneal link between the renal fascia and the posterior layer of the coronary ligament, sometimes referred to as the hepatorenal ligament). There may also be tensions in both layers of the coronary ligament itself. If the restrictions or blocks are felt to be more posterior, it may be useful to release the kidney or colon first, for example, before generally mobilizing the liver, or to address the falciform ligament before starting work with the liver directly.

If the liver is to be addressed specifically using this contact, then the practitioner usually applies a very gentle rhythmic lifting and dropping down movement to gradually relax to relevant tissue barriers, allowing a return to more normal swinging of the liver under the right dome of the diaphragm. If actual movement is uncomfortable or needs to be avoided, then a functional or indirect unwinding technique can be applied to relax the peritoneum, its ligaments and the liver capsule. The patient can be gently moved in various directions and the palpating hand can alter its directional focus subtly to change the emphasis onto different tissues at different times, without actually needing to move the subcostal contact very much at all. Sometimes the practitioner can ask the patient to breathe in and out to aid relaxation subcostally, to allow a slightly deeper contact. However, this can be counterproductive as when the patient breathes in, they often overinspire and force the practitioner's hands out of the subcostal region, thus compromising the basic technique.

This contact can be adjusted slightly to change the emphasis onto other parts of the suspensory apparatus of the liver. If the subcostal contact is placed quite laterally (lateral to the edge of rectus and the midclavicular line) then when the liver is eased superiorly, it will tend to focus on the right triangular ligament, which is found on the inside of the posterior wall of the diaphragm, inside ribs 10 and 11, lateral to the angle of the ribs. If the subcostal contact is placed slightly to the left of the midline, then the left lobe of the liver can be engaged and when the liver is lifted superiorly, the left triangular ligament is contacted. Note that the hand must palpate slightly more deeply under the left costal margin to engage the left triangular ligament than on the right, where the contact can remain quite superficial. Also note that the liver does not usually cross any more to the left than the left midclavicular line. The right lobe of the liver and the right triangular ligament are quite related to the right kidney and adrenal, and the left lobe and left triangular ligament are quite related to the heart and pericardial sac.

If a broad subcostal contact is utilized, with one hand on the right of the costal margin and the other just to the left of the midline, side-to-side movements of the liver can be created. Lifting superiorly first with one hand and then the other will swing the liver transversely under the diaphragm, and lead to engagement of the triangular ligaments as the main focus (rather than the coronaries which were engaged with the direct superior and inferior movement). Some traditional osteopathic liver techniques considered the impact of liver ptosis, where the right lobe of the liver was thought to slide laterally and inferiorly from under the right dome of the diaphragm, towards the right kidney and the ascending colon. If the practitioner considers that an element of ptosis is present (or an inferior drag on the liver from posture, gravity and lower abdominal peritoneal tensions, for example) then the broad liver contact just described can be used to address these problems. Scooping the liver from right to left in a superomedial direction will rebalance the liver suspensory mechanisms, allowing the liver to be resuspended more naturally and comfortably under the right dome of the diaphragm (and relieving pressure on surrounding structures as a result).

A broad subcostal contact can also be used to stretch or mobilize the lesser omentum, which passes from the underside of the liver to the lesser curvature of the stomach. If the practitioner maintains the subcostal contact hand alignment but now eases the hand inferiorly towards the patient's left hip, this will effectively compress onto the stomach and allow the lesser omentum to be gently stretched. This is not the easiest technique to apply and supine techniques discussed below may be more effective.

Taking a general contact onto the inferior border of the liver from the midline to the right side enables the practitioner to search for two notches located along the inferior border, which are localizing points for the gall bladder and the falciform ligament. The more medial notch, found between the edge of the rectus and the midline, is the locating point for the falciform ligament and the ligamentum teres (or round ligament) which runs in the inferior free border of the falciform. The lateral notch, usually found just lateral to the lateral edge of rectus, is where the gall bladder sac is located. It is surprising how soft the gall bladder sac can feel and it can be almost indistinguishable from the undersurface of the liver, even when there are known gall stones present. It is definitely not always possible to feel stones and too much searching for elusive lumps and bumps can irritate the tissues and is not advised. Once the notches are located, the falciform ligament can be stretched by moving the liver superiorly towards the patient's right shoulder or by easing the subcostal hand inferiorly towards the left hip to stretch the falciform in a downwards direction (the falciform passes to the umbilicus, where it links with the urachus from the bladder).

Gall bladder releases can also be performed from this position. Note: bile duct techniques are discussed below, with the small intestine/duodenum contacts. Once the lateral notch has been identified, the subcostal contact should focus on this region. The gall bladder lines the inferior surface of the liver from the lateral notch posteriorly and slightly medially, towards the porta hepatis. Remember that the inferior surface slopes superiorly as well as posteriorly, so the palpating hand must be sufficiently supinated to ensure that the gall bladder sac is followed accurately. Sliding the palpating contact against the inferior surface of the liver from outside to inside will longitudinally stretch the gall bladder sac. This should not be painful but if any tenderness is present, make much more subtle movements and pressures, and always only work within tissue comfort. This is one way in which old-fashioned 'milking' techniques can be applied. However, this description might encourage too active a technique to be performed and it is much better to gently longitudinally ease the tissues towards the porta hepatis than to think the gall bladder is being 'milked'. Usually the tissue will only allow a gentle longitudinal unwinding or balancing of the gall bladder sac, and direct stretching is only sometimes applied in suitable cases.

It should be remembered that any attempts to release the gall bladder sac must be done only after checking the sphincter of Oddi and the duodenum, and the rest of the bile duct, before attempting to unwind the sac. Duodenal and bile duct techniques are described later. Note: the contact in Figure 5.22 can also be used to address the gall bladder.

Releasing within the liver itself is also possible with these basic sitting subcostal techniques. The substance of the liver should be slightly soft and the surface should feel smooth and slippery. Because of the extensive connective tissue components of the liver, forming the sinusoids and other internal structures, the liver can become quite stiff and tense within itself. This is common in many pathological changes, as well as with a biomechanical torsion or restriction pattern, with no disease present. The practitioner should feel into the substance of the liver and gain some idea of the internal elasticity and compliance, and level of tissue comfort. Performing a general listening approach will guide the practitioner as to the best point of contact from which to start to release the liver. A functional, unwinding or other indirect technique can be very useful to relax the internal liver structures and improve compliance. At the end of the technique the liver should feel more supple and gently flexible.

Figure 5.22 shows a sidelying contact for work on the liver and gall bladder. When considering the liver in this position, the use of the hand covering the ribcage becomes quite important (gall bladder techniques are considered below). The ribcage hand should not compress down into the abdomen but should gently engage the ribs and underlying liver so as to overlap these tissues over the subcostally placed contact. The two hands effectively work in concert, creating a gentle rhythmic movement that moves all the tissues together, keeping them in constant, very slow, gentle motion. This is much more comfortable for the patient and creates a much more effective and easy release within the tissues than a static contact. The subcostal hand is cupping around the ribcage, taking care not to contact the costal margin directly. The inferior border of the liver is located and gently moved into various directions, to mobilize the different lobes, segments or ligaments of the liver in a similar manner to that described above. The patient can often relax more in this position and

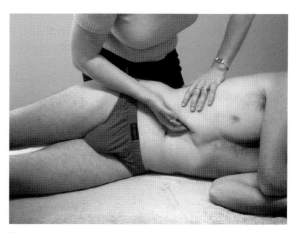

Figure 5.22   Sidelying liver release and gall bladder release.

preparatory work on the ribcage, intercostal and dorsal spine can easily be performed without having to move the patient's position. However, for a very global release of the liver, the sitting techniques are more effective.

With the patient in a supine position, as in Figure 5.23, several of the above techniques can be repeated. This contact shows a good position for lesser omentum releases, to improve either liver or stomach function. The abdominal hand is eased subcostally, using slack created by pushing the skin and superficial organs to the right and towards the costal margin, and by slightly 'overlapping' the right ribcage over the abdominal hand.

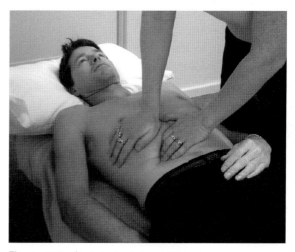

Figure 5.23   Lesser omentum contact.

The abdominal contact is between the midline and the right midclavicular line. The contact must also remain above a horizontal line drawn between the ends of the ninth ribs (this represents the transpyloric line). This ensures that the lesser omentum and lesser curvature of the stomach are contacted. If the contact is lower than the transpyloric line then although some of the stomach will still be engaged, the transverse colon and other organs will also be found and so the technique becomes much less effective for the lesser omentum. The lesser omentum can be stretched near its free border (the hepatoduodenal ligament) containing the bile duct, portal vein and other vessels and nerves. These structures will also be stretched or mobilized during the technique. It can also be stretched nearer its oesophageal and diaphragmatic insertion, by moving the abdominal contact slightly towards the midline and stretching in an inferior direction. This can help release the oesophagus.

The technique shown in Figure 5.23 can be adapted to work on the falciform ligament and ligamentum teres (round ligament). To affect these structures, a more midline contact must be taken (not completely midline or the technique affects the linea alba), just lateral and to the right of the midline, from where the medial notch on the undersurface of the liver is located. This is invariably behind the upper fibres of the rectus abdominis muscle and so this should be relaxed prior to performing the technique on the falciform. The technique is the same for the falciform and the ligamentum teres, as they are both part of the same structure, run in the same orientation and cannot be satisfactorily distinguished from each other to make individual techniques significantly different in description. The ligamentum teres runs in the free border of the falciform ligament, which is very slightly deeper (a few millimetres) than the main bulk of the ligament, which inserts along the inside surface of the rectus muscle to the umbilicus. Both structures are very superficial, being only just deeper than the abdominal wall and parietal peritoneum. The falciform is superficial to the greater omentum. It can usually be felt as a separate structure as it palpates like a loose cord when irritated or torsioned (it is not quite a centimetre wide). The lesser omentum, which runs in the same plane but a little deeper, is much wider and so will palpate quite differently.

TECHNIQUES FOR THE STOMACH

The stomach is suspended from the spleen, the underneath of the diaphragm and the inferior surface of the liver. The transverse colon adheres to the greater curvature, via the connection between the greater omentum and the mesocolon for the transverse. The body of the stomach is less affected by diaphragm and ribcage tensions in a direct sense (unlike the liver, which is very directly affected by this type of restriction). It is indirectly affected by the liver and is reflexly irritated throughout itself, when either the pylorus or cardiac sphincter/oesophageal hiatus is irritated or dysfunctional. Therefore the pyloric sphincter and the cardiac sphincter make good points to commence the exploration of the stomach. Once these areas are functioning more effectively, any remaining tension or irritation in the body and fundus of the stomach can be addressed by treating the smooth muscle layers more locally.

Running between the cardiac sphincter and the pylorus is the lesser curvature, which passes to the undersurface of the liver. The lesser omentum techniques to ease the lesser curvature of the stomach and improve lymphatic drainage to that and the pylorus have already been described above, under the section on liver techniques. They were shown in Figure 5.23.

Figure 5.24 shows an adaptation to the lesser omentum and falciform techniques for the liver. Here the contact is now onto the hinge of the

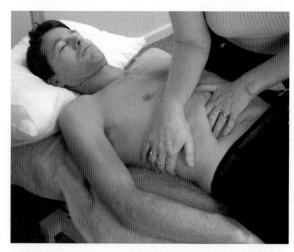

Figure 5.24   Duodenum, with liver/diaphragm contact.

beginning of the duodenum (between the duodenal cap/pyloric region and the descending part of the duodenum). In this contact, the pylorus can be scooped medially, thereby both relaxing it and opening the hinge of the first part of the duodenum. As with the flexure techniques, there is no need to stabilize the rest of the duodenum, as it is firmly attached to the posterior abdominal wall, on the side of the upper three lumbar vertebrae on the right. The contact with the ribcage is very useful as the liver can be gently 'rolled' over the top of the duodenum and pylorus, giving a deeper release to their relationship than by just engaging the duodenum alone. The ribcage hand also creates slack for the subcostal contact.

This pylorus articulation and hinging technique is a version of the contact for the hepatic flexure, shown in Figure 5.16. Instead of opening or hinging the pyloric/duodenal angle, the sphincter can be locally unwound using a functional approach, or inhibition, if required. Sphincters often seem to respond to slow, rhythmic rotatory (clockwise and anticlockwise) movements, though.

Figure 5.25 shows a sitting subcostal technique to release the bulk of the stomach, and to inferiorly stretch its superior ligamentous attachments with the diaphragm, spleen and splenic flexure. The posterior contact for this technique was described with Figure 5.17. The anterior contact aims to cups around the body of the stomach, to gain slight 'purchase' on this so that the stomach can be mobilized and stretched in different directions, to engage the different suspensory mechanisms and relations of

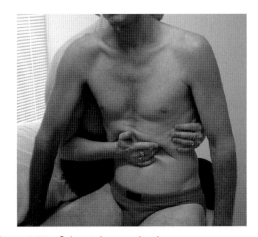

Figure 5.25   Subcostal stomach release.

the stomach. It is necessary to feel around the border of rectus and to pass deep to this; otherwise the stomach cannot be contacted sufficiently to create actual movement or proper engagement of the tissues. The abdominal contact can utilize pressure from the finger pads and the heel of the hand to gently 'grip' the stomach. The abdominal hand can also be slightly eased under the costal margin, to contact higher up on the stomach, depending on tissue tolerances. Again, the two hands/arms can work in concert, so that a gentle continuous rhythmic mobilization of the stomach can be achieved. Easing the stomach inferiorly directly to the pubis will stretch or affect the oesophageal ligaments (gastrophrenic) and cardiac portion of the stomach; easing inferiorly and to the patient's left hip will engage the diaphragmatic portion of the lesser omentum; easing inferiorly and to the patient's right hip will engage the splenic and colonic ligaments (the gastrosplenic, gastrocolic and lienorenal, between the spleen and the kidney).

This sitting contact is particularly useful for cases of reflux and hiatus hernia. One caution must be not to pull inferiorly too strongly, and certainly not with any speed. Techniques to 'reduce' a hernia are sometimes described but could be contraindicated, in the author's view. This is where the stomach is 'tugged' inferiorly, at the limit of a direct tissue barrier, to pull the stomach out of the oesophageal hiatus, so disengaging it from the thoracic cavity. Not only is the movement too violent in many cases, it can be difficult to limit the range of the movement and could very easily irritate or even damage the stomach tissues. When a hiatus hernia is present, there are often food contents lodged in the pocket of the stomach that protrudes into the thorax. This effectively creates a plug and it is not possible to pull this bulge through into the abdomen without causing tissue damage. It often provokes tissue irritation and further spasm of the diaphragmatic hiatus, which is exactly the outcome that is to be avoided when trying to manage these cases.

Additionally, with any condition accompanied by chronic inflammation or congestion around the upper gastrointestinal tract, there are often oesophageal varicosities. If these are stretched or stressed too directly they can rupture, which is a very serious complication requiring urgent hospital attention.

A more suitable way of managing cases of hiatus hernia and gastro-oesophageal reflux disease (GORD) is to use a gentle inferior traction. The stomach can be contacted as described in Figure 5.25 but this time, the aim is to imagine the stomach and any hernia as though it were a softly inflated balloon, with part of the balloon bulging above the diaphragmatic hiatus and into the thorax. If gentle traction is applied and the stomach/balloon very slowly and rhythmically coaxed downwards using a spiral swinging motion, it may be possible to reduce the hernia or bulge by slowly encouraging the tissues to ease into the abdomen. Performing the technique in such a gentle and slow way allows the local tissues to adjust to the changing forces and pressures, and to relax into the technique, allowing the stomach more freedom of movement. Any significant restriction can easily be felt (such as if there were a food plug blocking the stomach's descent), and so the technique can be halted at this stage. This approach to the technique is much safer and more easily applied and not contraindicated, as before.

Figure 5.26 shows another sitting approach to the stomach. This is an indirect technique using contact with the ribcage and subcostal techniques to 'feel through' the abdominal layers towards the upper portion of the stomach. Here, the cardiac sphincter and fundus can be unwound and indirectly released. In this contact, the posterior hand should be just medial to the angle of the ribs (but not on the transverse processes of the vertebrae)

and posterior to the midaxillary line. To affect the spleen, the posterior hand should be lateral to the angle of the ribs but still posterior to the midaxillary line. The anterior hand can be placed generally subcostally in both approaches. In fact, this type of contact is also useful for an indirect sitting release of the kidneys, with the posterior hand being near to ribs 10–12, rather than 9–11 (for the spleen and cardia).

The stomach can also be mobilized and the ligaments stretched inferiorly by using a slightly different sitting technique. This is useful if the practitioner needs to work on the diaphragm and liver as well, which is often the case when the stomach is not functioning properly. In the contact shown in Figure 5.27, the practitioner is standing behind the patient, with their arms passing under the arms of the patient. The practitioner is slightly to the right of the patient's spine and can use their forearm contact to aid torso movement, to help the technique. The contact should be gently placed under the subcostal region (slightly to the left of the midline but no more laterally than the midclavicular line). The hand cups under the costal margin and eases upwards to arrive near the inferior surface of the left lobe of the liver and the diaphragm. Again, the depth is achieved not by pushing the hard fingers upwards but by gently supinating the hand and wrist, keeping the fingers relaxed so that the patient effectively 'sinks' over the palpating contact. If the subcostal contact is gently eased towards the practitioner's lower belly, the posterior surface of their hand (i.e. fingernails and posterior fingers) will slightly compress onto the body of the stomach. This slight compression

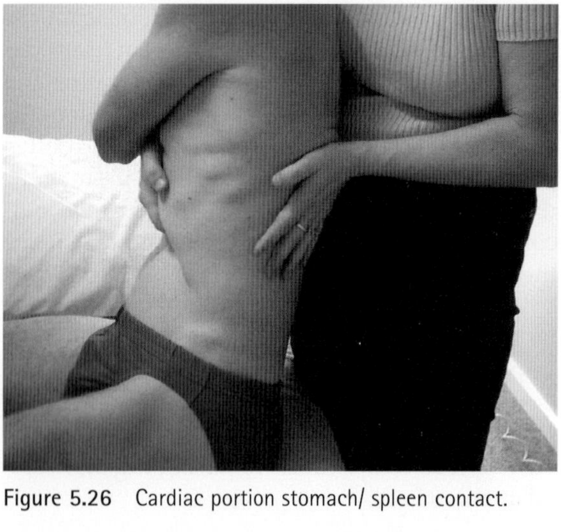

Figure 5.26 Cardiac portion stomach/ spleen contact.

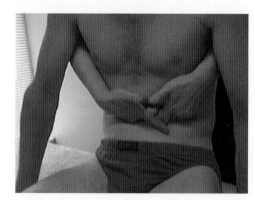

Figure 5.27 Stomach/left lobe liver release.

can then be used to traction or mobilize the stomach in a variety of directions. If an indirect, functional or unwinding approach is desired, this can be performed in this position also.

A final basic technique for the stomach can be to work on the greater curvature. In Figure 5.28, the abdominal hand is palpating just lateral to the midclavicular line, aiming to pass around the edge of the rectus muscle to locate the greater curvature of the stomach. If the contact is any more lateral than this, then the colon will be engaged instead. The stomach can also be percussed, and there should be an audible difference between the stomach area and the colonic area. When the greater curvature is located in this subcostal region, then it can be mobilized and released in conjunction with the splenic side of the transverse colon and the upper greater omentum. It is usually difficult to exactly palpate the lower border of the greater curvature, as this can be very variable in position. It can be found anywhere between the umbilicus and the symphysis pubis, and is often confused with other intestinal contents in the lower half of the abdomen. Hence, it is usually more effective to mobilize the greater curvature in its upper portions, to ensure accuracy of contact. If the abdominal contact in Figure 5.28 is moved slightly medially then the body of the stomach can be released, which is very good as a basic adjunct to mobilization and release of the surrounding ligaments. Any smooth muscle and connective tissue irritation or

contracture within the body of the stomach can interfere with the pacemaker activities and reflexes operating within this section of the gut tube, and can affect gastric function quite dramatically. Therefore, a general 'soft tissue' approach or a diffuse unwinding approach through the bulk of the stomach can be very useful.

TECHNIQUES FOR THE SMALL INTESTINE AND BILE DUCT

The small intestine is usually considered in three main sections: the duodenum, the root of the mesentery, and the ileum and jejunum as a separate collective mass. The bile duct can be treated alongside the duodenum, as the two are in very close proximity and are functionally interrelated.

The sitting techniques to release the underneath of the liver and the gall bladder sac, first illustrated in Figure 5.21, can be adapted to engage the bile duct and duodenum, as well as the liver. In this technique the upper bile duct (above its fixation behind the duodenum and pancreas) can be addressed as shown in Figure 5.29. The palpating hand can sweep down, towards the duodenum, stretching the upper bile duct by stretching the tissues as one descends. It is necessary to have reasonable depth for this technique, and to go very slowly and carefully as it is easy to create discomfort and irritation. It is a technique best performed after several preparatory sessions, to allow the tissue time to become supple enough to allow this depth of contact.

The rest of the common bile duct, in the lesser omentum and via its 'retroperitoneal' fixation, can

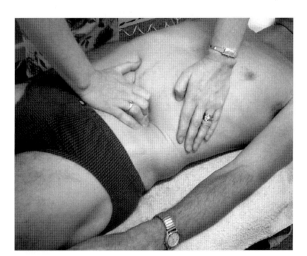

Figure 5.28   Greater curvature mobilization.

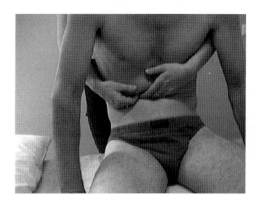

Figure 5.29   Liver/bile duct release.

be addressed by working through the descending part of the duodenum. Before working on these deeper techniques, a general release of the small intestine and root of the mesentery is advisable.

Figure 5.30 shows a general technique to release the small intestine. This sidelying position is useful as it allows a global mobilization without creating any pressure onto anterior lumbar structures such as the aorta. It also allows the knees to be bent and the patient often feels less vulnerable in this position than when supine (as the small intestine can be an area where many patients don't like to be touched, for psychological or emotional reasons, similar to the epigastric/diaphragmatic region). It also allows a general contact onto the posterior spine, which can support the lumbar column and use that as an indirect counterpressure to aid release of this section of the abdominal cavity. The abdominal contact is approximately between the two midclavicular lines, below the level of the umbilicus. The hand contact can be as low down as the symphysis pubis if necessary, as the coils of the small intestine often hang this low. The ileum and jejunum are considered as one 'large mass' and unwound and mobilized globally.

The contact shown in Figure 5.31 can then be used, to help 'scoop' the small intestine out of the lower abdominal and pelvic areas. This can improve pelvic congestion and relieve pressure on the pelvic structures. The patient's knees can be bent, as required. It is important for the ulnar borders of

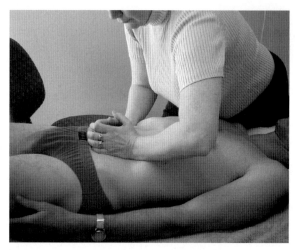

Figure 5.31   Inferior small intestine release.

the hands to remain between the two midclavicular lines, to ensure that the small intestine alone is mobilized, as contact lateral to this will also engage the ascending and descending colons.

Other techniques for the small intestine include direct work to the duodenum. The duodenum is classically separated into four sections, sometimes labelled D1–4 for technique purposes. The last parts of the duodenum are usually considered first, to allow the exit to the duodenum to be freed before working on more cephalic sections of the gut tube. Figure 5.32 shows a contact for the duodenojejunal junction (DJ junction/D4). This section of the

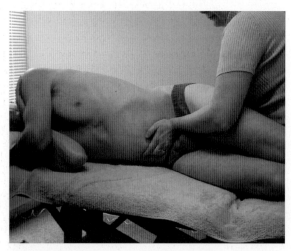

Figure 5.30   General small intestine release.

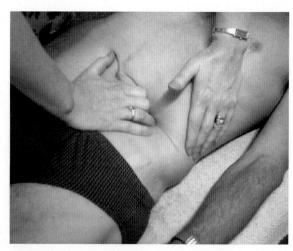

Figure 5.32   Duodenojejunal junction release.

duodenum acts like a sphincter and although there is no actual sphincter, the terminal part of the duodenum will hinge and the ileum as a whole will twist and rotate slightly about its fixation point, the ligament of Treitz. This hinging torsional function is very important and any restriction or tension in this area will disturb this and create dysfunction that can be reflected all along the gastrointestinal tract.

The DJ junction is usually located around the L2–3 vertebral body level, just above the umbilicus but just lateral to the edge of the rectus. It is best located by palpation, looking for a soft muscular clump of tissue, rather than by measuring. It can be masked or appear larger than it is if there is accompanying tension in the root of the mesentery or the left kidney, for example. The DJ junction is a locating point for the inferior pole of the left kidney in most people.

This technique can also be adapted to ease the DJ junction inferiorly, to engage and stretch the ligament of Treitz, which suspends the terminal duodenum from the posterior abdominal wall and crura of the diaphragm, and indirectly from the transverse processes of L1 and L2. To achieve this, the hand contact must be oriented inferiorly (the practitioner will move to be next to the patient's right hip) and the hands can then rotate around, so that the fingers can easily traction the DJ junction inferiorly to engage the ligament of Treitz.

Figure 5.33 shows a technique to release the root of the mesentery for the small intestine. This can also indirectly release the transverse part of the duodenum (D3), which crosses the anterior lumbar region at about the L3 vertebral body level, superficial to the transverse part of the duodenum. It is often said in osteopathic circles that there is a large biomechanical relationship between L3 and the root of the mesentery (ROM). The ROM runs obliquely across the midline, crossing the lumbar spine. The left section is higher than the right. It starts at the DJ junction and finishes at the ileocaecal valve area. If the ROM is tight, then the coils of small intestine it supports may also be tight and together they can palpate as a large, thick slab of tense tissue running across the midline. It contains the superior mesenteric artery and vein, and the lymphatics and nerves passing to the midgut. Release at this point can have a very beneficial effect throughout the whole small intestine

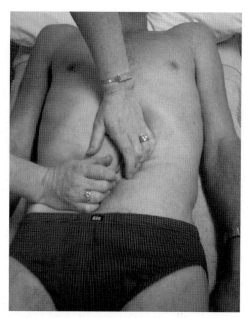

Figure 5.33   Root of mesentery.

and most of the large intestine. One caution is to avoid contact with the abdominal aorta when working on the ROM.

Figure 5.33 shows the contact from below the ROM. It is not usually contacted superiorly, as the pancreas and superior mesenteric plexus are located in that position and may be uncomfortable to work on (as many ROM techniques include direct stretches and recoil approaches). When contacting inferiorly, some degree of slack needs to be created, so that the fingers can then settle into the abdomen and move towards the posterior abdominal wall. The aim is to contact the base of the ROM nearest to the posterior abdominal wall. Having gained sufficient depth (or as much as the tissues permit), this should be maintained and a slow movement superiorly (perpendicular to the line of the ROM) introduced. This will stretch the ROM and mobilize its base. The practitioner can start at one end and gradually move along it, carefully repositioning the hands each time so as to work perpendicular to any particular section of the ROM. Remember that the abdomen is at its most shallow in the periumbilical region. A functional or indirect unwinding technique can also be applied. If required (and the tissues are not too sensitized) then a recoil technique, again applied perpendicular to the ROM, can be useful.

Figure 5.34 shows a contact to follow the line of the ROM and the transverse section of the duodenum (D3). The practitioner gently applies rhythmic compressive tension along the duodenum and ROM, to allow it to relax and decongest. This technique can be adapted slightly to incorporate the pancreatic duct and into the tissue of the pancreas itself. This is done by moving the abdominal hand slightly cephalically, roughly opposite the level of the umbilicus, but still contacting the descending part of the duodenum. As medial and superior pressure is created (along the line of the practitioner's hand as it is oriented in Figure 5.34), the movement must go 'up and over' the curve of the lumbar vertebral column to avoid compression on the sensitive structures at that point.

In Figure 5.35, the primary contact is the pisiform, which acts with cephalic pressure along the descending part of the duodenum, which is oriented vertically along the lateral mid and upper lumbar spine, on the right. The duodenum should be able to be gently 'buckled' along its length; if there is any tissue torsion or tension, it becomes stiff and resistant to this type of mobilization. The duodenum can be released by creating a wave-like repetition of gentle pressures that act along the length of the duodenum, designed to relax the walls of this section of the gut tube. This section of the duodenum needs a lot of careful work whenever there are any bile duct, gall bladder or pancreatic issues, as the sphincter of Oddi is located on the medial wall of the descending duodenum and it controls the flow of bile and pancreatic

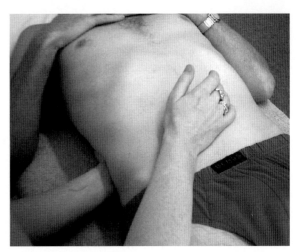

Figure 5.35   Descending duodenum release, with posterior support.

enzymes into the small intestine. The posterior contact in this technique is to place the finger pads on the transverse processes of the mid and upper lumbar vertebrae on the right (or just lateral to this, if the contact is tender or very stiff). The posterior hand can gently ease upwards (away from the table) and into the abdomen from behind, to engage the posterior surface of the descending duodenum. The two hands can therefore work in concert to achieve a more global release. This can be useful to release the right kidney as well, which lies deep to the duodenum this point. Note: the inferior angle of the duodenum is a locating landmark for the inferior pole of the right kidney in most people.

Figure 5.36 shows a contact on the lateral border of the descending part of the duodenum (D2). The practitioner stands on the opposite side of the patient and palpates into the sulcus between the ascending colon and the duodenum (the paracolic gutter, with the renal fascia and kidney acting as the floor of the gutter). The hand contact must be above the level of the umbilicus, to be on the duodenum. Note: it is not possible to palpate all the way up the lateral border of the duodenum without crossing the mesocolon for the transverse (as shown in Fig. 5.5). The sphincter of Oddi is found halfway up this section of the duodenum, approximately opposite L2. The tube of the duodenum can be gently sidebent/curved, so as to stretch the medial border and engage the sphincter. The duodenum can also be contacted anteriorly and

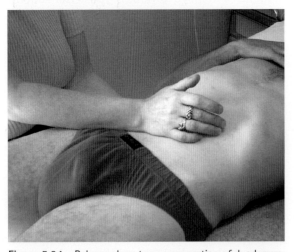

Figure 5.34   Release along transverse section of duodenum.

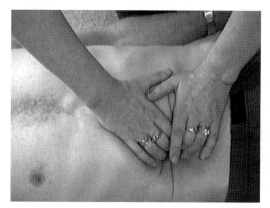

Figure 5.36   Descending duodenal and sphincter of Oddi release.

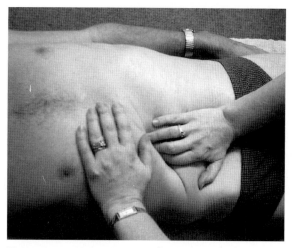

Figure 5.37   Alternative pyloric/duodenal contact.

inhibition applied to tense and restricted tissues, including the sphincter, as this is often easily identifiable when there is dysfunction. Again, functional releases and indirect balancing can be applied at this level, and rotatory (clockwise/anticlockwise) rhythmic movements may reintegrate sphincter function easily.

The adapted technique shown in Figure 5.37 is useful to emphasize lateral tissue tension that can be acting on the duodenum, such as the renal fascia and the mesocolon for the ascending colon (which bridges the paracolic gutter). With a contact onto the lateral duodenum, the ribcage contact can be released, allowing the ribs to slightly move away from the palpating hand, thereby indirectly stretching the tissues to the side of the duodenum. The palpating hand can contact over the anterior surface of the descending part of the duodenum and if slightly turned, the fingers can now pull gently inferiorly towards the patient's feet, stretching the duodenum longitudinally and also

engaging the lower part of the common bile duct where it is adhesed posterior to the duodenum and head of the pancreas.

TECHNIQUES FOR THE RECTUM

These are included with other pelvic techniques in Chapter 7.

TECHNIQUES FOR THE MESENTERIC BLOOD VESSELS AND AUTONOMIC PLEXI

It is important to release the connective tissues and peritoneal ligaments around the major blood vessels to the gut and around the autonomic plexi and ganglia located on the anterior lumbar region, in order to achieve integrated gut tube function and digestive balance. These techniques are discussed in Chapter 8.

References

1. Kwok H, Marriz Y, Al-Ali S, Windsor JA. Phrenoesophageal ligament re-visited. Clin Anat 1999;12(3):164-70.
2. Van Der Zypen E, Revesz E. Investigation of development, structure and function of the phrenicocolic and duodenal suspensory ligaments. Acta Anat (Basel) 1984;119(3):142-8.
3. Mirilas P, Skandalakis JE. Benign anatomical mistakes: right and left coronary ligaments. Am Surg 2002;68(9):832-5.
4. Kumar D, Phillips SF. The contribution of external ligamentous attachments to function of the ileocecal junction. Dis Colon Rectum 1987;30(6):410-16.
5. Barral J-P, Mercier P. Visceral manipulation. Seattle, Washington: Eastland Press; 1988.
6. Liebermann-Meffert D. The greater omentum. Anatomy, embryology, and surgical applications. Surg Clin North Am 2000;80(1):275-93, xii.

Chapter 6

Overview of urinary tract

 Note: some comments on the adrenal glands are also reviewed in Chapter 8. The prostate is also discussed in Chapter 7.

This chapter includes a basic anatomical overview for the urinary system and an introduction to the examination and treatment techniques that can be used. It gives an indication of the integration between the somatic and visceral systems, and of reflex relationships, which builds upon information in previous chapters. Patient management is discussed, together with the other body systems, in Chapter 9. All case management discussions are included in that integrated patient management chapter as it is important in osteopathy to remember that treating patients with urinary tract problems does not involve work to the kidneys and bladder alone.

SURFACE ANATOMY

Table 6.1 shows the musculoskeletal landmarks for the urinary system.

LIGAMENTS AND SUPPORTS

KIDNEYS

The kidney has various fascial coverings: the two layers of the renal fascia, the fatty capsule, and the fibrous capsule of the kidney itself. The kidney is surrounded by a dense layer of fat, which is preferentially preserved when the body as a whole loses weight, to help maintain sufficient physical support to the kidneys and adrenals. The general arrangement of the renal fascia is shown in Figure 6.1.

The renal fascia has two layers.

- *Posterior layer* – 'Zuckerkandl fascia', which relates to thoracolumbar fascia

Table 6.1 Musculoskeletal landmarks for the urinary tract

Urinary structure	Musculoskeletal landmark	Comments
Superior pole left kidney	T10–11 vertebral body supine and T11–12 standing	Note: the 12th rib generally bisects the left kidney such that half of the kidney is above and half below (the 11th rib crosses the top of the left kidney)
Inferior pole left kidney	L1–2 vertebral body supine and L2–3 standing	The visceral landmark is the duodenojejunal junction
Superior pole right kidney	T11 vertebral body supine and T12 standing	Note: the 12th rib generally bisects the right kidney such that two-thirds of the right kidney is below the rib and one third is above
Inferior pole right kidney	L2 vertebral body supine and L3 standing	The visceral landmark is the angle between the descending and the transverse sections of the duodenum
Renal pelvis	Around L1	This approximates to the transpyloric plane (bisecting the ends of the 9th ribs anteriorly)
Kidneys	Overlie the upper lumbar plexus of nerves	Renal dysfunction can irritate the subcostal, iliohypogastric and ilioinguinal nerves
Kidneys	Lie on psoas and quadratus lumborum, and the arcuates of the diaphragm	Renal dysfunction can affect lumbar spine, lower ribs, hips and sacroiliac joints
Lower sections of renal fascia	Overlies the femoral nerve as it emerges from beneath psoas	Represents an occasional link between the kidneys and femoral neuralgia
Upper ureter	The renal pelvis is opposite L2, and the ureter usually follows the line of the vertebral bodies, just next to the transverse processes of the lumbar vertebrae	Lumbar mechanics and the psoas muscle are particularly important for ureter function
Ureteric constrictions	There are three points of ureteric constriction: just after the renal pelvis, where the ureter crosses the pelvic brim (anterior to the sacroiliac joints) and just prior to its entry into the posterosuperior part of the bladder	These areas of constriction are often the site of renal stone impaction
Lower ureter	Crosses the area of the ischial spine, prior to its entry into the posterosuperior part of the bladder	Posterolateral tissue restrictions within the pelvic bowl can affect the lowest part of the ureter, which can be significant in cases of vesicoureteric reflux (relevant in recurrent renal infection, enuresis and other urinary disorders)
Bladder	Posterior to the symphysis pubis, and lying against the obturator internus muscle	There is a marked physical relationship between the hip and the bladder via the obturator tissues and problems with one will automatically transfer to the other
Urethra	Posterior to the symphysis joint line and ending slightly lower than the inferior arch	The urethra is bound to the symphysis pubis and is affected by its mechanics as well as those of surrounding organs and tissues
Prostate	Posterior and slightly inferior to the inferior pubic arch. Anterior to the two ischial tuberosities	The urogenital triangle (anterior pelvic floor) is important for prostate mobility
Bladder in the newborn	Suprapubic position	The bladder in the newborn is an abdominal organ

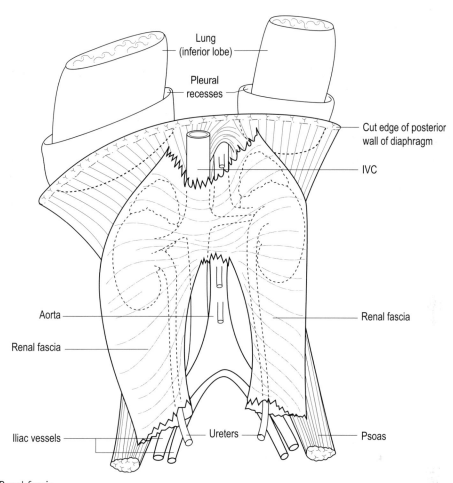

Lung
(inferior lobe)

Pleural
recesses

Cut edge of posterior
wall of diaphragm

IVC

Aorta

Renal fascia

Renal fascia

Iliac vessels

Ureters

Psoas

Figure 6.1   Renal fascia.

- *Anterior layer* – 'Gerota fascia', which relates to other retroperitoneal ligaments and some peritoneal structures

Inferiorly, the renal fascial 'bag' continues into the pelvic region (dissipates in front of the sacroiliac joints). It contains the kidneys, ureters, suprarenal glands and various blood vessels and communicates across the midline.

The anterior renal relationships are shown in Figure 6.2. Tension or restriction in any of these structures can affect renal (and adrenal) function, and vice versa. The cysterna chyli sits behind the right kidney, giving the kidney a lymphatic influence as well.

The main movements of the kidneys are as follows.

- Superior and inferior slide along the length of psoas.

- As psoas lies obliquely, the kidney will move laterally as it descends.
- As the belly of psoas is curved, at the lower part of the renal descent movement, there is an external rotation as the kidneys 'roll' over the external border of the muscle.
- These movements are induced by the excursion of the respiratory diaphragm.

URETERS

The bulk of the ureters is contained within the renal fascia. The pelvic part of the ureters passes underneath the peritoneum, wrapping the lower gastrointestinal tract, and in females passes deep to the posterior wall of the broad ligament, before arriving at the posterosuperior wall of the bladder. The ascending and descending colons attach to the anterior renal fascia in its lower sections,

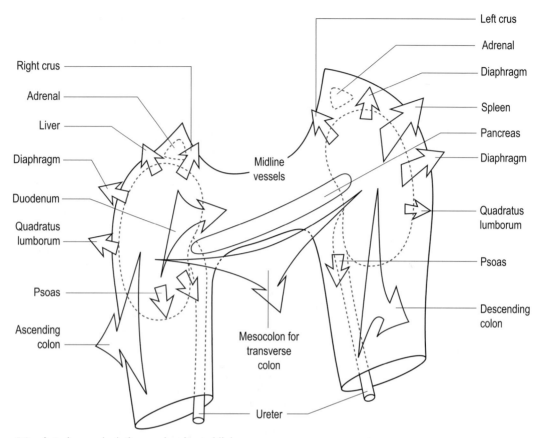

Right crus

Adrenal

Liver

Diaphragm

Duodenum

Quadratus
lumborum

Psoas

Ascending
colon

Left crus

Adrenal

Diaphragm

Spleen

Pancreas

Diaphragm

Quadratus
lumborum

Psoas

Descending
colon

Midline
vessels

Mesocolon for
transverse
colon

Ureter

Figure 6.2 Anterior renal relations and peritoneal links.

and the right ureter effectively passes behind the root of the mesentery. The left ureter passes behind the upper part of the mesocolon for the sigmoid.

The main movements of the ureters are as follows.

- The ureters should have a longitudinal elasticity.
- They should be able to twist and torsion slightly at the junction with the posterior wall of the bladder.

BLADDER

In the fetus, part of its circulation is maintained by the umbilical arteries, passing from the internal iliac arteries via the umbilicus to the placenta. After birth, these become obliterated and as a result, the fibrous cord that remains is sandwiched between the obturator internus muscle/internal

face of the pubis and the anterior wall of the bladder: the bladder effectively attaches to these fibrous cords. These cords are called the medial umbilical ligaments and they effectively give superior support to the bladder up to the umbilicus. This superior support aids that given by the urachus, which is the obliterated embryological remnant of the superior part of the bladder that also passed to the umbilical cord via the umbilicus. After birth, the apex of the bladder is suspended by the urachus to the umbilicus. The urachus is fused to the inner surface of the linea alba but has a slight degree of freedom of movement, to aid in a superior/inferior mobility of the bladder. The urachus can be disrupted after lower abdominal surgery and caesarean operations, for example. This may be relevant in cases of bladder prolapse and superior bladder wall irritation. The superior ligaments/ supports of the bladder are shown in Figure 6.3.

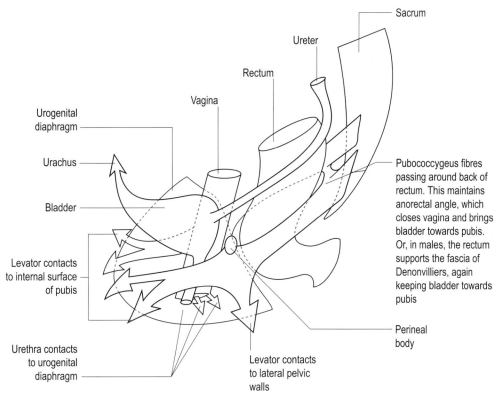

Sacrum

Ureter

Rectum

Vagina

Urogenital
diaphragm

Urachus

Bladder

Levator contacts
to internal surface
of pubis

Urethra contacts
to urogenital
diaphragm

Levator contacts
to lateral pelvic
walls

Pubococcygeus fibres
passing around back of
rectum. This maintains
anorectal angle, which
closes vagina and brings
bladder towards pubis.
Or, in males, the rectum
supports the fascia of
Denonvilliers, again
keeping bladder towards
pubis

Perineal
body

Figure 6.3   Supports of the bladder.

The other ligaments that support the bladder do so by attaching to the lower part of the bladder wall, prostate and/or urethra. They are part of the generalized pelvic connective tissue that supports the lower part of all the pelvic organs/structures.

The main movements of the bladder are as follows.

- Bladder neck mechanics in the female are very important. The bladder neck operates a little like a flap valve and can buckle or elongate, depending on the actions of the trigone or the vagina. It is also influenced by the pubocervical ligaments.
- Trigone mechanics in the female are influenced by the upper vagina, vaginal fornix and retrovesical pouch. In the male, they are influenced by the rectum and the retrovesical pouch.
- The bladder as a whole will move superiorly and inferiorly, in an arc that follows the curve of the internal face of the pubis.
- The bladder can slightly roll from side to side, 'suspended' from above by the urachus and the umbilical ligaments.

URETHRA/PROSTATE

Figure 6.4 shows the inferior supports of the bladder and the urethral/prostatic ligaments. These pass anteriorly and laterally from the lower part of the face of the bladder and prostate, and from the anterior part of the urethra. In females, the lowest part of the urethra and the external urethral sphincter are embedded in the urogenital diaphragm. In males, this is also the case but the mechanics of the urethra are intimately bound up with the prostate, making it more influential to the urethra than the urogenital diaphragm per se. These ligaments include the pubovesical, pubourethral and puboprostatic ligaments. Organ stability also arises from the fascial bands passing from the front of the lower pelvic bowl to the rear, supporting either side of the organs, called the pubogenito-rectosacral fascia. These bands are present in both males and females. This structure will be revisited in Chapter 7. There are also some bands of fascia extending laterally from the base of the bladder through to the internal iliac vessels (which enclose the vascular beds for the bladder).

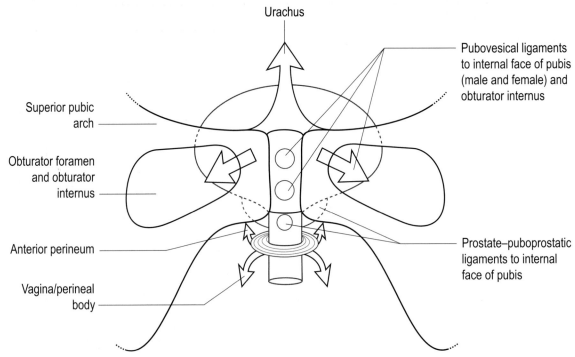

Figure 6.4   Inferior supports of the bladder and urethral/prostatic ligaments.

The main movements of the urethra/prostate are as follows.

- The female urethra is intimately linked with the vagina and should have longitudinal stretch, but lateral freedom, and an ability to torsion/spiral longitudinally, depending on the actions of the bladder neck.
- The upper male urethra is linked with prostate movements and is 'immobile' where it is embedded within the prostate. The horizontal section of the urethra depends on symphysis pubis mechanics.
- The prostate moves superiorly and inferiorly, between the two obturator foramina, depending on the flexibility of the pelvic floor muscles.

MOTILITY

Please refer to the appendix for illustrations of the motility patterns for the urinary system. The motility can be affected by tensions in any of the ligaments described above, by smooth muscle tension and tissue irritation within the organs themselves, or indirectly from somatic relations which are biomechanically affected or irritated.

REFLEX RELATIONSHIPS

Table 6.2 shows the reflex relationships for the urinary system.

VEINS, ARTERIES AND LYMPHATICS

Table 6.3 shows the main blood and lymph vessels relating to the urinary system. It is important to consider the visceral ligaments and fascial conduits that contain the blood vessels, as work on those structures will influence venous drainage, blood flow (as ligamentous torsion may affect the arteries/arterioles, and the sympathetic nerves that course along their length) and lymphatic drainage, all of which are important for organ health. The somatic relations also indicate where the musculoskeletal system may be engaged to aid fluid movement in the structures concerned.

Table 6.2 Reflex relationships for the urinary tract

Organ	Anatomical name	Somatic level/relationship
Kidneys		
Sympathetic – spinal cord	T10–11 mostly, can be to L1	Lower dorsal spine and dorsolumbar junction
Sympathetic – paravertebral chain ganglia	T10–11	Lower ribs
Sympathetic – plexus	Renal, from the aortic and coeliac plexi, the lowest splanchnic nerve and the first lumbar nerve	Dorsolumbar junction
Parasympathetic	No supply to kidney tissue	
Ureter		
Sympathetic – spinal cord	T10–L1	T10–L1
Sympathetic – paravertebral chain ganglia	T10–L1	Lower ribs and psoas muscle
Sympathetic – plexus	Fibres from the renal, aortic, superior and inferior mesenteric	Upper lumbar spine and dorsolumbar junction
Parasympathetic	Vagus (R>L) and S2–4 (lowest part of ureter)	Upper cervical spine and cranial base, and sacrum
Bladder		
Sympathetic – spinal cord	T11–L2	T11–L2
Sympathetic – paravertebral chain ganglia	T11–L2	Lower ribs and psoas muscle
Sympathetic – plexus	Vesical plexus, either side of bladder	Anterior lumbar spine fascia, for the hypogastric that leads eventually to the vesical plexus
Parasympathetic	S2–4	Sacral mechanics, piriformis and the coccyx (to affect the pelvic connective tissues and the lowest part of the dura)
Urethra		
Sympathetic – spinal cord	T11–L2	T11–L2
Sympathetic – paravertebral chain ganglia	T11–L2	Lower ribs and psoas muscle
Sympathetic – plexus	Vesical plexus, either side of bladder	Anterior lumbar spine fascia, for the hypogastric that leads eventually to the vesical plexus
Parasympathetic	S2–4	Sacral mechanics, piriformis and the coccyx (to affect the pelvic connective tissues and the lowest part of the dura)
Prostate		
Sympathetic – spinal cord	T11–L2	T11–L2
Sympathetic – paravertebral chain ganglia	T11–L2	Lower ribs and psoas muscle
Sympathetic – plexus	Pelvic plexus, either side of bladder	Anterior lumbar spine fascia, for the hypogastric that leads eventually to the vesical plexus
Parasympathetic	S2–4	Sacral mechanics, piriformis and the coccyx (to affect the pelvic connective tissues and the lowest part of the dura)

Table 6.3   Blood and lymph vessels

Organ	Anatomical name	Mesenteric or peritoneal ligament relation	Somatic relation, where applicable
Kidney			
Veins	Renal vein	Renal fascia. Note: ovarian/ testicular veins drain into left renal vein, giving a 'reproductive role' to the left kidney	Psoas, 12th ribs, dorsolumbar junction
Arteries	Renal artery	Renal fascia. The left renal artery is longer, and therefore prone to more torsional irritation, although the right is indirectly affected by liver restriction	Psoas, 12th ribs, dorsolumbar junction
Lymphatics	Para-aortic nodes	Crurae of diaphragm are important	Upper lumbar spine and 12th ribs
Ureter			
Veins	Renal, gonadal and vesical veins	Renal fascia	Lumbar spine and psoas mechanics
Arteries	Upper part supplied by the renal artery, the middle by the gonadal artery, and the lower by the vesical artery	Renal fascia	Peritoneal irritation or damage can impact on renal arterial supply and therefore tissue health
Lymphatics	Aortic nodes drain the upper ureter and common iliac nodes drain the lower ureter	Posterior abdominal wall	Lumbar spine, sacroiliac and hip mechanics are important for lymphatic drainage
Bladder			
Veins	Superior and inferior vesical veins, to the internal iliac vein	Deep pelvic fascia	Pelvic floor mechanics are important
Arteries	Superior and inferior vesical arteries, from the internal iliac artery	Deep pelvic fascia	Pelvic floor mechanics are important
Lymphatics	Main part drains into the external iliac nodes and nodes next to bladder, and the lower part drains into the internal iliac nodes	Deep pelvic fascia	Hip and pubic mechanics are important
Urethra			
Veins	Inferior vesical vein	Deep pelvic fascia	Perineal/urogenital triangle mechanics are important
Arteries	Inferior vesical artery	Deep pelvic fascia	Perineal/urogenital triangle mechanics are important
Lymphatics	Internal iliac nodes	Deep pelvic fascia	Pelvic floor mechanics are important
Prostate			
Veins	Inferior vesical vein	Deep pelvic fascia	Perineal/urogenital triangle mechanics are important
Arteries	Inferior vesical artery	Deep pelvic fascia	Perineal/urogenital triangle mechanics are important
Lymphatics	External iliac nodes	Deep pelvic fascia	Pelvic floor mechanics are important

SOMATIC AND VISCERAL INTERACTIONS

The kidneys are retroperitoneal organs and are placed close to the diaphragm, the 12th ribs, the psoas and quadratus lumborum muscles, and have several other organs 'overlaid' upon them. As a result, they are influenced by, and influence, many different body systems. The 12th ribs are the best locator for the kidneys, as indicated in Table 6.1. As at least half of each kidney is below the level of the 12th ribs, when the person is standing much more of the kidney is exposed 'below' the costal margin than most practitioners imagine. If the anterior projection of the 12th rib is drawn onto the anterior abdominal wall, the kidneys will be quite accessible below the costal margin, making abdominal palpation easier than might be thought.

The kidneys slide up and down the 'platform' formed by the psoas and quadratus lumborum muscles, and will pivot/hinge around their own blood vessels. As the position of the abdominal aorta is slightly to the left of the midline (the inferior vena cava being to the right), the right renal artery is long and the left relatively short. The left renal vein is long and the right relatively short. These vessels form the 'vascular pedicles' around which the kidneys move. The relationship between the kidneys and psoas is one of the most marked within whole-body mechanics and kidney tensions can therefore spread up to the cranial base or down into the sacroiliac joints, hip and lower limbs to the feet, as a result of the compromised psoas function.

Previous chapters illustrated the relationship between the respiratory system and the renal system, discussing the different cavity dynamics that operate between the lower thorax and the upper abdomen, and the way the lungs and the kidneys both slide up and down in their own 'respiratory' excursion. There is an 'overlapping' arrangement of the lungs and pleural layers, and the renal fascia and kidneys, separated only by the diaphragm – giving the two a strongly reciprocal relationship. The kidneys (and adrenals) were also identified as being in a transition zone as far as cavity dynamics and general visceral movement were concerned, which exposed them to a variety

of stresses and strains. Accordingly, in many cases, chronic dorsolumbar restriction requires evaluation and treatment to both the urinary and respiratory systems. And even if there is renal dysfunction that requires treatment, this may only be successful when combined with treatment of the ribcage, respiratory system, upper abdominal organs and dorsolumbar spine, for example.

> Renal restrictions must therefore always be put into context with the surrounding tissue and organ mechanics.

It is also interesting to note that many cervicobrachial restrictions may be related to renal dysfunction. The renal fascia can be supplied by the phrenic nerve and irritation within the kidney may therefore manifest as an irritation of the mid-cervical spinal cord and a referred pain/neural reflex into the C3–5 distribution affecting the skin and muscles of the neck and upper shoulder girdle.

EXAMINATION AND TREATMENT OF THE UPPER URINARY TRACT

When palpating the kidneys, it is important to remember that not only are they mobile (the renal fascia forming a type of 'sock' or 'pouch' within which they can slide up and down a couple of centimetres) but they rest on various muscles, including quadratus lumborum. This means that when pushing gently from an anterior abdominal contact, if there is no posterior support, the kidney will just be pushed against the quadratus which will bulge posteriorly, effectively making the kidney 'disappear' from the abdominal contact. Therefore, when palpating the kidney, a bimanual approach is very useful, enabling the posterior contact to continually support the quadratus, thereby maintaining the kidney in a relatively 'anterior' orientation.

Figure 6.5 shows a unilateral contact for the kidney. As stated above, it is important to maintain the posterior support via the quadratus lumborum and 12th rib, otherwise the kidney will 'sink' away from the abdominal contact as soon as anterior pressure is applied. Note: this technique can also be performed in a sidelying position, and

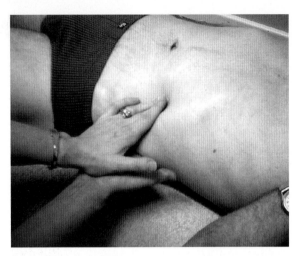

Figure 6.5   Unilateral renal palpation, supine.

the heels of the hands can be used as the palpating parts, rather than the fingers.

The anterior contact, which is the finger pads in Figure 6.5, is placed in the sulcus between the ascending colon and the duodenum (the paracolic gutter). On the right side, the thumb is first placed approximately opposite the umbilicus. On the left, the finger pads would first be placed an inch or so above this level. Note: the pisiform or heel of the hand can also be used. The posterior contact uses the flat palmar surface of the fingers, such that the middle finger is aligned with the 12th rib and the other fingers rest naturally either side of this. It is important that the finger tips do not pass more medially than the lateral border of the paravertebral muscle mass. This is so that they can support the quadratus lumborum muscle and lower ribs separately without engaging the lumbar muscles. This gives a more effective posterior support to the kidney. It also means that the posterior hand can be moved more effectively, to mobilize or release the posterior renal fascial ayer. The aim is to flatten the abdomen between the two hands, compressing it and trying to 'close' the opening of the inferior renal fascia. Now, maintaining this closure/compression of the lower abdomen, the hands are moved superiorly (and slightly medially) in order to 'slide' the kidney upwards within the renal fascial bag. The kidney should slide upwards a centimetre or two, before it 'runs out of space' and is blocked by the superior renal fascia and the liver (on the right) or the spleen (on the left).

Once the kidney has reached its superior limit, the hands will 'roll over' the inferior pole, which has been resting close to the abdominal contact throughout the technique. The two hands will be effectively 'pushed' or eased apart by the bulk of the kidney, and the abdomen will feel 'thicker' at the level of the inferior pole of the kidney than just below (where the hands are clamping down on the more easily compressible ascending or descending colon). Once the inferior pole has been identified, then the hand position can be adjusted slightly so that the main bulk of the kidney is palpated. Keeping the bilateral contact in place and utilizing a degree of compression between the two hands, the kidney can now be moved in a superoinferior direction, in a mediolateral direction or globally, to assess its freedom within the renal fascial bag. The kidney can be mobilized generally or the two layers of renal fascia can be somewhat separately released (by adjusting the influence of either hand/contact).

It may be necessary to work on those organs and peritoneal structures that attach onto the anterior surface of the renal fascia before a lasting release of the kidney can be achieved. Also, on the right, the influence of the liver is very important and so any problems there should also be addressed prior to evaluating the kidney. Note: this technique requires sufficient skin slack at the onset of the superior movement, and the hand contact begins lower on the right, as the right kidney is lower than the left.

This technique can be adapted to use the heels of the hands, rather than the finger tips, as shown in Figure 6.6. If desired, this technique utilizing

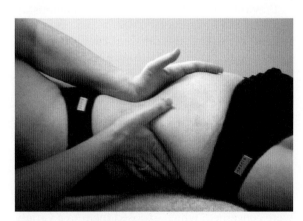

Figure 6.6   Alternative kidney mobilization.

the heels and palms of the hand can be performed with the patient sidelying, with the practitioner working on the uppermost side (and sitting facing towards the patient's head). This alternative position allows the practitioner to stabilize or engage the pelvis with their upper arm and chest, and be more global in their mobilization of the lateral abdomen.

Figure 6.7 shows a bilateral contact for the kidneys. The technique is similar to the unilateral contact, using the same principles of compression and slide of the kidney superiorly, except that the thumbs are used for the anterior contact and the fingers for the posterior contact around the 12th ribs/quadratus lumborum. Using both hands at once allows the practitioner to evaluate the whole of the renal fascial relationship, which crosses the midline. If the hands are moved slightly inferiorly, then the two ureters can be evaluated, if desired.

Figure 6.8 shows a sidelying contact for the kidney and the upper ureter. This allows a stronger general mobilization and stretch to the ureters. The practitioner uses a thumb contact near to the midaxillary line, on the lateral border of the quadratus lumborum muscle. This provides the posterior support and pressure in an antero-medial direction, to lift the kidney into the abdomen and slightly medially. The other fingers or other hand cup around the 'tube' of the descending colon (when the patient lies on their right) to reach into the paracolic gutter. The renal fascia and kidney are found on the 'floor' of the gutter, between the colon and either the duode-nojejunal junction/stomach (on the left) or the

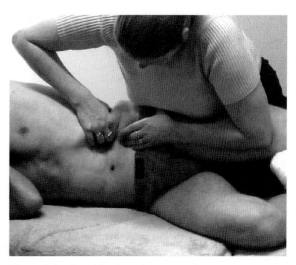

Figure 6.8 Renal fascia and upper ureter.

descending part of the duodenum (on the right). The two contacts now compress the abdomen, with the aim of closing the inferior renal fascia and moving the kidney upwards slightly, so that its position becomes more stable.

With the kidney now engaged, the practitioner can use both hands together and their abdominal contact on the side of the patient's ribcage to effect a global mobilization of the kidney and renal fascia. Strong focused movements can be introduced if required, with care taken to remain within tissue comfort. The ureter can be stretched by moving the kidney superiorly or by stretching the ureter/renal fascia inferiorly. The two hands can also be placed so that both contact the ureter, which can then be stretched by moving the hands away from each other. Many combinations are possible with this basic contact. It also makes a very useful position for a global balancing technique or a fascia or functional unwinding of the tissues in the region.

Figure 6.8 also shows one final component for this technique, which can be applied or not depending on how the tissues feel at the time. The upper leg of the patient is straightened out and the hip relatively extended. Care is taken not to tip the pelvis anteriorly, nor to induce too much lumbar lordosis. This is achieved by the practitioner using their flexed knee up on the couch, which supports the patient's leg, and the practitioner's hip/lower abdomen supports the patient's

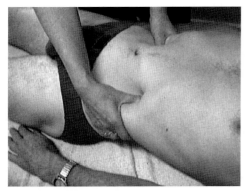

Figure 6.7 Bilateral kidney balancing.

posterior pelvis. The aim of easing the patient's leg posteriorly is to 'pre-stretch' the psoas muscle, to engage the renal fascia and ureters at the onset of the technique. During the technique the leg can also be eased further posteriorly, to aid in the release if required.

EXAMINATION AND TREATMENT OF THE LOWER URINARY TRACT

GENERAL

The lower section of the ureter, anterior to the sacroiliac joint and superior to the bladder, can also be examined and treated. This may be necessary after appendix operations or episodes of renal colic, for example. These stretches also release the suspensory ligaments of the ovary and the neurovascular bundle for the testes/gubernaculum remnants. The practitioner uses the fingers of both hands to palpate into the abdomen, in the iliac region. Care is taken to ensure sufficient skin slack between the two contacts, so that stretch is applied to the deeper tissues, not to the skin. This is shown in Figure 6.9.

MALE

Whenever the bladder is palpated via the suprapubic route, the rectus abdominis insertion must be

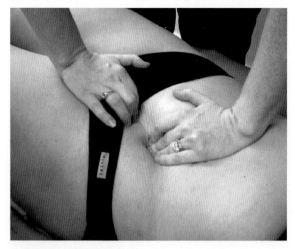

Figure 6.9   Lower ureter stretch and release (mimics suspensory ligament of ovary release).

considered, as this will directly overlie the bladder in the zone to be examined. This means that when the rectus is tight, some superficial block to palpating the bladder will be present, which needs to be addressed prior to commencing the technique. Patients can also be wary of bladder palpation, for the obvious reason that it can make them feel as though they want to micturate. They should always be offered the opportunity to empty the bladder prior to the technique being applied. A full bladder will not make the bladder more palpable.

The bladder is situated just deep to the pubis and it is important not to palpate too deeply, otherwise other structures (such as the small intestine or sigmoid) will be evaluated rather than the bladder. It is also important to note that the bladder does not rise above the symphysis and this means that the practitioner must pass their finger contact deep and inferior to the top of the symphysis.

The bladder cannot be directly stretched nor the ligaments released effectively unless a close contact is achieved. In males this creates a problem as the penis often overlies the area that is to be examined. The practitioner must ask the patient to move his genitals across slightly or lower his underwear (to push the genitals a little lower *whilst keeping them covered by the underwear*) in order to gain access to the bladder area. For this reason, although the rectus muscles are firmer in the male, performing the technique with the knees bent to relax them is not usually recommended, as it brings the genitals over the pubis. However, bent knees may be necessary if the rectus is particularly involved, and the patient should be asked to position his genitals accordingly.

Figure 6.10 shows a general contact to release the bladder. The anterior hand is cupping either side of the insertions of rectus, to pass around them, to contact the superior part of the bladder. The posterior hand can contact either the sacrum or the coccyx, in order to engage the deep pelvic connective tissue or the pelvic floor, as required.

Figure 6.11 shows a contact which passes either side of the superior pubic arch, with one hand below the arch, in the obturator foramen region, and the other contact above the arch, in the inguinal region. In this technique, one hand is contacting onto the obturator membrane area,

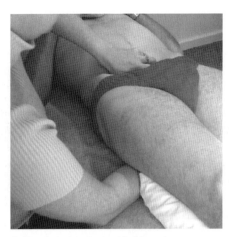

Figure 6.10   Anteroposterior bladder release.

just posterior to the adductor tendon, and the other hand is just above the superior pubic arch. Note: some authors describe a technique to palpate the obturator membrane by passing anterior to the adductor muscle, and pressing through it to reach the obturator area. This is usually uncomfortable and not recommended as femoral vascular compression often occurs.

In this technique (and in all suprapubic techniques in the male), the practitioner may elect to wear gloves for hygiene purposes. Check that the patient does not have a latex allergy prior to using this type of glove.

The aim of the technique is to have the contacts reach onto one side of the bladder, one from above and one from below. If the obturator membrane is supple, then quite close contact between the two hands/palpating fingers can be achieved, which places the effect of the technique close to the lateral bladder wall and prostate in men or the bladder neck in women. It may be necessary to release the obturator area first before attempting this technique.

With the hands now placed around the superior pubic arch, the practitioner can apply a rhythmic pumping action which will help to lift the bladder up and down, via alternate suprapubic and obturator membrane pressure. This rhythmic motion makes a very effective general release of the bladder and can begin to achieve a deeper release in the interior pelvic bowl. A functional or unwinding balancing release can also be performed.

i Note: lower bladder and prostate releases in the male can be performed via a contact with the perineum. These techniques are described in Chapter 7. The bladder lifting techniques and release of the urachus discussed below can also be used in males.

FEMALE

The techniques for females are mostly similar to those for males, with some additions in relation to the urethra, which is directly accessible in females. All the techniques discussed above (excluding those incorporating the prostate, obviously) can be performed on female patients, in addition to those discussed below.

A sitting 'lift' technique to the bladder can affect the urachus, the pubovesical and medial umbilical ligaments. Figure 6.12 shows the practitioner standing behind the patient, reaching around to the suprapubic region. It is important to remember that the bladder is behind and inferior to the symphysis pubis and unless the fingers contact deep to and inferior to the pubis, the bladder will not be sufficiently affected. The fingers must use some slack in the lower abdominal muscles, to ease these behind the internal face of the pubis.

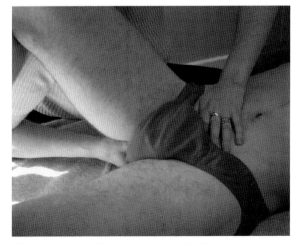

Figure 6.11   Combined obturator and bladder release – male.

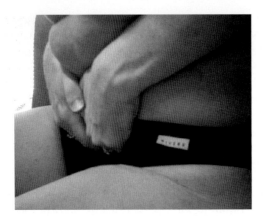

Figure 6.12 Sitting 'lift' of bladder.

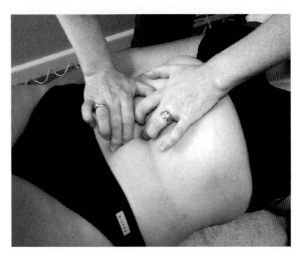

Figure 6.13 Umbilical release for urachus.

The aim of the technique is to pass between the pubis and the anterior wall of the upper part of the bladder. In male patients it may be necessary to ask them to move the genitals clear of the suprapubic region prior to starting the technique. The practitioner must also remember not to palpate 'backwards' towards the sacrum/coccyx area, as this usually results in a contact that slides posteriorly over the top of the bladder and ends up affecting the small intestine/ rectum.

When the fingers are properly placed and the initial movement is inferior, the practitioner aims to use very slight finger pad compression of the top of the bladder, in order to slightly 'grip' it, so that it can then be 'lifted' superiorly. This lift is a difficult procedure to perform correctly without quite a lot of practice, as often the fingers merely slip off the bladder. Gaining sufficient grip on the bladder without pressing too deeply into the lower abdomen is the key. Once the bladder can be eased superiorly, the practitioner feels for the amount of suppleness in the top of the bladder, and the degree of superior movement. This can be quite a strong technique and the available range of movement when performed correctly is only a few millimetres. If more movement is created, the practitioner has usually lost the bladder contact and is working on the general peritoneal sliding surfaces between the lower abdominal wall and the small intestine or sigmoid.

Please note that after suspensory surgery for bladder and/or uterine prolapse, the dynamics of the tissues in the area can be quite altered and this technique may be difficult to apply (in many cases

suspensory surgery is only partially successful and the prolapsed condition may revert over time).

Figure 6.13 shows a technique to evaluate the urachus with respect to the umbilicus and linea alba. This is particularly useful in children (when trying to balance liver and pelvic torsion patterns, for example, in cases of enuresis). The practitioner takes a light contact into the umbilicus and also onto the anterior surface of the linea alba. Now, using a local 'listening' technique or small active testing/ stretching movements, the practitioner can evaluate torsion or tension within the urachus. There is also a link with the falciform ligament (passing from the liver to the umbilicus) which can also be evaluated as part of the technique, by slightly adapting the direction of testing and using palpation above the umbilicus as well as below it. Often the liver and the bladder benefit from being released 'together' via these links.

Figure 6.14 shows a two-handed contact superior to the pubis, to affect the top of the bladder wall. If the practitioner's hands are particularly large in relation to the patient, a unilateral contact can be used. Note that if the patient's knees are bent, the practitioner must make sure that they continue to palpate just deep to the face of the pubis (which rests at a more horizontal level when the patient's knees are flexed, compared to a more oblique angle with the knees straight). This technique is useful for many bladder conditions where the detrusor muscle is irritated.

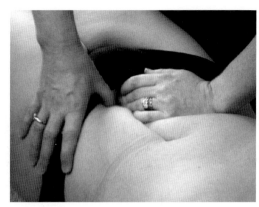

Figure 6.14 General suprapubic release of bladder wall and superior pubovesical ligaments.

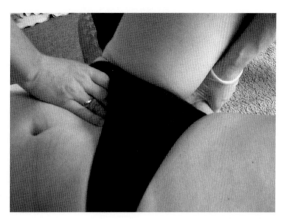

Figure 6.15 Combined obturator and bladder release – female.

It is particularly useful after lower abdominal surgery and caesarean operations, for example, and can also be relevant after hernia repair.

The fingers gently create some slack in the superficial tissues, to allow the contact to ease down between the anterior wall of the bladder and the pubis. This is very similar to the sitting contact shown in Figure 6.12. In the supine technique, the aim is not to 'lift' the bladder (although this can be done) but to stretch/mobilize the upper wall of the bladder and to ease tissue tension within the pubovesical ligaments, between the anterior bladder and the pubis. The practitioner can 'scoop' and stretch from side to side, and can effectively test the way the bladder can roll from side to side against the pubis. This rotatory/ sideshifting movement is quite important and is often reduced when there is chronic bladder irritation, cystitis or recurrent infection, for example. Functional and unwinding techniques can also be used rather than direct stretch.

Figure 6.15 shows a combined release using a contact onto the obturator foramen area and the bladder, using a lateral suprapubic contact. Here, the two hands can be brought quite close together to access the tissues deep to the superior pubic ramus. The bladder and its ligaments insert in this area, onto the obturator internus muscle. A stretch, inhibition or rhythmic mobilization can be performed, or a functional or unwinding/ balancing approach utilized.

> *i* Note: perineal release for the lower urethra and per vaginal techniques for the urethra, bladder neck, trigone and various ligaments and pelvic floor links are discussed in Chapter 7 where internal techniques and those to sensitive areas are reviewed. Retrovesical pouch techniques (useful for postcaesarean cases, for example) are also discussed in Chapter 10.

Chapter 7

Overview of reproductive system

This chapter includes a basic anatomical overview for the reproductive system and an introduction to the examination and treatment techniques that can be used. It gives an indication of the integration between the somatic and visceral systems, and of reflex relationships, which builds upon information in previous chapters. Patient management is discussed, together with the other body systems, in Chapter 9. All case management discussions are included in that integrated patient management chapter as it is important in osteopathy to remember that treating patients with reproductive tract problems does not just involve work to the uterus or prostate.

SURFACE ANATOMY

Table 7.1 shows the musculoskeletal landmarks used to locate the reproductive system.

Table 7.1   Musculoskeletal relations for the reproductive system

Reproductive structure	Musculoskeletal landmark	Comments
Ovaries	On the internal face of the lateral pelvic walls, on the posterior layer of the broad ligament	The ovaries are effectively suspended from the face of the sacroiliac joints and the lateral pelvic walls, via the broad ligament
Suspensory ligament of ovaries	Paracolic gutter	These pass down from the renal fascia, which is attached to the lumbar fascia, and links the highest point of ovarian support to approximately the L3 vertebral body height either side
Uterus	In normal anteflexed and anteverted position, the uterus is palpable above the pelvic brim. This brings the fundus into the first third of the space between the umbilicus and pubis. This makes the uterus usually palpable above the pubis, although it remains below the pelvic brim when not pregnant	The pelvic brim is inclined at an angle. The pubis is level with the sacrococcygeal joint. If the space between the pubis and the umbilicus is divided into thirds, the sacrum is located in the middle third when the patient stands, and the lumbosacral joint is approximately at the level of a line drawn between the two anterior superior iliac spines
Round ligament	Passes through the inguinal canal over the face of the pubis to the labia	It can easily be palpated over the face of the pubis, and any inguinal or symphysis problem can affect the round ligament, creating cyclical spasm and pain, for example
Prostate	Posterior and slightly inferior to the inferior pubic arch. Anterior to the two ischial tuberosities	The urogenital triangle (anterior pelvic floor) is important for prostate mobility
Seminal vesicles	Posterior to the bladder	Sacral and deep pelvic mechanics are important for the seminal vesicles
Spermatic cord	Passes over the top and sides of the bladder, to pass through the inguinal canal and rings, over the face of the pubis, to descend into the scrotum, attaching to the epididymis and testis	Inguinal and pubic symphysis mechanics are important for the spermatic cord which contains the vas deferens and related vessels and nerves

LIGAMENTS AND SUPPORTS

Apart from the broad ligament and the fascia of Denonvilliers (both peritoneal structures), the pelvic floor organs are mostly supported by ligaments formed from generalized pelvic connective tissue and are all 'subperitoneal' structures. Exceptions are the round ligaments and ovarian ligaments which are formed from the remnants of the female gubernaculum. This balancing act by tissues of multiple origins gives the urogenital system a unique set of benefits, and consequently problems.

UTERUS

Figure 7.1 shows the uterine ligaments. The two broad ligaments are peritoneal structures and as such are continuous with the parietal peritoneum that lines the abdominal walls and the inside of rectus and passes over the psoas and other lumbar structures. This may serve as a reminder that the gastrointestinal tract is very influential to uterine function: not only does the peritoneum form a mesentery for the uterus, but it gives the small intestine and sigmoid a horizontally orientated sliding surface on which to move. The broad ligaments effectively represent the floor of the abdominal

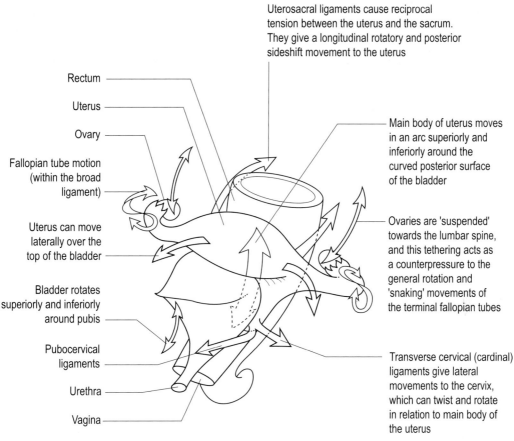

Uterosacral ligaments cause reciprocal tension between the uterus and the sacrum. They give a longitudinal rotatory and posterior sideshift movement to the uterus

Rectum

Uterus

Ovary

Fallopian tube motion (within the broad ligament)

Uterus can move laterally over the top of the bladder

Bladder rotates superiorly and inferiorly around pubis

Pubocervical ligaments

Urethra

Vagina

Main body of uterus moves in an arc superiorly and inferiorly around the curved posterior surface of the bladder

Ovaries are 'suspended' towards the lumbar spine, and this tethering acts as a counterpressure to the general rotation and 'snaking' movements of the terminal fallopian tubes

Transverse cervical (cardinal) ligaments give lateral movements to the cervix, which can twist and rotate in relation to main body of the uterus

Figure 7.1   Uterine ligaments.

cavity as far as the gastrointestinal tract is concerned. The folds of the broad ligaments behind the uterus, in front of the rectum, in front of the uterus and behind the bladder form pouches that give particular mobility to the uterus and surrounding structures. They are called the pouch of Douglas and the retrovesical pouch, respectively, and are shown in Figure 7.2.

The uterosacral ligaments, pubocervical ligaments and cardinal (transverse) ligaments are all formed from the general pelvic connective tissue called the pubogenito-rectosacral fascia, which was introduced in Chapter 6 when the fascial supports of the bladder were being discussed. The uterosacral and pubocervical ligaments support the lower uterus and vagina between the sacrum and the pubis. The transverse cervical or cardinal ligaments form a lateral stabilizing influence to the lower uterus and cervix, attaching to the lateral

pelvic walls. This arrangement of ligaments makes the cervix one of the more stable sections of the reproductive tract.

The uterosacral ligaments are the conduits for the autonomic nerves that pass into the pelvic bowl serving most local structures. They are definite bands of tissues, which can be palpated per rectum, and contain smooth muscle cells as well as being hormonally receptive and responsive. They insert onto the lower sacrum, coccyx, sacroiliac ligaments and the piriformis muscle, and as such are intimately involved in sacral, lumbopelvic and hip mechanics.

The round ligaments are separate structures that arise from the gubernaculum and as such are akin to the spermatic cord in the male. They are continuous with the ovarian ligaments (round ligaments of the ovaries), which are discussed below. They pass from the 'shoulders' of the uterus, where the

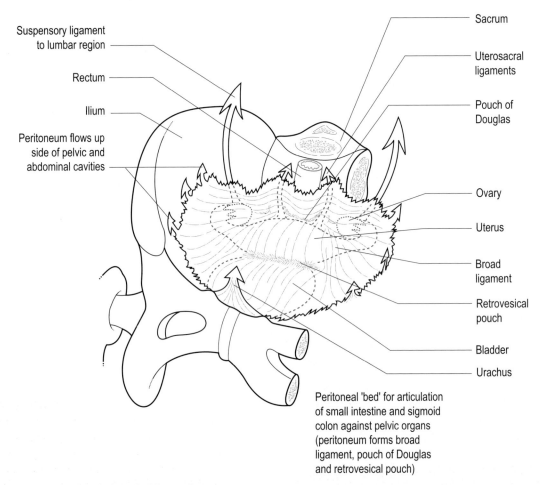

Suspensory ligament to lumbar region

Rectum

Ilium

Peritoneum flows up side of pelvic and abdominal cavities

Sacrum

Uterosacral ligaments

Pouch of Douglas

Ovary

Uterus

Broad ligament

Retrovesical pouch

Bladder

Urachus

Peritoneal 'bed' for articulation of small intestine and sigmoid colon against pelvic organs (peritoneum forms broad ligament, pouch of Douglas and retrovesical pouch)

Figure 7.2 Pouches and visceral sliding surfaces.

fallopian tubes join the uterus, and course anteriorly to the deep inguinal ring. From there, they pass through the inguinal canal, out of the superficial inguinal ring and over the face of the pubis to insert into the labia. They provide anterior stabilization to the uterus. They contain some smooth muscle fibres and can 'contract'.

All the above ligaments are found beneath the peritoneal broad ligaments and as such are 'subperitoneal' structures. The mechanical interrelatedness of the 'peri-peritoneal' spaces was introduced in Chapter 3.

Figure 7.3 indicates that the broad ligament influences the body of the uterus, and therefore some particular movement dynamics, whereas many of the other ligaments influence the cervix and lower body of the uterus in a different way, leading to different movement dynamics in that

section of the reproductive tract. This is often reflected in a highly individualized 3D torsion pattern within the pelvic tissues. This is added to by the fallopian tubes, which are influenced by the broad ligaments and the ovarian and round ligaments (which are indirectly related, as they originally arose from the same embryological structure, the gubernaculum, which is mesenchymal in origin). These latter tend to give an anteroposterior influence from the lumbar region to the pubis (along the suspensory ligament of the ovary, the ovarian ligament, and along the round ligament). One way of visualizing all these relationships is to imagine the uterus as a hot air balloon, with the cervix as the basket and the various ligaments acting like the ropes connecting to the balloon. The balloon and basket can move 'independently' yet in a related or reciprocal manner. Torsion and tension

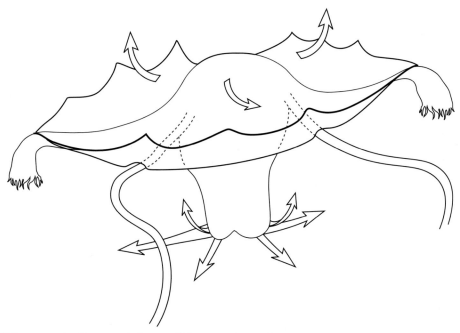

Figure 7.3   Different uterine ligaments influence different uterine torsions.

in one part will be transferred to the other and can adversely impact on general movement dynamics of the whole reproductive tract.

> **Balloon and basket**
>
> **Uterosacral ligaments**
> - Relate to sacral mechanics
> - Influence the lower segment of the uterus
>
> **Round ligaments**
> - Relate to mechanics of the groin, pubis and perineum
> - Influence the fundus
> - Normal sidebending and rotational torsion of uterus in pregnancy are influenced by the dynamics of the round ligaments
>
> **Fallopian tubes, broad ligaments**
> - Relate to the mechanics of the lateral abdomen, sigmoid, small intestine and caecum
> - Influence the fundus

All together, the arrangement of the uterine ligaments gives some interesting movement dynamics

to the uterus as a whole, and also within the uterus itself. It is best to consider that the cervix and uterus move as two independent organs, and effectively this is what they are in a functional sense. The uterine body and cervix move in their own patterns and 'articulate' against each other. The fallopian tubes can also act as separate organs and this is particularly so when it comes to concepts relating to fertility and conception. The fallopian tube is a sensitive, supple structure that is highly mobile and it takes very little to disturb the natural peristaltic waves that cyclically operate along its length. The isthmus at the junction between the tube and the uterus acts like the glenohumoral joint and local torsion can effectively mimic rotator cuff distortions of the shoulder girdle. The fimbriae are also delicate structures that 'feel, touch and stroke' over the ovary, ready to 'gather up' the ovum and direct it towards the tubal opening. The tubes can be so mobile that it is not unknown for one side to collect the ovum from the opposite ovary. It is also interesting to note that the fallopian tubes are open at the ovarian end (ampulla) to the abdominal cavity, as there is a small opening in the peritoneum which allows peritoneal fluid to enter into the fallopian tube.

The main movements of the uterus (in its anteverted and anteflexed orientation) are as follows.

1. Body of uterus
   - Side-to-side movement, over the top of the bladder.
   - Lower uterine body should not be held too posteriorly and should have ability to flex and torsion along its length

2. Cervix
   - Local 'gear-stick' type of mobility (in multiple planes) underneath the uterus.

3. As a whole
   - Superior and inferior arc movement, over the curved surface of the bladder (upwards towards the abdominal wall and down to the pelvic floor).
   - Should be able to tip back and forwards as though hinging on top of the vagina.

4. Vagina
   - Longitudinal elasticity, with the posterior wall following rectal mechanics and the anterior wall following bladder mechanics.

   - Superior suspension aided by the levator ani muscles.

5. Fallopian tubes
   - Sinuous movements as part of broad ligament mobility.
   - Articulate with body of uterus like the glenohumeral joint.
   - Fimbriae act like fingers on the end of the 'wrist' of the tube.

OVARIES

Figure 7.4 shows the ovarian ligaments. The suspensory ligament of the ovary links the ovary to the lumbar and renal fascia and runs down the front of the sacroiliac joints, before passing under the broad ligaments to reach the lateral aspect of the ovary. From the medial end of the ovary, a ligament passes to the fundus of the uterus, next to the isthmus of the fallopian tube. This is called the ovarian ligament or round ligament of the ovary. The ovary and its two supportive ligaments either side are all enveloped in the mesovarium, a small fold of the posterior wall of the broad ligament.

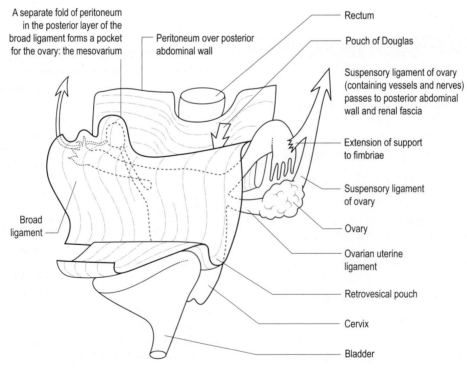

Figure 7.4   Ovarian ligaments.

This makes the ovary independently mobile but related to the mechanics of the lower lumbar region, the sacroiliac joints and the uterus. Remember that the lumbar links relate to the renal fascia, in which the suspensory ligament of the ovary is located.

The main movements of the ovaries are small pendular movements over the posterior layer of the broad ligament.

PROSTATE AND SEMINAL VESICLES

The prostate is embedded in the pubogenito-rectosacral fascia previously outlined in Chapter 6. The seminal vesicles are embedded in the base of the bladder via a dense fibromuscular sheath. Note: they cannot be palpated per rectum unless inflamed, enlarged or tender. Between the base of the rectum and the posterior part of the prostate is the fascia of Denonvilliers – the male equivalent of the peritoneal pouch of Douglas found in females. The fascia extends inferiorly towards the perineal body, to which it is attached. The anterior part of the prostate is linked to the inside of the pubis and the obturator foramina by the puboprostatic ligaments. The membranous portion (horizontal part) of the urethra is linked to the underneath of the symphysis pubis where it emerges from the prostate and passes through the perineum. Figure 7.5 shows the prostatic ligaments and supports.

The main movements of the prostate and seminal vesicles are superior and inferior movements, following the perineum and levator ani mechanics.

VAS DEFERENS AND TESTES

The vas deferens is about 50 cm long and arises from the epididymis next to the testis and

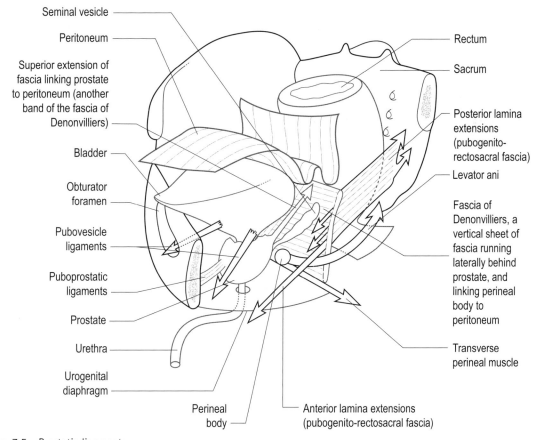

Figure 7.5   Prostatic ligaments.

passes upwards. It enters the abdominopelvic cavity via the superficial inguinal ring, the inguinal canal and the deep inguinal ring, and passes inferior to the peritoneum and the gastrointestinal tract organs. It passes over the superolateral parts of the bladder and descends behind it to join in with the seminal duct, to form the ejaculatory duct. It is part of the spermatic cord and is the male remnant of the gubernaculum, along which the testes migrate from the thoracolumbar region of the posterior body wall, around the inner aspect of the lateral abdominal wall, and through the inguinal canal to the scrotum. The vas deferens, testes and relations are shown in Figure 7.6.

The main movements of the testes and vas deferens are as follows.

- Spiral movements suspended from the lower face of the pubis.
- The spermatic cord should be slightly elastic longitudinally and be mobile against the face of the pubis.

MOTILITY

Please refer to the appendix for illustrations of the motility patterns for the reproductive system. The motility can be affected by tensions in any of the ligaments described above or by smooth muscle tension and tissue irritation within the organs themselves, or indirectly from somatic relations which are biomechanically affected or irritated.

REFLEX RELATIONSHIPS

Table 7.2 shows the reflex relationships for the reproductive system.

VEINS, ARTERIES AND LYMPHATICS

Table 7.3 shows the major blood and lymph vessels for the reproductive system. The visceral ligaments

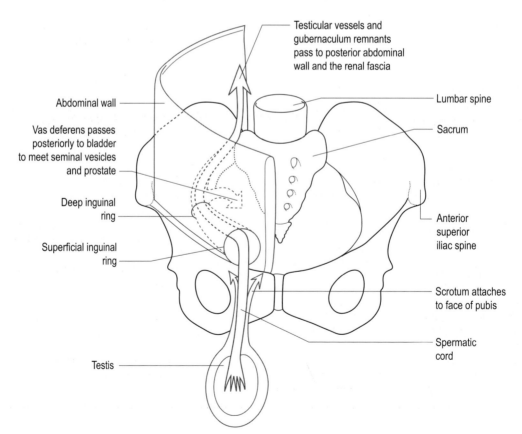

Figure 7.6 Testicular and spermatic cord relations.

Table 7.2 Reflex relationships for the reproductive system

Organ	Anatomical name	Somatic level/relationship
Ovaries		
Sympathetic – spinal cord	T10–11	T10–11
Sympathetic – paravertebral chain ganglia	Lumbar splanchnics	Lower ribs
Sympathetic – plexus	Ovarian, via the hypogastric	Lumbar mechanics and psoas
Parasympathetic	S2–4 but there may be some vagal fibres involved	Sacral mechanics
Fallopian tubes		
Sympathetic – spinal cord	T10–11	T10–11
Sympathetic – paravertebral chain ganglia	Lumbar splanchnics	Lower ribs
Sympathetic – plexus	Ovarian and pelvic via the hypogastric	Lumbar mechanics and psoas
Parasympathetic	S2–4	Sacral mechanics
Uterus		
Sympathetic – spinal cord	T12–L2	Dorsolumbar and upper lumbar spine
Sympathetic – paravertebral chain ganglia	T12–L2	Rib 12 and medial arcuate ligament
Sympathetic – plexus	Pelvic/uterine plexus via the hypogastric plexus	Anterior lumbar spine fascia, for the hypogastric that leads eventually to the pelvic plexus
Parasympathetic	S2–4	Sacral mechanics, piriformis, hip and lumbosacral junction
Testes		
Sympathetic – spinal cord	T10–11	T10–11
Sympathetic – paravertebral chain ganglia	Lumbar splanchnics	Lower ribs
Sympathetic – plexus	Testicular, via the hypogastric	Lumbar mechanics and psoas
Parasympathetic	S2–4, but there may be some vagal fibres involved	Sacral mechanics
Prostate and seminal vessels		
Sympathetic – spinal cord	T12–L2	T12–L2
Sympathetic – paravertebral chain ganglia	Pelvic splanchnics	12th rib and psoas muscles
Sympathetic – plexus	Vesical plexus	Anterior lumbar spine fascia, for the hypogastric that leads eventually to the pelvic plexus
Parasympathetic	S2–4	Sacral mechanics, piriformis, hip and lumbosacral junction
Vas deferens		
Sympathetic – spinal cord	T10–11	T10–11
Sympathetic – paravertebral chain ganglia	Lumbar splanchnics	Lower ribs
Sympathetic – plexus	Via the hypogastric plexus	Lumbar mechanics and psoas
Parasympathetic	S2–4, but there may be some vagal fibres involved	Sacral mechanics

Table 7.3 Blood and lymph vessels

Organ	Anatomical name	Peritoneal/fascial ligament relation	Somatic relation, where applicable
Ovaries			
Veins	Ovarian vein	Renal fascia, mesovarium (broad ligament)	The right ovarian vein passes to the inferior vena cava, and the left to the left renal vein, making it more prone to poor drainage and the influence of any adverse renal/left dorsolumbar mechanics
Arteries	Ovarian artery	Renal fascia, mesovarium (broad ligament)	Psoas and lumbar spine mechanics are important
Lymphatics	Drain into the inferior vena caval and aortic nodes		General pelvic mechanics are important
Fallopian tubes			
Veins	To the ovarian and uterine veins	Broad ligament and renal fascia	Sacroiliac mechanics are important
Arteries	From the ovarian and uterine arteries	Broad ligament	General pelvic mechanics are important
Lymphatics	Drain into the inferior vena caval and aortic nodes		General pelvic mechanics are important
Uterus			
Veins	Uterine vein, draining to the internal iliac vein. Some veins anastomose with the superior rectal veins	Retrovesical pouch mechanics are important	Sacral mechanics are influential
Arteries	Uterine artery, which has considerable anastomoses with the ovarian artery	Vaginal mechanics are important	Pelvic floor is influential
Lymphatics	Fundus drains into the caval and aortic nodes, the body drains into the internal iliac nodes, the cervix into the internal iliac or nodes next to the cervix, and the cornu into the superficial inguinal nodes		General pelvic mechanics are important
Testes			
Veins	Testicular vein	Renal fascia, and spermatic cord	The right testicular vein passes to the inferior vena cava, and the left to the left renal vein, making it more prone to poor drainage and the influence of any adverse renal/left dorsolumbar mechanics. As the spermatic cord passes through the inguinal canal, those tissues can constrict the vascular structures and cause problems
Arteries	Testicular artery, from aorta		
Lymphatics			Inguinal region mechanics are important

Continued

Table 7.3 Blood and lymph vessels—cont'd

Organ	Anatomical name	Peritoneal/fascial ligament relation	Somatic relation, where applicable
Prostate and seminal vessels			
Veins	Inferior vesical vein		
Arteries	Inferior vesical artery		
Lymphatics	Prostate drains into the external and internal iliac, and the seminal vesicles drain into the external iliac nodes		General pelvic mechanics are important
Vas deferens			
Veins	Vesical and prostatic veins		
Arteries	Vesical arteries		
Lymphatics	External iliac nodes		Hip mechanics are important

and fascial conduits that contain the blood vessels are important to consider, as work on those structures will influence venous drainage, blood flow (as ligamentous torsion may affect the arteries/arterioles and the sympathetic nerves that course along their length) and lymphatic drainage, all of which are important for organ health. The somatic relations also indicate where the musculoskeletal system may be engaged to aid fluid movement in the structures concerned.

SOMATIC AND VISCERAL INTERACTIONS

PELVIC FLOOR AND GAIT

The relationships between bony pelvic biomechanics and the pelvic floor have been introduced earlier. It is important to remember that changing the bony dimensions of the pelvis will lead to alterations in pelvic floor tone. For example, standing with heels raised (plantarflexion) will result in lower pelvic floor tone/decreased mean resting tone, compared to standing on the heels (dorsiflexion) which leads to an increased tone of the pelvic floor.[1] Pelvic joint stability is also related to pelvic floor function, as the relative stiffness of the pelvic ring (the ligamentous ring passing from the pubis along the inferior pubic rami, along the sacrotuberous and sacrospinous ligaments to the sacrum, and the interosseous and iliolumbar

ligaments of the posterior pelvis) depends on pelvic floor strength.[2] Conversely, sacroiliac joint injury alters lumbopelvic load transfer, alters thoracic diaphragmatic (respiratory) function and decreases pelvic floor tone.[3] Hence, whenever pelvic floor dysfunction is relevant to a patient's presentation, the mechanics of the bony pelvis need evaluation.

Many cases of repetitive sacroiliac or iliolumbar strain or lumbosacral facet articular dysfunction may be maintained by pelvic floor contracture and/or weakness. Strain to the sacroiliac joint (through sports, for example) can lead to compensatory changes in the pelvic floor muscles, such as contracture and stiffening. Subsequent movement dynamics of the ilium may remain adapted if the pelvic floor component does not return to normal. Subsequent ischial tuberosity movements may be diminished, leading to increased torque at the sacroiliac joints. This can create pain and dysfunction within the above-mentioned sacroiliac and lumbosacral structures. Treatment of the pelvic floor component can improve the overall management of these conditions and may reduce rates of recurrence.

PELVIC FLOOR AS SUPPORTIVE SLING

Figures 7.7 and 7.8 show views of the pelvic floor which indicate the 'sling' arrangement of the muscular fibres. The levator ani muscle is paired and

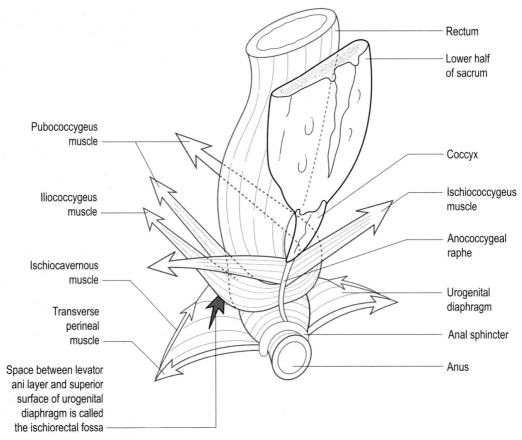

Rectum

Lower half
of sacrum

Coccyx

Ischiococcygeus
muscle

Anococcygeal
raphe

Urogenital
diaphragm

Anal sphincter

Anus

Pubococcygeus
muscle

Iliococcygeus
muscle

Ischiocavernous
muscle

Transverse
perineal
muscle

Space between levator
ani layer and superior
surface of urogenital
diaphragm is called
the ischiorectal fossa

Figure 7.7   Rear view of pelvic floor sling.

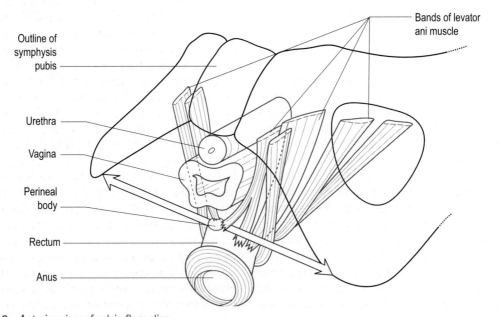

Bands of levator
ani muscle

Outline of
symphysis
pubis

Urethra

Vagina

Perineal
body

Rectum

Anus

Figure 7.8   Anterior view of pelvic floor sling.

the two muscles meet at several points in the midline. Effectively, the fibres pass backwards from the pubis and obturator foramen area on one side, looping around the lower part of the rectum (with some insertion to the anococcygeal raphe/coccyx or sacrum) and then continue forward around the other side of the rectum, to end up on the pubis/obturator area on the other side. Some fibres start more laterally from the edge of the foramen area, pass around the back of the rectum and then forwards to the other side. Some fibres also start on the lateral walls of the pelvis, pass around and then join to the lateral pelvic wall on the other side. As can be seen in Figure 7.7, this creates various bands or layers for the levator ani muscle group. Layers that attach most laterally on the pelvic walls pass around the rectum higher up and those that attach to the pubis pass around the rectum lower down. As a result of the natural resting tone in the levator ani muscles, the rectum is naturally bent at an angle – the anorectal angle – and this will increase when the levator ani muscles are contracted further and the rectum is moved anteriorly.

Some of the fibres that start on the pubic/medial obturator foramen area pass around the side of the urethra and vagina (like the rest of the fibres) but then turn and insert into the perineal body, which is situated between the rectum and vagina. From there, the fibres pass forwards again to the pubis. These fibres form a sling around the back of the vagina, rather than the rectum. When these fibres contract, the perineal body is moved anteriorly. Figure 7.8 shows an inferior view of the levator ani muscle group, indicating the looping fibres around the vagina and the rectum. The urogenital diaphragm (not shown) would cover over the space between the two inferior pubic arches and reinforce the more vulnerable anterior section of the pelvic outlet. The free border of the posterior section of the urogenital diaphragm is shown in Figure 7.7 and the different slants/positions of these two sections of the pelvic floor can be seen. The urogenital diaphragm is approximately horizontal when the person stands. There is a gap between the two layers of the pelvic floor, either side, between the top of the urogenital diaphragm and the inferior surface of the levator ani muscle. This space is filled with fatty connective tissue and is called the ischiorectal fossa.

The pelvic floor (levator ani muscles) is not in fact a 'floor' – implying that it lies horizontally – but rather it is a funnel that spirals around the lower pelvic organs and pelvic tissues and gradually closes them into a tight 'neck' or tube below the funnel. The closure mechanisms of the levator ani on the urethra, vagina and rectum are shown in Figure 7.8. In the male, some of the lower fibres of the levator ani (the pubococcygeus) will sling around the base of the penis and pass around the back of the urethra, which will aid ejaculation and sexual function. In the female, the pubococcygeus is largely responsible for sensation during intercourse.

Organ prolapse

This sling and loop arrangement helps to demonstrate how organ prolapse can occur in the pelvic region. Setting aside congenital differences in collagen content (and therefore tensile strength of the pelvic connective tissues), the actions of the pelvic floor are the most important guard against pelvic organ prolapse. In Chapter 10 on obstetrics, the actions of the pelvic floor on the sacrum, coccyx and ilia will be discussed in more detail but basically, contraction of the pelvic floor brings the coccyx and lower sacrum forwards and closes the pelvic outlet, while pelvic floor relaxation allows the coccyx and lower sacrum to move posteriorly and the pelvic outlet to enlarge. This basic forwards-and-backwards motion of the sacrum is also transmitted to the organs. For women, with the lower rectum naturally bent at an angle, this forms a sort of 'lap' that the vagina can 'sit back on'. The pelvic floor fibres passing around the back of the rectum do so 'behind its knees' and muscle contraction will pull the 'knees' of the rectum forwards, closing the vagina forwards against the back of the bladder. The bladder is effectively sitting on the straight legs of the vagina, which is sitting back on the knees of the rectum. With pelvic floor contraction, the bladder is compressed against the inner surface of the pubis and continence in all three organs is maintained. The uterus stays in position flipped forwards on top of the bladder, because the vagina is kept closed beneath it, leaving it nowhere to 'escape to' despite being exposed to abdominal pressure from the gastrointestinal organs above.

As the sacrum moves posteriorly the rectum follows, as it is attached to the anterior surface of the sacrum. As the rectum moves posteriorly, so too does the posterior wall of the vagina. The anterior wall of the vagina would follow, together with the posterior wall of the bladder to which it is attached. There should be a little give in the anterior attachments of the bladder to the pubis to allow the anterior wall of the bladder to move posteriorly as well. The vagina will remain closed in all of this because of surrounding organ pressure but if the rectum moves too far posteriorly through pelvic floor weakness, and/or if the bladder does not move sufficiently posteriorly during pelvic floor relaxation, then the two walls of the vagina will effectively move in opposite directions and begin to gape open. Once this occurs, there will be nothing to prevent the uterus bulging down in response to abdominal pressure and to escape this, the vagina actually starts to turn inside out as the uterus first tips vertically and then slips down within the open vaginal canal, leading to prolapse. The bladder and rectum can both follow, leading to cystocoele and rectocoele respectively.

Men tend not to suffer from pelvic organ prolapse mainly because their pelvises are smaller and they are not exposed to obstetric trauma. As a gross oversimplification, male pelvises suffer from being too tight and female pelvises suffer from being too loose (although spastic conditions of the female pelvic floor can also occur). The osteopathic management of pelvic floor problems and organ prolapse are discussed in Chapter 9.

FUNCTIONAL EXPRESSIONS OF PELVIC FLOOR ACTIVITIES

Traditional anatomical illustrations of the pelvic floor do not give an 'active' sense of pelvic floor function. The levator ani and urogenital diaphragm together perform many varied tasks and are involved in micturition, parturition, visceral support, defaecation and sexual function. The pelvic floor can hold various tensions and reflect a person's emotional well-being: it can be tense and resistant, elastic and accommodating, rigid and unwelcoming, weak and unresponsive, and so on. There is a whole range of 'conversations' that the pelvic floor complex has during the course of a person's life and whenever it is palpated, the practitioner can gain some sense of 'communication' with the patterns of tensions, torsions and disorders

that are being expressed within it. This is very valuable during the treatment and management of various pelvic organ problems (as will be discussed later).

Engaging the pelvic floor with the right 'language' (recognizing the validity of various palpatory findings) will help treatment immensely. The image of the 'face' of the pelvic floor in Figure 7.9 gives an idea of the possible variety of pelvic floor expressions, and how these can be influenced by movements and torsions within the organs that attach into it and within the bony pelvis at its periphery.

EXAMINATION AND TREATMENT – FEMALE REPRODUCTIVE SYSTEM

UTERUS

The abdominal palpation of the uterus is generally simple, although various factors need to be borne in mind. The surface projection of the pelvic bowl in which all the pelvic organs are contained is quite small. Many practitioners make the mistake of taking too broad a contact and one too far away from the symphysis pubis to effectively explore the pelvic organs. The pelvic inlet is bounded by the pubis below, the two medial borders of the psoas muscle either side and the line drawn between the two anterior superior iliac spines superiorly. This space approximates to the size of the patient's clenched fist placed just above the pubis in the midline. The pelvic organs are covered over by coils of the small intestine and quite often the sigmoid, making uterine palpation sometimes confusing via the abdominal route.

Gentle palpation in the suprapubic space should reveal a sense of thickness deep into the pelvic bowl, which is the resistance offered by the muscular uterine fundus if placed in its anteverted and anteflexed position. In cases where there is retroversion, hysterectomy or prolapse, this space appears 'empty' on palpation as though there is a 'hole' in the middle of the pelvic space. The hands will sink in too readily, as the uterus is either missing or has moved further posteriorly into the pelvis, or slipped lower down towards the pelvic floor. If several patients with known hysterectomy (without accompanying adhesive or other complications)

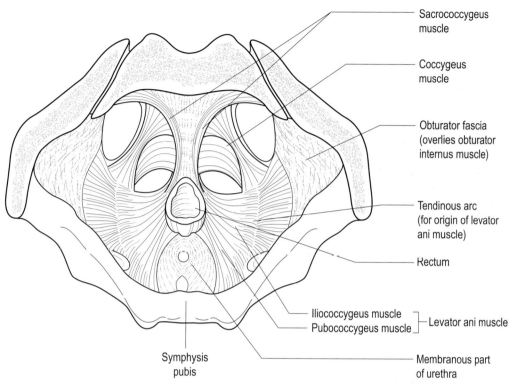

Sacrococcygeus
muscle

Coccygeus
muscle

Obturator fascia
(overlies obturator
internus muscle)

Tendinous arc
(for origin of levator
ani muscle)

Rectum

Iliococcygeus muscle ⎤
Pubococcygeus muscle ⎦ ⎱ Levator ani muscle

Symphysis
pubis

Membranous part
of urethra

Figure 7.9   Pelvic floor 'expressions'.

are compared with women with the uterus intact, the difference in palpation is soon appreciated. With practice, it is quite easy to palpate the uterus via this abdominal route. If the small intestine is irritated or the sigmoid is restricted and tense, for example, there may be several 'thick, dense or resistant' areas that can mimic uterine palpation. It is necessary to compare these palpatory findings with a general examination of the gastrointestinal tract to gain confidence in recognizing actual uterine palpation findings.

Generally, the uterine findings will be on a deeper level than the intestinal ones. A note of caution, though: increasing abdominal palpating pressure will not increase the chances of palpating the uterus – quite the opposite, in fact. Too much suprapubic pressure will block the technique, be uncomfortable and cause the uterus to bulge towards the pelvic floor away from the palpating fingers. Another caution is if the woman has an interuterine coil fitted: it is best to avoid much direct evaluation and treatment in this case and a 'listening' or functional technique should be

used instead. Uterine palpation is also easier in the first half of the menstrual cycle after the menses, as the tissues are less sensitive and oedematous and more responsive at this time. If the woman is in the first trimester of pregnancy, specific work on the uterus should be mostly avoided, although this does not mean that a pregnant woman cannot be treated, nor that local work to the uterus is absolutely contraindicated at this time. Direct uterine work in obstetric care in the first trimester is quite specialized and has many cautions, and should not be performed without specialized osteopathic training.

Figure 7.10 shows a global pelvic contact, with one hand contacting the sacrum from behind and the other palpating through the lower abdomen. The abdominal hand is placed so that the heel of the hand is just above the pubis. In this way, the two hands can 'come together' slightly and get a general sense of deep pelvic torsions and tensions. Often this contact is useful to relax general tensions through the lower abdomen prior to more specific uterine palpation and treatment.

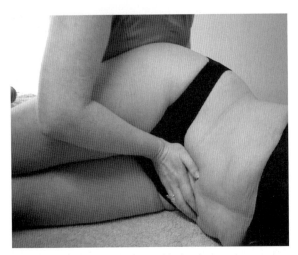

Figure 7.10   General uterosacral balancing.

Figure 7.11 shows a basic contact for local uterine examination. The two hands are placed just above the pubic area and will first gently press downwards, to test for the surface projection of the uterus. It will feel like a small area of increased resistance, usually in the midline, just below the level of a line drawn between the two anterior superior iliac spines. This initial testing is necessary as the uterus is often slightly to one side or the other, as a result of uneven tension in its supporting ligaments or surrounding tissues. Once the actual position of the uterine fundus is more clear, this then becomes the starting point of contact for further uterine exploration.

From the identified starting point, the hands move the superficial skin a little to create some slack and then try to ease down to the left, the right or just below the fundus of the uterus. The uterus is moved gently from side to side, cephalically and caudally, and slightly up and down (deep into the pelvis and then allowed to rebound anteriorly again). This tests the basic uterine mobility and relative tension/elasticity in surrounding ligaments. With this relatively superficial contact, side-to-side movement tests the broad ligaments/fallopian tubes; lifting the uterus cephalically tests the retrovesical pouch; and moving it into the pelvis and letting it spring back tests the round ligaments and, to a lesser extent, the uterosacral ligaments. The round ligaments resist movement towards the sacrum and the uterosacral ligaments resist the rebound movement away from the sacrum, when irritated or disturbed. The uterus itself should not be stiff or tense and should feel like the supple, muscular 'bag' that it is. The depth used in this basic test is not sufficient to test the deeper uterine ligaments or the above ligaments when the uterus is retroverted.

Figure 7.12 shows a contact for the round ligament as it passes over the face of the pubis. One hand palpates over the pubis at the level of the superficial inguinal ring (just lateral to the pubic tubercle and the insertion of rectus on the pubic bone). The other hand stabilizes the iliac crest. It can also be placed over the inguinal canal (approximately superior to and following the line of the inguinal ligament) to release that to indirectly affect the round ligament as it passes through it.

To test (or treat) the uterosacral ligaments, more depth is required in order to pass along the length

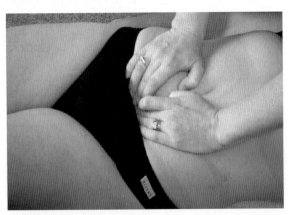

Figure 7.11   Uterine/bladder contact.

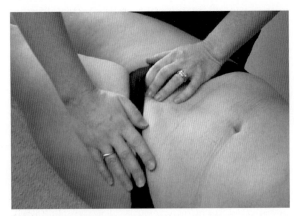

Figure 7.12   Round ligament and inguinal ring examination.

of the uterus towards the cervix. Only by engaging at the level of the cervix will there be sufficient contact to actually mobilize and stretch the ligaments as necessary. More superficial 'listening' tests will identify torsions within the uterosacral ligaments and enable a general release of the ligaments but chronic contracture and adhesions may need actual mobilization or stretching. This deeper palpation can be done with the patient supine (in which case it is performed as above but with more depth of contact) but is often easier in a sidelying position, to allow greater slack in the superficial tissues. The sidelying contact is shown in Figure 7.13.

In this technique, the contact remains close to the pubis and not too close to the lateral pelvic wall. The practitioner can use one hand to stabilize the pelvis and move it in several directions (through a contact onto the iliac crest) to help create slack and local tissue relaxation around the palpating contact. If necessary, one hand can be used to 'support' the other, to help maintain sufficient depth to palpate the desired ligaments. Usually this contact tests or treats the uterosacral ligament on the side closest to the table. A less deep contact will of course, test the broad ligament and the fallopian tube if required. It can also be used to ease problems and adhesions with the small intestine, which should slide freely around the superior surface of the uterus, prior to performing the deeper techniques. The hands can also be swapped so that the practitioner's other hand is the abdominal contact, if desired. One hand can

also contact the sacrum to work through to the uterosacral ligaments from behind, if desired.

OVARIES AND FALLOPIAN TUBES

The techniques described above which move the uterus from side to side will test the broad ligaments and therefore the fallopian tubes, as mentioned. If there is a problem, a more specific release may be required, as may work on the ovary.

Figure 7.14 shows a unilateral contact for the fallopian tube or ovary area. This will also release one broad ligament, in which both of the above are enveloped. The practitioner uses one contact onto the iliac crest and anterior superior iliac spine, and fairly strongly pulls this bony contact medially, to create tissue slack in the iliac region of the lower abdomen. The abdominal hand now commences its contact just inferior to the anterior iliac spine, having first eased some skin slack from medial to lateral, so that as the fingers are then eased down medial to the anterior spine, there is sufficient skin slack to allow this. Once the finger has descended past the medial border of psoas (taking care not to place pressure on the iliac vessels in the process), the contact arrives at the level of the ovary and fallopian tube and the fingers can now be very gently eased back medially whilst ensuring that the depth of contact is not lost. If desired, the abdominal contact can be kept still at this point and the iliac crest can be allowed to

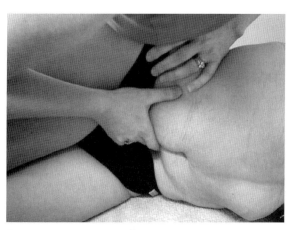

Figure 7.13 Deep uterine/ovarian release.

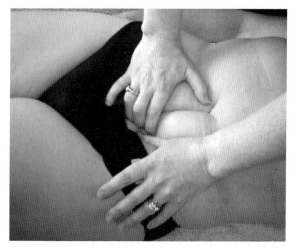

Figure 7.14 Unilateral contact for the fallopian tube or the ovary.

slowly 'spring back' laterally to create the required stretch on the fallopian tube or broad ligament. This is sometimes useful if the abdominal contact is a little sensitive for much direct mobilization.

> ⓘ Note: a technique for the lower portion of the ureter was discussed in Chapter 6, which can be replicated here for the suspensory ligament for the ovary as this runs in the same plane and position as the ureter (both are contained within the renal fascia and both emerge from this as it peters out at the front of the sacroiliac joint level). They both run under the posterior leaf of the broad ligament, one finally passing to the ovary and the other passing to the back of the bladder.

PELVIC FLOOR AND OBTURATOR CONSIDERATIONS

Pelvic floor work is essential to reproductive health in males and females. Direct perineal and levator ani contacts are very useful and are easily performed using an external contact. Techniques that incorporate the obturator foramen are also very useful as the levator ani muscles insert onto the obturator internus muscle, which covers the foramen on its internal surface.

Figure 7.15 shows a perineal contact using the ischial tuberosity and the inferior pubic ramus as a guide. The contact is medial to the ramus and lateral to the labia. The practitioner first locates the ischial tuberosity and then cups the hand around the inner posterior thigh and locates the inner surface of the tuberosity. From here, they must allow the hand to follow along the inner surface, towards the perineum. The hand must not grip the bone and the fingers should be pointing directly to the patient's head and not slightly medially, as this would take them too medially in towards the vagina. The hand should be flexible at the level of the wrist so that any straightening of the wrist will bring the fingers inside the tuberosity and onto the perineum. Many practitioners initially make the mistake of not palpating deeply enough (far enough around) and stay located just on the inferior medial surface of the tuberosity. This will not contact onto the perineum and the hand must be moved around much further so that the fingers can feel the inferior pubic arch and then pass medial to it. In Figure 7.15, the practitioner's hand can pass up into the perineum more than is shown – the fingers are at the starting point of the technique, not the finishing point. The fingers can effectively 'walk up and down' the inferior pubic ramus, palpating and treating all along the urogenital diaphragm and perineum.

Figure 7.16 shows a contact for the obturator foramen. Note that the thumb contact onto the obturator passes posterior to the adductor muscle mass. The practitioner's hand on the patient's thigh is to lift the superficial skin and tissues up towards the knee before the thumb is placed. Whilst holding the skin of the thigh up, the thumb is placed into the obturator area and behind the bulk of the adductor muscle. Note: there is a large 'sulcus' in

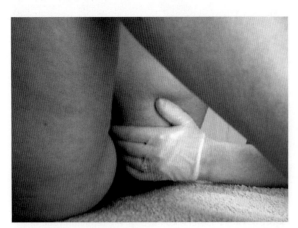

Figure 7.15   Perineal contact.

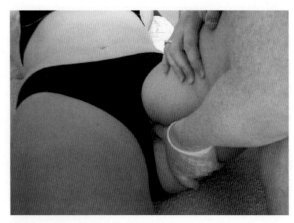

Figure 7.16   Obturator contact.

this section of the thigh between muscles and the thumb and thenar eminence slot nicely into this. The thumb should not be just behind the adductor tendon, as this makes the technique uncomfortable and insufficient contact onto the obturator foramen area will be achieved.

Having placed the thumb, the skin of the thigh can be relaxed and as this settles inferiorly, the thumb can now gently descend (along the line of the leg) onto the pubic bone. The thumb must first contact the bone, to ensure that it is placed far enough along the leg towards the inner hip for the final technique to be successful. Once the bone is located, lift the thumb very slightly and move it laterally, into the neck of the femur area (by easing the whole of the thenar eminence and hand into the flesh of the inner thigh). This gets the thumb contact just lateral to the pubic arch and now the thumb can be gently pushed against the obturator foramen area, which will now be right next to it. From here, inhibition, functional work or other balancing or soft tissue techniques can be employed. This is also the basic contact when a combined obturator/bladder or pelvic organ technique is discussed (whether in the male or the female).

> *i* Note: some techniques for the pelvic floor are also described in Chapter 10. A combined technique for the obturator foramen area and bladder in the male was shown in Chapter 6.

INTERNAL PER VAGINAL AND PER RECTAL TECHNIQUES

Osteopaths can use per rectal and per vaginal techniques for a variety of purposes, which can differ from the traditional medical application of these procedures. Be aware that pelvic pathology and pelvic surgery can radically alter palpatory findings during per rectal and per vaginal examinations.

Patients usually present with a unique set of torsions and tensions and it is not possible to describe the subtle variations in directions needed to manage these tissue dysfunctions; it all depends on how it feels during the examination. As with all osteopathic techniques, a good knowledge of anatomy and pathology will allow the osteopath to categorize

and identify the tissue dysfunctions, enabling the manual treatment to be individualized to the patient. Tissue response is everything during osteopathic treatment and no set protocol can be developed to describe the exact techniques used. The application of standard osteopathic principles will ensure that appropriate management is given.

Latex allergy and informed consent

It is important to establish whether the patient has a latex allergy prior to commencing these techniques, and an alternative type of glove must be available in such cases (even if not used internally, latex can cause irritation to external tissues such as skin, which should be avoided).

The issue of informed consent is also important. Many regulatory bodies have their own protocols for obtaining informed consent for internal techniques or examination and treatment of sensitive areas by osteopaths. The use of deferred examination after explanation (allowing time to consider the proposal), chaperones (although some patients prefer not to have them), and written consent (although not legally foolproof) is usually best practice. It is also worth remembering that many patients may feel comfortable at the time, having listened to various explanations and experienced various tendernesses or tensions when the osteopath performs a general external examination, but may change their view when they discuss the matter with friends or partners (who have not had the benefit of listening first hand or feeling the physical aspects of the external examination). Given careful consideration of the above, most patients are happy to proceed with an internal technique, especially if initial attempts to rectify the problem using external treatments have not achieved the desired outcomes.

The relevant hygiene and waste disposal considerations in the practitioner's own regulatory locale should be adhered to.

PER VAGINAL TECHNIQUES

Figure 7.17 shows a mock internal contact onto the uterus. For this technique, the patient does not need both knees wide apart, as this creates stress and strain at the hips and pubic area. With the patient supine, the feet can be comfortably placed

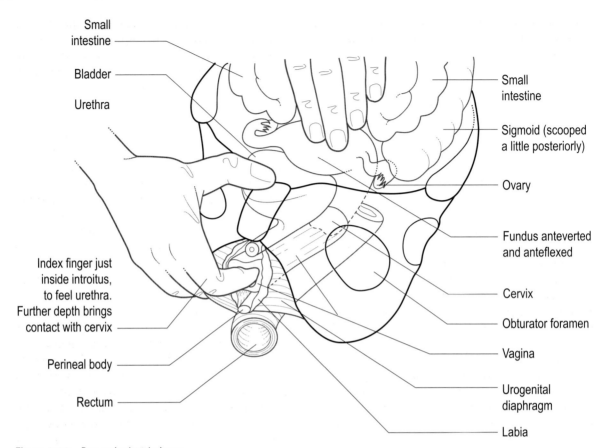

Figure 7.17   Per vaginal techniques.

hip width apart, with the knees above the position of the feet. Usually the practitioner can hold the knee/leg closest to them between their side and their palpating arm. This stabilizes the leg, allows some movement to be induced at the hip and helps create slack. The patient often finds this more comfortable than holding up their own leg. The other leg can remained flexed, can rest down on the table or can be held (by the patient) tucked up against the patient's chest. This latter is useful to allow greater depth of vaginal penetration which may be required if there is retroversion or significant tension in the uterosacral ligaments, for example.

Uterine considerations

One finger is usually inserted into the vagina first. If the vagina is supple enough, two may be introduced but when there is tension or pain in the vagina and internal pelvic region, this may be too

much pressure for patients initially. A two-finger contact allows the cervix to be gently gripped between the two fingers, for better control. However, if only one finger is inserted, then sufficient uterine contact can usually be maintained to allow reasonable release of tissues. The practitioner's other hand is most commonly placed externally on the suprapubic region, to apply some gentle compression onto the fundus of the uterus, to 'stabilize' the internal contact. Once the uterus is held 'between' the two hands, then some gentle movements can be introduced.

Firstly, the overall consistency of the uterus is evaluated; it should feel like a supple and elastic muscular bag. Internal pelvic palpation should not be painful but often is, so proceed with caution and only work within patient tolerances and tissue reaction limits. When feeling between the internal contact and the abdominal hand, the 'articulation' between the cervix and the body of the uterus can be evaluated. The cervix should be pointed posteroinferiorly but may be torsioned into a number of directions. The uterus as a whole should be free to move slightly up and down, forwards and backwards, and side to side. Any restriction should be noted and it is always most helpful to get the patient to compare the sensations and movements in each of the different directions as, if they can perceive differences, they have a much clearer idea of the aim of the technique and how to judge for themselves if change has been achieved.

The abdominal hand can be placed lateral to the uterus so that a general lateral stretch can be applied to the fallopian tube/broad ligaments. Do not forget that a functional or balancing/unwinding technique can also be applied within any of these techniques. This lateral contact is useful to explore the vaginal fornixes and any adnexal restrictions, if sufficient depth can be obtained during the examination. If a posterior or posterolateral cervical contact can be achieved, the cervix can be eased anteriorly or anteromedially/laterally. This will engage the uterosacral ligaments, which connect the lower uterus and cervix posteriorly to the anterior sacrum, piriformis and sacral ligaments. In some women with uterosacral spasm or tension, adhesions or retroversion, it may be very difficult to reach the cervix, as it can be located very deeply or may be twisted in such a position that makes taking a good hold of it difficult. This is also the case if the practitioner has very short fingers. In these situations, the practitioner must be satisfied with a general release. Sometimes a rectal examination may be of value, as discussed below.

Ovarian considerations

The ovaries are not readily palpable unless there is a problem. They are located towards the lateral pelvic walls, slightly further back than the position of the uterus, and often require both hands (internal and external) to work closely together, as they need to engage the sweep of the broad ligament, to find the ovary nestled on its posterior surface. Once located, a local listening/functional or balancing/unwinding technique is often best to ease any surrounding torsions. Much like the kidney, the ovary can 'slip away' from any mobilizing contact due to the arrangement of peritoneal folds that surround it (making it quite mobile in the absence of adhesions).

A per vaginal contact can also be very usefully applied to the bladder, urethra, pelvic floor, rectum and coccyx.

Pelvic floor considerations

When exploring the pelvic floor, the internal contact is first applied just inside the entrance (introitus) where contact is made laterally against the pubococcygeus muscle either side. The finger can be rotated anteriorly, so that the fibres next to the bladder can be palpated, or posteriorly, so that the fibres either side of the rectum can be palpated. In fact, the palpating finger usually sweeps the pelvic floor fibres from front to back, testing the elasticity and tension all around. It may be necessary to swap sides and use the other hand to palpate the contralateral side of the internal pelvic floor (unless the practitioner's wrist is very flexible).

The finger(s) can also be placed in a neutral position in the lower vagina whilst the patient attempts to contract the pelvic floor, to explore weakness due to pudendal nerve damage or other perineal trauma. This contact is useful to help guide the patient to a better appreciation of her pelvic floor, which will help her perform the exercises more effectively (and can encourage her to do so, as patients often find it difficult to tell if they are doing the exercise, and can cease trying due to lack of sensory feedback). A weak pelvic floor can feel very thin and sagging, and the surrounding tissues and vagina can be gaping or feel 'ballooned' out. A tense pelvic floor can feel quite rigid and quite 'disjointed', i.e. patchy tension or spasm is quite common, interspersed with thin 'straggly' sections and quite lumpy or fibrotic scarred sections, especially following episiotomy or other perineal repair.

In cases of prolapse, the pelvic floor can feel as though the levator ani is mimicking a pair of curtains, which have been drawn outwards towards the lateral bony pelvic walls, thereby leaving the midline gaping open. It is as though the folds of the pelvic floor have been 'glued together' so that they now cannot be drawn together to close the vaginal entrance and support the pelvic organs (a bit like adhesive capsulitis not allowing glenohumeral abduction). In such cases, the pelvic floor needs to be drawn medially so that the fibres are 'separated out' again, allowing a more natural closure mechanism to operate.

The pelvic floor can also be helped by work on the perineal body, which is contacted directly posteriorly, on the lowest part of the posterior vaginal wall in front of the rectum. Often an inhibition against this is useful, or a functional unwinding, to help balance all the varied fibres of the pelvic floor in their different alignments to reestablish a better resting position. Per vaginal and per rectal coccyx techniques are discussed below, which can also be very useful for pelvic floor dysfunctions.

Bladder considerations

When testing the bladder, the abdominal hand is usually placed a little lower than for the uterus, this time just above the symphysis pubis. It may be necessary to work 'around the edges' of the rectus in order to feel sufficiently retropubically to gain a good release of the bladder.

When feeling anteriorly, the tube of the urethra and the bulge of the external urethral sphincter are very easily palpated through the anterior wall of the vagina (the vagina does not palpate like a thick muscular coat over these structures – they bulge into the vaginal 'space'). The finger only needs to be a centimetre or two inside the vagina to feel the urethra and sphincter up against the inside of the symphysis pubis joint. Passing any deeper will mean that when the finger presses against the pubis, the bladder neck and trigone (midsection of the posterior wall of the bladder) will be felt. This deeper contact can, of course, be used to palpate these structures, as required. The urethra should be elastic longitudinally and should be able to be 'rolled' from side to side. It should not feel buckled, twisted or shortened. The bladder neck is also tested for lateral freedom, and for a supple flexibility underneath the main part of the bladder. Contacting just either side of the bladder neck and pressing into the obturator muscle/face of the pubis makes a very good release for the pubovesical ligaments, especially if coupled with a good abdominal hand contact from the outside (just above the superior pubic arch, near the medial inguinal ligament).

The side walls of the bladder can be explored by progressively passing slightly deeper into the vagina and continuing to 'walk up' the internal

face of the obturator area and pubis. Indeed, this particular variation can be adjusted to allow exploration of the superficial inguinal ring area, which is very useful for round ligament treatment and cases of hernia. This area is also often compromised after caesarean section or other lower abdominal surgery. Beware that bladder or uterine resuspension surgery will create some very individualized tense bands of suturing, scarring or tension, which are not resolvable (only their consequences). Also note that weak pelvic tissues are not very responsive in general and even a small change should be of benefit to the patient. In cases of cystocoele, the aim of any treatment is not so much to just lift up the bladder directly but to ensure there is nothing tethering the bladder in an inferior direction, and to create better tissue balance and feel so that more 'normal' tissue activity is reestablished, allowing the body to draw up the bladder and support it better from below by itself.

Feeling superiorly and anteriorly within the vagina will enable the practitioner to explore the retrovesical pouch, and feeling posteriorly and superiorly will allow exploration of the pouch of Douglas. Feeling posteriorly will allow examination of the coccyx and rectum, which is discussed below.

Coccyx and rectal considerations

Feeling posteriorly in the vagina will explore the rectum, posterior pelvic floor and coccyx. The rectum will feel like a firm, flexible tube, which is much larger in diameter than the urethra. The curve of the rectum can be followed by moving the internal finger from side to side, whilst rotated to face posteriorly. Direct treatment can be applied to the rectum if required. If the finger passes either side of the bulge of the rectum, it will arrive in the posterior fold of vagina that is lateral to the rectum, allowing the finger to come up against the lateral rectal ligaments, the posterior attachments of the levator ani, and the lateral coccyx and sacrococcygeal ligaments. In fact, this per vaginal coccyx examination is often preferable to a rectal contact, especially if there are haemorrhoids, spasm of the rectum or posterior pelvic floor or marked coccygeal inflammation, or where the patient does not wish a rectal examination for other reasons.

The practitioner's other hand can now be moved so that it can palpate the coccyx from outside, from the back. Whilst the internal finger maintains its position, ask the patient to gently and slightly rotate the pelvis (lifting one buttock up off the table a little), allowing the practitioner to slide their free hand under the back of the lower pelvis. The finger tips should be placed on the external surface of the coccyx and the patient asked to resettle the pelvis back on the table. Now the practitioner has a very effective contact on both sides of the coccyx and can apply a focused functional or unwinding/balancing technique, a direct inhibition technique or a strong stretch and mobilization as required. Stretching the pelvic floor in a posterior direction is very easy in this variation, as is mobilizing the coccyx in a backwards arcing direction (restoring more normal pelvic tissue alignment, support and action).

PER RECTAL TECHNIQUES – FEMALE

Figure 7.18 shows a mock per rectal examination. The prone position is the most common, although

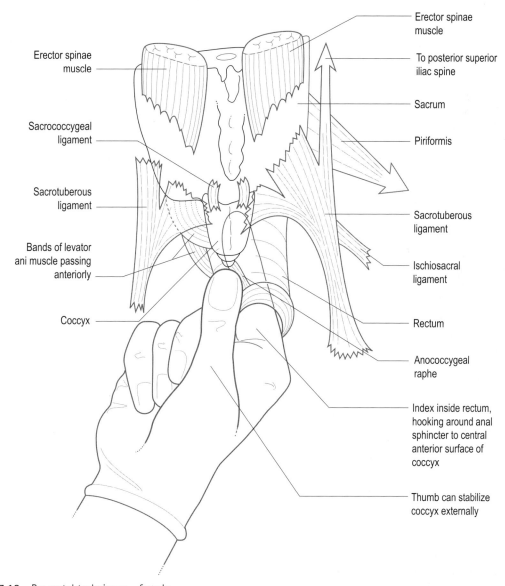

Figure 7.18 Per rectal techniques – female.

it can be performed sidelying, with some adaptation. When performing per rectal examination, warn the patient in advance that gas may be released as the finger is withdrawn and that some of the tissues could be quite tender or painful. If a highly sensitive area is touched without any warning, then the patient often lifts their pelvis and the rectal sphincter can spasm, and they find it difficult to relax through the rest of the technique. Discussing this in advance means the reactions are usually less severe, thus enabling the technique to be more efficiently applied. Haemorrhoids are usually a caution and if they are anything other than small and unobtrusive, the per rectal technique should be avoided (unless strong coccygeal torsions cannot be released any other way). Some light bleeding may occur after per rectal examination where haemorrhoids are present. Rectal examinations can detect masses or other palpatory findings that are not usual, and if present, the patient should be referred for medical examination, as indicated.

When entering the rectum, use sufficient lubrication and remember that initially the rectum is angled towards the head and the table (when the patient is lying on their front). The practitioner's palm can face the ceiling to begin with but if this does not allow easy access past the anal sphincter, start inserting the finger with the palm facing the table, which will allow some pressure to be exerted towards the perineal body and can make entry more comfortable. In this situation, having passed into the rectum a few centimetres, the finger should be rotated so that the practitioner's palm is now facing the ceiling.

Either way, the internal finger can then start to hook around the thick bulk of the anal sphincter and be eased towards the coccyx. The rest of the rectum is at an opposing angle to the very lowest part so, having passed deep to the anal sphincter, the rectum is now oriented towards the sacrum (ceiling when the patient is lying prone). Try to avoid direct contact onto the tip of the coccyx as this can be quite painful; try to contact on the face or on the sacrococcygeal joint line. The practitioner can mobilize the coccyx to and fro against the sacrum and can also perform soft tissue stretches or releases by gently moving the internal finger slightly to one side of the coccyx or the other. If required, the practitioner's other hand can take a contact (with one or two finger tips) on the external surface of the back of the coccyx, which will allow a bimanual mobilization or balancing of the coccyx and surrounding tissues.

If the internal finger is now rotated again so that it faces towards one side or the other, the uterosacral ligaments can often be explored. (Note that, unless the practitioner's wrist is very flexible, it may be necessary to change hands and reenter the rectum whilst standing on the other side of the patient to explore the contralateral pelvic floor or other tissues.) These feel like bands running either side of the rectum and can be quite tense. Often one side is more torsioned or tense than the other. If the finger is rotated fully anteriorly, then it can press into the posterior wall of the vagina, where the lower part of the uterus and cervix can sometimes be explored. The cervix can be eased anteriorly and released in cases of retroversion or posterior torsion. In retroversion, the fundus of the uterus sometimes pushes directly into the anterior wall of the rectum and can easily be palpated. Otherwise, the fundus of the uterus and the ovaries are not palpable per rectum.

> (i) Note: many of the pelvic floor and sacro-coccygeal techniques discussed below under the male reproductive system can also be used on women. Release of any pelvic floor tensions or imbalances is essential when any pelvic organ work is performed, and management of general pelvic problems in women is not complete without an accurate and detailed exploration of the pelvic floor and perineum.

EXAMINATION AND TREATMENT – MALE REPRODUCTIVE SYSTEM

PROSTATE AND PELVIC FLOOR

There are many contacts for the pelvic floor and only a few are shown here. Often, the bony parts of the pelvis and the general pelvic soft tissues need to be rebalanced when work on the pelvic floor is performed, and Figures 7.19 and 7.20 show sacral or sacroiliac contacts to achieve this. In Figure 7.19, one hand is covering the sacrum and the other is placed over the lower abdomen, for countercontact on the

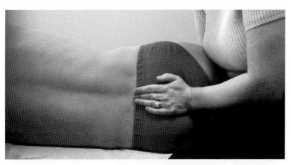

Figure 7.19   Sacral contact for general pelvic organ and pelvic floor release.

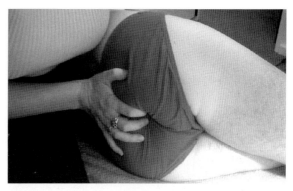

Figure 7.21   Coccyx contact.

pelvic tissues. It can also be placed directly onto the superior pubic arch and symphysis pubis, although in males in this sidelying position the genitals may get in the way. In females, it makes a very good way of balancing the superior pelvic ring. Once the bilateral contact is in place, the two hands slightly compress together to engage the deeper pelvic tissues. A general unwinding and release of the sacrum will balance out and ease any tissues attaching to it (be it dura, muscles, thoracolumbar fascia or pelvic floor, for example).

Figure 7.20 shows an adaptation where the posterior contact changes so that the index and thumb can palpate along the sacroiliac joint line. This makes a very useful 'entry' into the sacroiliac joint space, which can help to address general pelvic torsions quite effectively. Again, a functional or unwinding/balancing approach is best with this contact. The anterior hand can remain the same as before or be placed onto the lateral

buttock, greater trochanter or iliac crest, to engage slightly different aspects of the hip or pelvis as required.

Figure 7.21 shows a contact for the coccyx. Two fingers are placed either side of the coccyx and can engage its bony margins or move very slightly laterally to engage the sacrococcygeal ligaments. The palm can rest against the bulk of the sacrum. The anterior contact is suprapubically, as before (given that the practitioner is now facing the other way and so the fingers will point to the pubis). The aim is to follow the torsions and tensions local to the coccyx and to balance any adverse soft tissue tensions acting at this point. The anterior contact will help focus the technique towards the pelvic floor (if it contacts onto the pubic arch) or the pelvic organs (if it remains suprapubically).

Figures 7.22 and 7.23 show a simple technique to access both sides of the pelvic floor, without moving the practitioner or the patient. Examination gloves

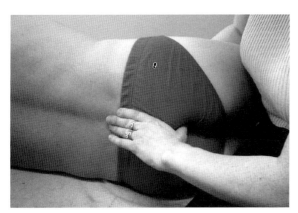

Figure 7.20   Thumb and index contacting along line of sacroiliac joint.

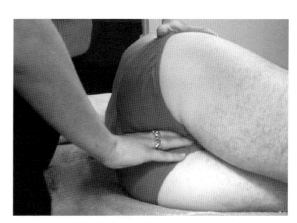

Figure 7.22   Pelvic floor release, lower side.

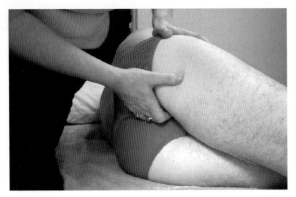

Figure 7.23 Pelvic floor release, upper side.

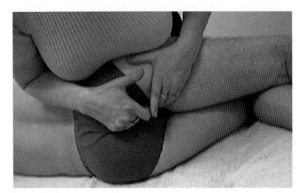

Figure 7.24 Global ilial and pelvic floor release.

can be worn as required. Initially the practitioner can palpate the pelvic floor on the lower side of the pelvis, by finding the medial border of the ischial tuberosity and then sliding the index fingers directly across its surface so that the finger sweeps over the inferior pubic arch and into the pelvic floor tissues. The finger pads can stay in close proximity to the bone and can be moved in and out and up and down, to work through various sections of the posterior pelvic floor, as shown in Figure 7.22.

Now the practitioner can swap the contact and this time palpate on the medial/inner surface of the ischial tuberosity on the side of the patient's pelvis facing the ceiling. This time the third, fourth and fifth fingers are used as the palpating contact and the technique is the same in that the hand moves either up or down the inferior pubic arch, and swings inwards to the pelvic floor as required. In both techniques, the practitioner's other hand can stabilize the rest of the pelvis by contacting the lateral hip/iliac crest. This hand can also be used to move the pelvis 'over' the palpating hand if this is best kept static (where the pelvic floor is very tender, for example).

Figure 7.24 shows a version of a pelvic floor technique that is also discussed in Chapter 10. This technique employs a 'floating' articulation of the ilium on the sacrum to create a different set of tension patterns and releases in the pelvic floor. The practitioner's hands are contacting around the posterior inferior iliac spine and the posterior aspect of the ischial tuberosity. The practitioner's diaphragm area is gently compressed against the anterior iliac crest, to help mobilize and orient the ilium, thereby allowing the palpating hands to do that rather than have to shift the ilium as well.

This contact can be adjusted to allow the practitioner to 'flare' the ischial tuberosity 'upwards and away from' the other side, giving a sort of spreading and opening to the inferior pelvic bowl. This can be used to stretch the sacroiliac and ischiosacral ligaments or indirectly act on the pelvic floor, as required. Fairly strong compression on the anterior iliac crest aids the stretch element at the posterior inferior pelvis. This type of stretch is particularly useful in males, and where there have been chronic coccygeal injury and pelvic congestion, or haemorrhoids, for example.

Having explored a variety of posterior pelvic floor techniques, one for the perineum should also be described, as this contact is more influential on the prostate. The others will all help prostatic problems indirectly but the supine technique shown in Figure 7.25 is far more effective and can be used for routine prostatic mobilization and massage, saving repeated per rectal techniques for this purpose.

Figure 7.25 shows the patient supine and the practitioner contacting onto the anterior perineum, lateral to the base of the penis but medial to the inferior pubic arch. It is often best to allow the knee of the patient to rest against the practitioner's shoulder so that the leg can relax, and the practitioner can use their own body movements to control leg and therefore hip/pelvic alignment as required. The perineal contact is initially a little complex to get right but after some practice is very efficient.

SPERMATIC CORD, TESTES, INGUINAL RINGS

There is often a need to examine and treat the spermatic cord and/or testes. The spermatic cord

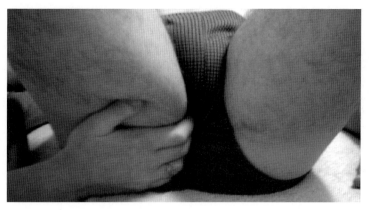

Figure 7.25   Supine release of the urogenital diaphragm and prostate.

contact is performed at the level of the superficial inguinal canal or over the face of the pubis, as shown in Figure 7.26. The spermatic cord will palpate like a thick venous cord over the face of the pubis and should not be tender, contracted, swollen or bound down. Care should be taken not to press very firmly or the cord will be irritated and the contact become painful. Gentle mobilization can be applied or a functional/balancing unwinding applied to the cord directly or through the inguinal canal area (if the palpating contact is shifted to the lower abdomen, accordingly). Testicular unwinding can be performed, again after explanation to and consent from the patient. The practitioner will gently take one testis in the fingers and thumb of one hand and gently unwind or release

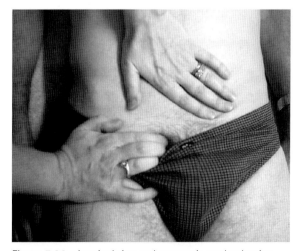

Figure 7.26   Inguinal ring and spermatic cord palpation.

any torsion patterns found. This also can be accompanied by a contact on the spermatic cord in the inguinal region, or suprapubically (to affect down to the posterior/inferior bladder, prostate and seminal vesicles), for example.

PER RECTAL TECHNIQUES – MALE

Per rectal techniques can be used to examine and treat the rectum, coccyx, pelvic floor and prostate. The seminal vesicles are not readily palpable but can be released by working on any anterior rectal or prostatic tensions present. Similar cautions as discussed for females apply to males when considering the use of per rectal techniques. Sometimes the per rectal techniques can be performed with the patient bent over the couch or table, so that the hips are flexed but the patient is not in a sidelying position (or the patient can lie prone over some pillows). Using a sidelying technique can be more awkward as it does not allow easy access to both sides of the pelvic floor or prostate without strain on the practitioner's wrist or hand. Take care to advise the patient in advance that some discomfort may be experienced after prostatic massage if circulation and drainage are improved and the tissues start to decongest. Usually, any per rectal techniques are performed only so long as required to release the tissues involved and should not persist to the point of pain. In most cases, the patient is relieved of symptoms following a per rectal examination and treatment.

Figure 7.27 shows a mock per rectal examination on the male pelvis. The descriptions given

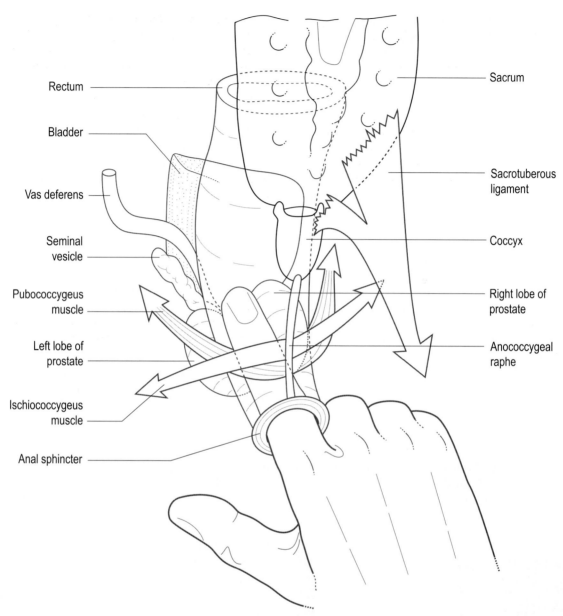

Figure 7.27 Per rectal techniques – male.

above for the use of this technique in women also apply to men regarding angle of entry into the rectum and the initial direction that the palpating finger points in (towards the ceiling or to the table). Once the palpating finger is within the rectum, it can be adjusted to enable work on the coccyx or posterior pelvic floor (aided by an external coccyx or sacral contact as desired). The finger can also explore the prostate, when it is pointed towards the pubis (table, with the patient prone).

Palpating anteriorly through the wall of the rectum allows access to the prostate. The two lobes and their intervening groove should be easily felt and the prostate should be slightly firm but smooth, as though the surface is slightly slippery. It is not normally tender. Care should be taken not to press too firmly. The finger can pass to one side of the prostate or the other, and then try to gently push or move the prostate into the midline, so as to mobilize it between the two inferior pubic arches.

There should be a small amount of give, and the prostate should not feel tense or stiff. Gentle rhythmic mobilization often eases prostatic tensions after a moment or two, and can also relax surrounding tissues.

Direct massaging of the prostate can be performed which is useful in cases of benign hypertrophy or with chronic prostatitis, for example. To massage the prostate, the finger is usually swept in lateral to medial movements across one lobe (repeating this from the top to the bottom) and then the other. Care should be taken not to overstimulate the prostate or to fatigue or irritate prostatic or anal tissues. The practitioner can also ease the palpating finger towards the pubis, against the perineal body to stretch the pelvic floor away from the coccyx (rather than to create any further penetration by the finger). This stretching of the pelvic floor and perineal body away from the coccyx can be very effective in diffusing hyperstimulated pelvic floor problems, with a high resting tone and chronic pain and dysfunction. This can be coupled with the use of respiratory assistance by the patient, if desired.

References

1. Chen CH, Huang MH, Chen TW, Weng MC, Lee CL, Wang GJ. Relationship between ankle position and pelvic floor muscle activity in female stress urinary incontinence. Urology 2005;66(2):288-92.
2. Pool-Goudzwaard A, Van Dijke GH, Van Gurp M, Mulder P, Snijders C, Stoeckart R. Contribution of pelvic floor muscles to stiffness of the pelvic ring. Clin Biomech (Bristol) 2004;19(6):564-71.
3. O'Sullivan PB, Beales DJ, Beetham JA, et al. Altered motor control strategies in subjects with sacroiliac joint pain during the active straight-leg-raise test. Spine 2002;27(1):E1-8.

Chapter 8

Overview of vascular, endocrine and immune systems

CHAPTER CONTENTS

Chapter contents continues

This chapter includes the vascular (blood and lymph) systems, as well as the endocrine and immune systems. These are all highly interrelated functionally and physiologically and should be considered as extensions of each other. The nervous system clearly has a huge influence on these systems as well, which should not be overlooked.

VASCULAR SYSTEM

Most people first contemplating the subject of visceral osteopathy would probably imagine that it relates to the management of such things as asthma, irritable bowel syndrome and possibly postsurgical adhesion pain and discomfort. Not many would initially consider the vascular system as an organ and therefore might think that it would lie outside the interest of a 'visceral osteopath'. Nothing could be further from the truth. In fact, all osteopaths need to incorporate fluid mechanics within their overall patient management, whether they are treating patients with sprained ankles or ligamentous strain of the knee, or working with carpal tunnel and other fluid retention problems, let alone any 'visceral conditions' including oedema and/or varicosities, for example. Blood and lymph circulation is essential for homeostasis, healing and immunity, and therefore is a central part of patient management, whatever the presentation.

Many visceral conditions are influenced by local and general fluid mechanics and it is essential for homeostasis that efficient blood and lymph transport and circulation are maintained. This is true of whole-body fluid circulation as well as local organ circulation. In previous chapters, neural and postural influences on fluid movement have been introduced and any patient needing a 'circulatory' treatment should have those general factors investigated and treated where necessary. Such problems could include pelvic venous congestion, ischaemic bowel problems (representing an imbalance in total blood flow distribution, i.e. not enough reaching gastrointestinal vascular beds), portal venous circulation problems, any condition with fluid congestion and oedema, such as chronic lung diseases and endometriosis, for example.

General examination and treatments could include:

- global postural assessment
- calf pumps
- thoracic diaphragm function
- pelvic floor function
- thoracic inlet and mediastinal releases
- work to relevant affected areas of the spinal column for neural reflex components (listed below).

Circulatory problems also include conditions affecting the cardiovascular and renal systems and there are many hypotheses about how osteopaths may influence such factors as essential hypertension or cardiac arrhythmias (in particular situations). Management of patients suffering chest discomfort following cardiac surgery may also be supported by contributing osteopathic techniques to the patient's care routine. There are many other scenarios where lymphatic and circulatory management would be beneficial and this chapter will give a basic outline of the examination and treatment of vascular structures.

Many of the examinations and treatments for the blood vascular system are based on the principle that to maintain laminar flow (as opposed to turbulent flow, this being very damaging and stressful to artery linings), vessels must be evenly supported, not torsioned along their length or externally compressed or irritated by soft tissue tensions and restrictions. Maintaining an even soft tissue environment for the vessels not only helps to maintain the patency of the arterial and venous system but also reduces local neural irritation to sympathetic fibres travelling with and serving the arterial tree.

SURFACE ANATOMY

Table 8.1 shows musculoskeletal landmarks for the larger components of the vascular system.

Heart

The major component of the vascular system is the heart. Standard anatomical texts give sufficient descriptions of the location of major arteries and veins so these will not be repeated here.

The heart develops embryologically as a consequence of mechanical influences caused by increasing fluid flow through the early vascular system. The heart originates as a tube, which then twists and spirals in a pattern established by those flow mechanics. Eventually, the heart chambers form and fetal circulation, with its unique links to the placenta, integrates the activity of the heart into existing flow dynamics. The heart also starts in the throat and has to descend as the embryo develops. This descent is the cause of the looping

Table 8.1 Musculoskeletal landmarks for the vascular system

Vascular structure	Musculoskeletal landmark	Comments
Carotid sinus and Body	Cervical fascia, superior to the upper border of the middle of sternocleidomastoid	Neck and throat mechanics, and those of the thoracic inlet are important for the fascia in which the carotid vessels are enclosed, and hence important to these baroreceptors
Mesenteric baroreceptors	Posterior abdominal wall	Posterior abdominal wall mesocolon, Toldt's fascia and the root of the mesentery are important sites for proposed mesenteric baroreceptors
Heart	The heart is retrosternal and projects slightly to the left of the midline. Its superior extent is level with the space between the 2nd and 3rd costal cartilages; the right side of the heart follows the line of the right costochondral articulations, between cartilage 4 and 7; the inferior border of the heart is level with the xiphisternal articulation; the left–hand extent of the heart is at the midclavicular line, in the 5th and 6th intercostal spaces	Chest mechanics and throat – mediastinal tension patterns are important
Valves	Aortic valve – midline sternum, between the insertions of the 3rd and 4th costal cartilages Pulmonary valve – left border of sternum at level of 3rd costal cartilage Mitral valve – left side of sternum, near insertion of 4th costal cartilage Tricuspid valve – right side of the sternum, near the insertion of the 4th costal cartilage	Mediastinal tensions and the dynamics of the posterior wall of the heart are important (note: levels given in previous box are for the anatomical surface landmarks, not where the valve sounds are best heard. This is to enable more appropriate hand placement during techniques)
Axillary region	Between the pectoralis major and latissimus dorsi muscles	Axillary fascia supports the axillary vessels and this, coupled with clavicular and thoracic inlet mechanics (for the subclavian vessels), is important for upper limb vascular function

Continued

Table 8.1   Musculoskeletal landmarks for the vascular system—cont'd

Vascular structure	Musculoskeletal landmark	Comments
Femoral triangle region	Superficial to adductor magnus, lateral to pectineus and inferior to the inguinal canal	Hip and groin mechanics are important for the femoral triangle mechanics and lower limb vascular function (as are, to a lesser extent, those of the pubis and sacroiliac joint)
Aorta	Median arcuate ligament of the thoracic diaphragm	Tension in this region can potentially impede or disrupt aortic flow
Coeliac trunk	Median arcuate ligament of the thoracic diaphragm	Midline diaphragmatic torsions can be important for coeliac trunk function
Superior mesenteric artery and vein	Root of mesentery anterior to the mid lumbar spine	Upper and mid lumbar spinal tensions are also important for mesenteric circulation
Deep leg veins	Calf muscles	The venous 'calf pump', foot, knee and general lower limb-pelvic girdle mechanics are influential

arrangements of some of the autonomic fibres serving the heart which, as it descends to be located in the chest just above the diaphragm, drags its nerves and the phrenic nerves with it (which pass to the diaphragm). The heart is situated posterior to the sternum, as described above in Table 8.1 which also lists the anatomical surface anatomy points for the heart valves.

LIGAMENTS AND SUPPORTS

Heart

The fascial and pericardial arrangements for the heart were introduced in Chapter 4. The major ligaments are the vertebropericardial ligament, the sternopericardial ligament, the pericardial attachments to the diaphragm, and the superior mediastinal fascial attachments of the pericardium to the thoracic inlet and cervical fascias (linking ultimately to the cranial base via the pharyngobasilar fascia).

Upper limb vascular structures

Axillary fascial mechanics are important. Understanding the compartment anatomy of the upper limb will give an understanding of how the vessels within the upper limb, wrist and hand can become physically compromised and therefore dysfunctional. For example, carpal mechanics and those of the interosseous membrane

(including radial and elbow mechanics) will influence vessel dynamics in the forearm. Shoulder girdle, clavicular and axillary mechanics as well as those of the upper ribs will influence the vessel dynamics of the upper arm.

Lower limb vascular structures

Femoral triangle fascial mechanics are important. Understanding the compartment anatomy of the lower limb will give an understanding of how the vessels within the leg, ankle and foot can become physically compromised and therefore dysfunctional. For example, arch mechanics, the subtalar joint, ankle and interosseous membrane dynamics (including fibular and knee mechanics) will influence the lower leg vessel dynamics and function. Hip, knee and pelvic mechanics will influence the upper leg vessel dynamics.

REFLEX RELATIONSHIPS

Table 8.2 shows the reflex relationships for the vascular system.

VEINS, ARTERIES AND LYMPHATICS

Table 8.3 shows blood and lymph vessels to the heart and vasculature. The visceral ligaments and fascial conduits that contain the blood vessels are important, as work on those structures will influence venous drainage, blood flow (as ligamentous

Table 8.2 Reflex relationships for the vascular system

Organ	Anatomical name	Somatic level/relationship
Heart		
Sympathetic – spinal cord	T1–4	T1–4
Sympathetic – paravertebral chain ganglia	Mostly via cervical chain ganglia	
Sympathetic – plexus	Superficial cardiac plexus – inferior to arch of aorta receives fibres from the left sympathetic trunk and vagus	Pericardial and mediastinal mechanics are important
	Deep cardiac plexus – behind the arch on the bifurcation of the trachea receives fibres from both sympathetic trunks and both vagus nerves	
Parasympathetic	Vagus – right vagus serves the AV node, and the left serves the SA node	Upper cervical spine and cranial base
Cerebral circulation		
Sympathetic – spinal cord	T1–4	T1–4
Sympathetic – paravertebral chain ganglia	Via cervical chain ganglia	Upper ribs are important, as is thoracic inlet and upper cervical spine
Sympathetic – plexus	Fibres follow vertebral and carotid arteries to circle of Willis and other cranial vessels	Cranial base mechanics and movements of upper cervical spine are important
Parasympathetic	Vascular control mostly influenced by sympathetics	Upper cervical spine and cranial base
Upper limb vascular beds		
Sympathetic – spinal cord	T2–8	T2–8
Sympathetic – paravertebral chain ganglia	Rib 2–8	General chest mechanics are important
Sympathetic – plexus	Fibres follow upper limb arteries	Axillary fascia is important, as are arm fascial compartments
Parasympathetic	Vascular control mostly influenced by sympathetics	Upper cervical spine and cranial base
Lower limb vascular beds		
Sympathetic – spinal cord	T11–L2	T11–L2
Sympathetic – paravertebral chain ganglia	Lower 2 ribs	Dorsolumbar junction and arcuate ligament mechanics are important
Sympathetic – plexus	Fibres follow lower arteries	Femoral triangle fascia is important, as are lower limb fascial compartments
Parasympathetic	Vascular control mostly influenced by sympathetics	Upper cervical spine and cranial base
Gut vascular beds		
Sympathetic – spinal cord	T5–L2	T5–L2
Sympathetic – paravertebral chain ganglia	Mid to lower ribs	General chest and diaphragm mechanics are important
Sympathetic – plexus	Coeliac, superior and inferior mesenteric	Lumbar spine and posterior abdominal wall mechanics are important (especially psoas and the root of the mesentery)
Parasympathetic	Vascular control mostly influenced by sympathetics	Upper cervical spine and cranial base
Renal vascular bed (kidney)		
Sympathetic – spinal cord	T10–11 mostly; can be to L1	Lower dorsal spine and dorsolumbar junction

Continued

Table 8.2   Reflex relationships for the vascular system—cont'd

Organ	Anatomical name	Somatic level/relationship
Sympathetic – paravertebral chain ganglia	T10–11	Lower ribs
Sympathetic – plexus	Renal, from the aortic and coeliac plexi, the lowest splanchnic nerve and the first lumbar nerve	Dorsolumbar junction
Parasympathetic	No supply to kidney tissue	

torsion may affect the arteries/arterioles and the sympathetic nerves that course along their length) and lymphatic drainage, all of which are important for organ health. The somatic relations also indicate where the musculoskeletal system may be engaged to aid fluid movement in the structures concerned.

IMMUNE SYSTEM

This section includes the general lymphatic vessels, bone marrow, spleen and thymus. The tonsils and adenoids were included in Chapter 4.

Osteopaths often become involved in the management of patients with a variety of allergic problems, such as asthma and eczema, and patients with compromised immune systems, such as with cancer and immunodeficiency syndromes, for example. Often the osteopathic role in these cases is supportive and is not designed to replace orthodox care but to complement it, to support the patient's body in their own self-healing and self-regulatory attempts. There are many techniques where the osteopath can hypothesize that they are removing barriers to efficient lymphatic and immune function, which may be of benefit in a number of clinical presentations. This section will give a basic review of some of those.

SURFACE ANATOMY

Table 8.4 shows musculoskeletal landmarks for the immune system.

Spleen

The spleen is an immunological blood filter and red blood recycling unit. One or more small splenic masses may develop in one of the peritoneal folds early in fetal life. An accessory spleen is present in about 10% of individuals, commonly situated near

Table 8.3   Blood and lymph vessels for major vascular structures

Organ	Anatomical name	Fascial/ligamentous relation	Somatic relation, where applicable
Veins	Coronary veins – collecting together in the coronary sinus, lying between the left atrium and ventricle, and opens into the right atrium	Pericardial mechanics and vertebropericardial and sternopericardial ligaments	Cervical, throat and mediastinal mechanics through to the diaphragm and upper gastrointestinal tract are all important
Arteries	Coronary arteries, off the aorta, just beyond the ventricular outlet	Pericardial mechanics and vertebropericardial and sternopericardial ligaments	Cervical, throat and mediastinal mechanics through to the diaphragm and upper gastrointestinal tract are all important
Lymphatics	Anterior and posterior mediastinal nodes	Mediastinal fascia	Chest and thoracic inlet mechanics are important

Table 8.4 Musculoskeletal landmarks for the immune system

Immune structure	Musculoskeletal Landmark	Comments
CNS		
Perivascular spaces	Throughout the skull	Please refer to standard anatomy text
Subarachnoid space	Throughout the skull	Please refer to standard anatomy text
Arachnoid villi	Throughout the skull	Please refer to standard anatomy text
Dural venous sinuses	Throughout the skull	Please refer to standard anatomy text
Systemic		
Right and left thoracic ducts – venous entry	Just above the medial end of the clavicles, about one-third of the way from the sternal end	Entry into the venous system is at the junction between the jugular and subclavian/brachiocephalic veins
Thoracic duct	Runs along the front of the dorsal spine	Emerges from the abdominal cavity through the medial arcuate ligament (aorta) or the medial arcuate ligament (psoas), making diaphragmatic and mediastinal mechanics important
Cysterna chyli	Anterior to the psoas and other muscle of the posterior abdominal wall, posterior to the renal fascia and the duodenum	Influenced by the mechanics of the upper lumbar region of the posterior abdominal wall and associated viscera
Regional lymph nodes	Distributed widely	Influenced by local articulatory and soft tissue dynamics (refer to standard anatomical texts)
Spleen	Along the axis of the 10th rib on the left, no more anteriorly than the midaxillary line	Extends from the 9th to the 11th ribs and is usually lateral to the posterior equivalent of the midclavicular line. Lower rib mechanics are important
Thymus	Superior mediastinum, retrosternally	In a child the thymus extends superiorly to the thyroid gland, and it shrinks with age to be confined within the mediastinum

the hilum of the main spleen or adjacent to the tail of the pancreas. However, an accessory spleen may also occur along the splenic vessels, in the gastrosplenic or splenorenal ligaments, within the pancreatic tail, in the wall of the stomach or bowel, in the greater omentum or the mesentery or even in the pelvis and scrotum.[1]

Thymus

This is involved in the maturation of T-cells and is located is the superior mediastinum. It is very large in the child (and envelops the upper heart and major blood vessels in the superior mediastinum) and can extend as superiorly as the bottom of the thyroid cartilage. As it shrinks during adolescence and adulthood, it comes to reside retrosternally and is much smaller in relation to heart than before.

Bone marrow

This is concerned with the production of immune system cells. At birth and in childhood, all bones contain red marrow. At maturity and after, the red marrow is mainly contained only in certain bones (vertebrae, cranial bones, sternum, clavicles, ribs, ilium, scapulae, proximal humeri and femurs).

Nutrient foramina (passage of nutrient artery and vein)

- *Humerus* – medial border, about halfway down, just below the insertion of coracobrachialis.
- *Clavicle* – posterior surface (facing root of neck), about halfway along, where the curve of the bone changes, lateral to the insertion of sternohyoideus.
- *Ilium* – on the inner surface of the ala, towards the middle of the lower part of the iliac fossa,

just above the arcuate line and at the lower border of the insertion of iliacus.

- *Scapula* – on the inferior portion of the spine of the scapula, in the centre of the infraspinatus fossa, covered by insertion of infraspinatus.
- *Ribs* – posterior surface of the neck of the ribs (near the transverse process articulation).
- *Femur* – about halfway down the medial aspect of the shaft, just medial to the linea aspera and the insertion of vastus medialis.

Lymph nodes

These are an immunological filter and are found extensively through the body. Main collections are at the proximal limbs (axilla and hip), the pelvis, posterior abdominal wall, abdominal mesenteries, mediastinum and neck.

LIGAMENTS AND SUPPORTS

Spleen

The spleen develops in the top of the greater omentum, between the upper part of the greater curvature of the stomach and the posterior abdominal wall. It is surrounded by the peritoneum and it is effectively suspended from the stomach, diaphragm and the renal fascia, and the splenic flexure of the colon is suspended off the spleen. These peritoneal relations make up four principal ligaments of the spleen: the gastrosplenic ligament, the colicosplenic ligament, the phrenocolic ligament (where this extends beyond the flexure of the colon's attachment to the diaphragm, onto the spleen) and the phrenosplenic (splenorenal/lienorenal) ligament. There are two portions to the gastrosplenic ligament: upper and lower, with the upper portion containing more collagen fibres and appearing more dense.[2]

Thymus

The thymus can extend superiorly as far as the thyroid and inferiorly as far as the fourth costal cartilages, in the child. The thymus is arranged in two lobes which drape over the heart, in between it, the sternum and the lungs. It is embedded in the fascia of the anterosuperior mediastinum and as such is linked with the mechanics of the transversus thoracis, the sternum and manubrium, the superior extensions of the pleural costomediastinal recesses and the superior extensions of the sternopericardial ligament, the heart and the lungs, the larynx, thoracic inlet and the thyroid cartilage, tongue and temporomandibular joint.

REFLEX RELATIONSHIPS

Table 8.5 shows reflex relationships for the immune system.

VEINS, ARTERIES AND LYMPHATICS

Table 8.6 shows blood and lymph vessels of the immune system. The visceral ligaments and fascial

Table 8.5 Reflex relationships for the immune system		
Organ	Anatomical name	Somatic level/relationship
Spleen		
Sympathetic – spinal cord	T5–9	T5–9
Sympathetic – paravertebral chain ganglia	Mid ribcage	Mid ribcage/chest mechanics are important
Sympathetic – plexus	Coeliac and superior mesenteric plexi	Subdiaphragmatic mechanics are important
Parasympathetic	Vagus	Upper cervical spine
Thymus		
Sympathetic – spinal cord	T1–4	T1–4
Sympathetic – paravertebral chain ganglia	Inferior cervical/stellate ganglion	Thoracic inlet mechanics are important
Sympathetic – plexus	Direct fibres 0from ganglion	Thoracic inlet mechanics are important
Parasympathetic	Vagus	Upper cervical spine

Continued

Table 8.5 Reflex relationships for the immune system—cont'd

Organ	Anatomical name	Somatic level/relationship
Lymph nodes		
Sympathetic – spinal cord	Via local sympathetic innervation channels	Depends on which organ/body area is concerned; review Table 8.2 on vascular reflexes above
Sympathetic – paravertebral chain ganglia	As above	As above
Sympathetic – plexus	As above	As above
Parasympathetic	Not applicable	

Table 8.6 Blood and lymph vessels for the immune system

Organ	Anatomical name	Fascial/ligamentous relation	Somatic relation, where applicable
Spleen			
Veins	Splenic vein, joins the mesenteric veins to give the portal vein	Passes behind the pancreas, vessels contained within the lienorenal ligament	Renal and right lower thoracic mechanics are important
Arteries	Splenic artery, off the coeliac trunk		Renal and right lower thoracic mechanics are important
Lymphatics	Splenic lymphatics drain the splenic capsule and trabeculae, and lymphocytes therefore pass directly into the bloodstream	Lienorenal ligament	Renal and right lower thoracic mechanics are important
Thymus			
Veins	Veins drain into the brachiocephalic, internal thoracic and inferior thyroid veins	Mediastinal fascia and throat/cervical fascia	Neck, shoulder girdle and upper chest mechanics are important
Arteries	From the internal thoracic and the inferior thyroid arteries	Mediastinal fascia and throat/cervical fascia	Neck, shoulder girdle and upper chest mechanics are important
Lymphatics	Brachiocephalic, tracheobronchial and parasternal lymph nodes	Mediastinal fascia and throat/cervical fascia	Neck, shoulder girdle and upper chest mechanics are important
Bone marrow			
Veins	Medullary vein	Passes into bone via nutrient foramina	See above for site of foramina
Arteries	Medullary artery	Passes into bone via nutrient foramina	See above for site of foramina
Lymphatics	No marrow lymphatics identified		
Lymph nodes			
Veins	Local nodular vein	Local fascial tissues	Local soft tissue mechanics are involved
Arteries	Local nodular artery	Local fascial tissues	Local soft tissue mechanics are involved
Lymphatics	Afferent and efferent lymph vessels to lymph nodes are part of the general lymphatic network	Lymph nodes are most numerous in the thoracic mediastinum, posterior abdominal wall, abdominal mesenteries, pelvis, neck and proximal ends of limbs (axilla and hip region)	Local mechanics are important, as are distal drainage points, such as the thoracic duct entries into the venous system (thoracic inlet) and the cysterna chyli (upper right abdomen)

conduits that contain the blood vessels are important, as work on those structures will influence venous drainage, blood flow (as ligamentous torsion may affect the arteries/arterioles and the sympathetic nerves that course along their length) and lymphatic drainage, all of which are important for organ health. The somatic relations also indicate where the musculoskeletal system may be engaged to aid fluid movement in the structures concerned.

ENDOCRINE SYSTEM

Many endocrine organs may seem 'out of reach', in a physical sense, of osteopathic manual work but there are ways of indirectly influencing structures such as the hypothalamus and pituitary which will be introduced below. Orthodox medicine remains highly sceptical of the relevance of osteopathic intervention in many clinical presentations and this is particularly the case when endocrine dysfunction and pathology are present. In fact, there are many ways in which osteopaths can support the endocrine system and help reduce neural irritation or improve circulation and drainage that could hypothetically improve endocrine function, even in the presence of pathology. It is important to state again that osteopaths do not aim to replace medical management in pathological presentations; this would, of course, be unethical. However, that is a long way from stating that osteopathic management is contraindicated in these patients (which it isn't) or that it would not be helpful (which it seems to be, empirically).

As the endocrine system utilizes blood transport for many of its components, the osteopathic management of local and general vascular components is key to an overall approach to endocrine problems. Also, as the endocrine organs work in concert, they should all be examined whenever any single one is expressing symptoms. This chapter does not include an overview of endocrine physiology or pathology, as these are found in many standard texts. It will instead focus on those parts of the anatomy (musculoskeletal, fascial, neural and visceral, for example) that can impact on endocrine function and are amenable to osteopathic examination and treatment where tensions, restrictions and adapted movement dynamics are found.

SURFACE ANATOMY

Table 8.7 shows musculoskeletal landmarks for the endocrine system.

LIGAMENTS AND SUPPORTS

Hypothalamus

This is not a distinct structure but a collection of several nuclei in the wall and floor of the third ventricle of the brain. It is the autonomic control centre, integrating afferent inputs and sending out appropriate efferent signals. The hypothalamus coordinates the actions of the nervous and endocrine systems by secreting hormones to the pituitary (as bloodborne elements or via neural connections).

Pituitary

The pituitary is a multifunctional endocrine gland located beneath the brain, linked to the brain by the pituitary stalk. The pituitary is divided into anterior and posterior lobes. The anterior pituitary is also known as the adenohypophysis or anterior lobe, and the posterior pituitary is also known as the neurohypophysis or neural lobe. The pituitary is connected to the hypothalamus by the pituitary portal system (pituitary stalk). The anterior pituitary is located between the posterior pituitary and the pars distalis. In humans, this lobe is poorly developed compared with other mammals. The posterior pituitary lies behind the anterior pituitary in the sphenoid depression in the base of the skull (sella turcica). The posterior pituitary is a continuation of the paraventricular and supraoptic nuclei of the hypothalamus.

Osteopathically, the pituitary is thought to be influenced by tensions and torsions within the fascia in and around the sella turcica (in which the pituitary is embedded).

The relevant fascial structures are the tentorium and the diaphragma sellae (which is in fact an extension of the tentorium), which both link with contiguous dural structures lining the skull and covering the brain. The diaphragma sellae is suspended between the four clinoid processes of the sphenoid, forming a membrane through which the pituitary stalk passes to link the hypothalamus

Table 8.7   Musculoskeletal landmarks for the endocrine system

Endocrine structure	Musculoskeletal landmark	Comments
Hypothalamus	Third ventricle	Situated between the two halves of the thalamus
Pituitary	Sella turcica	In the middle cranial fossa (behind the middle of the top of the eyes, halfway back along the skull)
Pineal	Just below the posterior end of the corpus callosum of the brain (effectively just above the beginning of the cerebellum)	No longer considered a vestigial organ
Thyroid and parathyroids	Anterior to and wrapped around the thyroid cartilage in the throat	Throat mechanics and cervical fascial tensions are important for the thyroid and parathyroids
Adrenals	Superior to the kidneys and therefore located deep to the diaphragm and angles of ribs 8–10	Lower rib and diaphragm mechanics are important for the adrenals
Pancreas	Draped across the front of the upper lumbar spine, roughly along a line drawn between the anterior ends of the 9th ribs (the transpyloric line)	Upper lumbar mechanics are important for pancreatic function
Gonads	Testes are suspended inferior to the pubis, and the ovaries are located on the posterior broad ligament, next to the lateral pelvic walls	Pubic mechanics and inguinal canal dynamics influence testicular suspension. Sacroiliac and internal pelvic mechanics influence ovarian suspension

with the posterior part of the pituitary, making those mechanics important as well. Reflex relationships are listed below.

Pineal

The pineal gland is located just below the posterior end of the corpus callosum of the brain (roughly in front of the upper beginning part of the cerebellum). It is organized into lobules of specialized cells, separated by septa containing unmyelinated nerves and blood vessels. A common age-associated change in the pineal is the presence of calcium particles ('brain sand') which enables the gland to be used as a radiological landmark. The gland is innervated by the sympathetic and parasympathetic nerve systems and signals arrive indirectly from the retina.

The pineal was once thought to be a phylogenetic relic – the vestigial remains of a dorsal third eye and an organ of little functional significance. However, it is now considered to be an endocrine gland of major importance, modulating the function of the anterior and posterior pituitary, the pancreas, parathyroids, adrenals and gonads.

Thyroid

The thyroid gland is composed of two lobes either side of the thyroid cartilage and upper trachea in the anterior portion of the neck. It develops from a downgrowth of endoderm arising near the root of the tongue called the thyroglossal duct. The mechanics of the thyroid cartilage and anterior throat and the neck are important for thyroid gland mechanics, as are those of the tongue, temporomandibular joint and thoracic inlet/upper mediastinum.

Reflex relationships are listed below.

Parathyroids

The parathyroid glands are associated with the thyroid gland in the neck and there are at least four and sometimes up to eight clustered around the thyroid gland. Any mechanics influencing and supporting the thyroid will be relevant for parathyroid function. In terms of osteopathic examination and local treatment techniques, they should be considered together with the thyroid gland mechanics and reflex relationships.

Adrenals

Also called the suprarenal glands, the adrenals are located on the upper poles of the kidneys and are divided into cortical and medullary regions. The mechanics of the adrenal glands mimic those of the kidneys and any technique aimed at resolving renal restrictions will influence the adrenals.

Pancreas

The pancreas is a large, rather diffuse gland with both exocrine and endocrine functions.

The endocrine components are found scattered within the exocrine and duct components of the pancreas. The pancreas is a retroperitoneal structure and is mainly affected by techniques that explore the root of the mesentery of the small intestine, the duodenum, sphincter of Oddi and the mesocolon for the transverse colon.

Gonads

The primary function of the gonads is to produce male and female gametes but the testis and ovary also act as endocrine glands. These glands are discussed in Chapter 7.

REFLEX RELATIONSHIPS

Table 8.8 shows reflex relationships for the endocrine system.

Table 8.8   Reflex relationships for the endocrine system

Organ	Anatomical name	Somatic level/relationship
Hypothalamus		
Sympathetic – spinal cord	T1–4	T1–4
Sympathetic – paravertebral chain ganglia	Via inferior cervical ganglion to middle cervical ganglion	Thoracic inlet and cervical mechanics are important
Sympathetic – plexus	Direct fibres via the ganglia	Thoracic inlet and cervical mechanics are important
Parasympathetic	Vagus	Upper cervical spine and cranial mechanics
Pituitary		
Sympathetic – spinal cord	T1–4	T1–4
Sympathetic – paravertebral chain ganglia	Via superior cervical ganglion to the posterior pituitary	Thoracic inlet and cervical mechanics are important
Sympathetic – plexus	Direct fibres via the ganglia	Thoracic inlet and cervical mechanics are important
Parasympathetic	Vagus gives fibres to nodose ganglia which pass to anterior pituitary	Upper cervical spine and cranial mechanics
Pineal		
Sympathetic – spinal cord	T1–4	T1–4
Sympathetic – paravertebral chain ganglia	Via inferior cervical ganglion to middle cervical ganglion	Thoracic inlet and cervical mechanics are important
Sympathetic – plexus	Direct fibres via the ganglia	Thoracic inlet and cervical mechanics are important
Parasympathetic	Sphenopalatine and otic ganglia	Upper cervical spine and cranial mechanics

Continued

Table 8.8 Reflex relationships for the endocrine system—cont'd

Organ	Anatomical name	Somatic level/relationship
Thyroid		
Sympathetic – spinal cord	T1–4	T1–4
Sympathetic – paravertebral chain ganglia	Via inferior cervical ganglion to middle cervical ganglion	Thoracic inlet and cervical mechanics are important
Sympathetic – plexus	Direct fibres via the ganglia	Thoracic inlet and cervical mechanics are important
Parasympathetic	Vagus	Upper cervical spine and cranial mechanics
Parathyroid		
Sympathetic – spinal cord	T1–4	T1–4
Sympathetic – paravertebral chain ganglia	Via middle cervical ganglion and superior cervical ganglion	Thoracic inlet and cervical mechanics are important
Sympathetic – plexus	Direct fibres via the ganglia	Thoracic inlet and cervical mechanics are important
Parasympathetic	Vagus	Upper cervical spine and cranial mechanics
Adrenals		
Sympathetic – spinal cord	T8–11	T8–11
Sympathetic – paravertebral chain ganglia	Lower ribs	Lower ribs
Sympathetic – plexus	Splanchnic nerves, passing through the coeliac plexus	Diaphragm and dorsolumbar mechanics are important
Parasympathetic	Most adrenal innervation is sympathetic	
Pancreas		
Sympathetic – spinal cord	(T5–9, but especially T7)	T5–9
Sympathetic – paravertebral chain ganglia	Greater splanchnics	Ribs 5–9
Sympathetic – plexus	Coeliac	Dorsolumbar spine
Parasympathetic	Left vagus	Upper cervical spine (left > right)
Gonads		
Sympathetic – spinal cord	T10–11	T10–11
Sympathetic – paravertebral chain ganglia	Lumbar splanchnics	Lower ribs
Sympathetic – plexus	Testicular or ovarian plexus, via the hypogastric	Lumbar mechanics and psoas
Parasympathetic	S2–4, but there may be some vagal fibres involved	Sacral mechanics

VEINS, ARTERIES AND LYMPHATICS

Table 8.9 shows blood and lymph vessels to the endocrine system. The visceral ligaments and fascial conduits that contain the blood vessels are important, as work on those structures will influence venous drainage, blood flow (as ligamentous torsion may affect the arteries/arterioles and the sympathetic nerves that course along their length) and lymphatic drainage, all of which are important for organ health. The somatic relations also indicate where the musculoskeletal system may be engaged to aid fluid movement in the structures concerned.

SOMATIC AND VISCERAL INTERACTIONS

General postural influences on whole-body circulation have been introduced in Chapter 3.

Table 8.9 Blood and lymph vessels for the endocrine system

Organ	Anatomical name	Fascial/ligamentous relation	Somatic relation, where applicable
Hypothalamus			
Veins	Hypothalamic veins	Dural and CNS mechanics	Cranial base mechanics
Arteries	Hypothalamic arteries	Dural and CNS mechanics	Cranial base mechanics
Lymphatics	Cerebrospinal fluid in the third ventricle	Dural and CNS mechanics	Cranial base mechanics
Pituitary			
Veins	Via portal vessels between the two parts of the pituitary; to the hypothalamus; and to systemic circulation via the dural venous sinuses	Dural and CNS mechanics	Cranial base mechanics
Arteries	Branches of the internal carotid artery	Dural and CNS mechanics	Cranial base mechanics
Lymphatics	Cerebrospinal fluid in the third ventricle	Dural and CNS mechanics	Cranial base mechanics
Pineal			
Veins	Local blood vessels	Dural and CNS mechanics	Cranial base mechanics
Arteries	Local blood vessels	Dural and CNS mechanics	Cranial base mechanics
Lymphatics	Cerebrospinal fluid in the third ventricle	Dural and CNS mechanics	Cranial base mechanics
Thyroid			
Veins	Thyroid plexus drains into the jugular veins	Superficial cervical fascia and soft tissue of throat	Cervical spine, jaw and throat mechanics are important
Arteries	Superior and inferior thyroid	Superficial cervical fascia and soft tissue of throat	Cervical spine, jaw and throat mechanics are important
Lymphatics	Right and left thoracic ducts	Thoracic inlet region	Thoracic inlet mechanics are important
Parathyroids			
Veins	Inferior thyroid veins	Superficial cervical fascia and soft tissue of throat	Cervical spine, jaw and throat mechanics are important
Arteries	Inferior thyroid arteries	Superficial cervical fascia and soft tissue of throat	Cervical spine, jaw and throat mechanics are important
Lymphatics	With the thyroid and thymus drainage routes	Thoracic inlet region	Thoracic inlet mechanics are important
Adrenals			
Veins	Right gland drains to the inferior vena cava and the left drains to the left renal vein	Renal fascia	Diaphragm and arcuate ligament mechanics are important
Arteries	Branches from the inferior phrenic artery, abdominal aorta and the renal artery	Renal fascia	Diaphragm and arcuate ligament mechanics are important
Lymphatics	Aortic and inferior vena caval nodes	Subdiaphragmatic, renal fascia and posterior liver relations/peritoneal ligaments are important	Diaphragm and arcuate ligament mechanics are important

Continued

Table 8.9   Blood and lymph vessels for the endocrine system—cont'd

Organ	Anatomical name	Fascial/ligamentous relation	Somatic relation, where applicable
Pancreas			
Veins	Pancreaticoduodenal veins, draining to the portal vein	Posterior abdominal wall, root of mesentery and mesocolon for the transverse colon	Upper gastrointestinal tract visceral dynamics are important
Arteries	To the head: the superior and inferior pancreaticoduodenal arteries; to the neck, body and tail: the splenic artery	Posterior abdominal wall, root of mesentery and mesocolon for the transverse colon	Upper gastrointestinal tract visceral dynamics are important
Lymphatics	Pancreatic nodes and superior mesenteric nodes	Posterior abdominal wall, root of mesentery and mesocolon for the transverse colon	Upper lumbar spine
Gonads			
Veins	Ovarian or testicular vein	Renal fascia, mesovarium (broad ligament) or inguinal/pelvic fascia for the testes	The right ovarian vein passes to the inferior vena cava and the left to the left renal vein, making it more prone to poor drainage and the influence of any adverse renal/left dorsolumbar mechanics
Arteries	Ovarian or testicular artery	Renal fascia, mesovarium (broad ligament) or inguinal/pelvic fascia for the testes	Psoas and lumbar spine mechanics are important
Lymphatics	Drain into the inferior vena caval and aortic nodes	Posterior abdominal wall fascias	General pelvic mechanics are important

This chapter includes factors related to local cardiac or vascular mechanics and function.

GENERAL VASCULAR ISSUES

Circulation has two major roles.

1. It is effectively a communication network, delivering hormones and other substances so they can work at distal points of the body.
2. It provides a nutrition delivery and waste product removal system. Circulatory (venous) return systems include muscle pumping and venous valves.

There are various 'special circulations' operating through life.

Coronary
- The role of coronary artery circulation/blood flow depends on aortic valve function and the actions of the left ventricle.

Osteopaths can consider this when providing supportive osteopathic care for coronary patients, for example (through the influence of the chest and pericardial mechanics on heart function; see below).

Cutaneous
- Involved in temperature control.
- Arteriovenous shunts can be created.
- Has extensive sympathetic innervation.

This is of interest to osteopaths as soft tissue massage techniques which affect skin circulation are thought to reflexly affect the circulation in segmentally related deep tissues such as the organs.

Skeletal muscle
Blood flow is determined by contractile activity (demand) and muscle type:

- red (slow twitch), high blood flow
- white (fast twitch), low blood flow.

Osteopaths utilize this concept when considering such things as compartment syndromes and local sympathetic vasoconstriction to a muscle or other structure irritated by somatovisceral reflex, for example.

Cerebral

- Via the internal carotid and vertebral arteries.
- Arterial inflow and venous outflow must match within very narrow limits.
- Total cerebral flow is relatively constant.
- Venous sinuses drain the skull and brain.
- Cerebrospinal circulation is the lymphatic component within the skull.

Osteopaths have developed many methods of influencing fluid flow dynamics within the enclosed cranial cavity and spinal vertebral canal spaces (within the dural and other membranous sleeves), which incorporate an appreciation of he principles of tensegrity and reciprocal tension as well as the mechanics of general fluid flow (e.g. autonomics).

Intestinal

- Small mesenteric arteries form extensive vascular beds in the submucosa of the GIT. Branches of these penetrate the longitudinal and circular muscular layers, making soft tissue contracture within the gut tube influential to gut circulation. At low flows, blood is shunted from arterioles to venules near the base of the villus, which can result in necrosis.
- Neural control of gut blood flow is almost exclusively sympathetic.

Osteopaths often work on segmentally related tissue to influence visceral function (e.g. gut circulation) through the effects of somatovisceral reflexes mediated through spinal articular soft tissues, as well as working on local soft tissue and fascial tensions that could impact on gut circulation.

Fetal

- Circulation in fetus.

  - Right and left ventricle pump in parallel into the aorta.
  - Very little pulmonary blood flow.
  - Low pressure in aorta due to low total peripheral resistance because of placenta-umbilical arteries.
  - Blood returning from the placenta via the umbilical veins bypasses the liver and flows directly into the inferior vena cava via the ductus venosus.

Osteopaths utilize the fibrosed embryological remnants of these blood vessels in their management of other problems such as bladder and upper gastrointestinal tract dysfunction, later in life.

- Circulatory readjustments at birth.

  - Increased blood flow through lungs and liver. Pulmonary vascular resistance decreases (decreased right ventricular pressure and pulmonary arterial pressure).
  - Loss of blood flow through the placenta. Doubles the systemic vascular resistance (increased left atrial pressure, left ventricular pressure and aortic blood pressure).
  - Closure of foramen ovale, ductus arteriosus and ductus venosus.

- Closure of foramen ovale. Due to reversal of pressure between the right atrium and left atrium the flap closes.
- Closure of ductus arteriosus. Reversal of flow from aorta to pulmonary artery, and increased oxygen levels cause constriction of smooth muscle.
- Closure of ductus venosus. Cause unknown. Allows portal blood to perfuse liver sinuses.

Osteopaths are interested in all the above changes to fetal circulation as those involved with paediatric care often see patients who have had corrective surgery or who retain various congenital anomalies within cardiovascular structures. It is important to incorporate these elements within the osteopathic care of that patient.

Control of blood pressure

1. Concepts of contents versus container.

   - Contents – blood volume.
   - Container – blood vessels.

2. Control of blood pressure is accomplished by affecting either vascular tone or blood volume.

Note: the kidney is involved in blood volume control and the sympathetics relate to vascular tone control (affecting the total size of the container, and peripheral resistance).

Cardiac output (CO) is related to heart rate (HR) and stroke volume (SV) where $HR \times SV = CO$. Heart rate control is neural (via sympathetics and parasympathetics) and stroke volume control is influenced by the balance between preload and afterload and is mainly neurally controlled. Preload is the amount of venous return pressure ie; the more blood coming back to the heart, the greater the stroke volume. Afterload is the amount of arterial pressure against which the heart is pushing (which is in itself related to peripheral resistance). If total peripheral resistance increases, stroke volume will go down.

The heart is a reactor to rather than an initiator of changes in cardiac output. It is a highly responsive organ and is not the prime controller of blood pressure. The sympathetic control of circulation through various vascular beds throughout the body is highly influential as that directly influences peripheral resistance (afterload) acting upon the heart.

Early osteopathic theories considered the reactive nature of cardiac function and the influence of the sympathetics on circulatory (blood volume) distribution. They worked on the principle that if the practitioner wanted to interact with the mechanisms controlling blood pressure, then the parts of the spine segmentally related to the level of sympathetic output for, say, the upper limb, the lower limb or the gut should be examined. If the spinal tissues and articulations were restricted or compromised, this indicated a possible irritation onto the sympathetics to that particular vascular bed (via a somatovisceral reflex), which would lead to increased peripheral resistance in that body area. Hence, the heart could not readjust itself until that peripheral resistance changed and so work to that section of the spine to influence the vascular bed concerned would be applied, and the theory was that the heart could then re-adapt and ultimately blood pressure would re-equalise at a more appropriate level. If renal-related spinal areas were also compromised, these would also be worked on to influence the mechanism for the control of blood volume (where relevant).

Any research looking at the influence of manual spinal treatments on blood pressure may well be misguided if the protocols involve the application of treatment solely to cardiac-related spinal segments (especially if the patient does not express spinal restriction at that level). This would also be true of research where the protocol would be to treat upper cervical articulations only, to influence the parasympathetic control to the heart, in isolation.

ARTERIAL ISSUES

Changes in the diameter of arteries and arterioles are under sympathetic control, which mostly induces vasoconstriction except in the brain, heart and lungs, where the opposite occurs. Small-diameter arterioles are the major determinants of peripheral resistance, which is a major component of the control of blood pressure, as stated above. Increased peripheral resistance will increase blood pressure and cause decreased blood flow within the local tissues served by those arterioles. However, long-term increases in blood pressure will lead to mechanical stress on arterioles and the rest of the vascular tree, including the heart.

Arteries have various mechanical properties which are important to their function. They must have non-linear elasticity and must also be distensible to smooth out the pulse before blood arrives at the capillaries, and to provide capacitance to aid cardiac function.[3] The arteries are resistant to damage from laminar blood flow but any factor that increases turbulence (such as increased blood pressure) will result in mechanical stress on the artery wall and often lead to atherosclerotic changes over time. Osteopaths consider that altered posture and altered movement dynamics of the whole abdomen, the upper limbs, the hip girdle and lower limbs, for example, can affect the physical environments of the arterial and vascular structures passing through those areas. This is considered to affect vessel flow and potentially lead to mechanical stress to the arteries involved.

This potential component of vascular strain seems underresearched but examples of how osteopaths would incorporate it clinically would be work on the axillary region, shoulder girdle and clavicle mechanics, in cases of thoracic outlet syndrome where the subclavian artery was compromised, and within the abdomen, where mesenteric artery torsion is thought to arise following tensions and restrictions developing in the peritoneum or viscera, or after adhesion or other surgical intervention. This mesenteric torsion would not be enough to block arterial flow (as in sclerotic occlusion) but may be sufficient to induce a mild ischaemia, similar to an 'abdominal migraine' type of problem or a type of 'compartment syndrome' where circulation is insufficient for tissue needs. This may manifest in myriad gastrointestinal symptoms which appear functional in nature (i.e. non-pathological).

HEART

Some of the relationships between the somatic and cardiac systems have been introduced in previous chapters, as has some of the general visceral interrelatedness. In particular, there is a very high degree of interrelatedness between the heart and lungs. Not only are the shape and orientation of the heart and lungs dynamically interrelated but the lungs will also dynamically support the heart as a result of their being wrapped around it. The mechanics of the lungs are designed to allow lung expansion all around the heart whilst accommodating heart volume changes. Embryologically, as the lungs grow out from the developing foregut, they pass either side of the heart. In doing so, they appear to place particular pressure onto the developing heart (from the relatively incompressible fluid-filled lung tissues) which helps to determine how the heart grows and develops. Some research even seems to indicate that lung lobar mechanics and strain patterns (which change as the fetus/child develops) will affect the orientation of the cardiac muscle fibres as the heart itself develops.[4]

Clinical osteopathic hypotheses would therefore consider that lung restriction on one (or both) side(s) may affect the heart. For example, if the sliding surfaces operating between the lower lobe on the left and the left ventricle are restricted or torsioned, this may cause cardiac mechanics to

adapt, which may have long-term consequences for cardiac function. This influence would be reciprocal.

Within the heart itself, mechanical perspectives are also important. The heart is an incredibly complicated dynamic structure which is a self-adjusting, self-regulating and self-maintaining muscular bag. The heart's internal electrical activity will keep adjusting itself depending upon the forces (mostly fluid pressures) acting within and upon it.[5] The heart reacts to influences around it and, as stated before, heart activity depends on blood flow in the periphery, which is under separate autonomic control to the heart.

The heart is not just a basic pump. In general terms, during the cardiac cycle the heart rotates itself along an axis from the back wall of the heart (where the atria are) through to the tip of the left ventricle.[6] This leads to a longitudinal rotation and also an AP shortening of the heart. The longitudinal rotation of the left ventricle twists up with systole and untwists with diastole, and provides a type of elastic recoil and stored potential energy within the ventricle[7] which is important for cardiac function. Uneven torsion and rotation mechanics within the heart can also adversely affect electrical activity in the heart, which can then impact on function.

The back wall of the heart is anchored deep in the mediastinum and to the anterior aspect of the upper dorsal spine, and the front of the pericardium is attached to the inside of the sternum. So, if there are any changes to chest mechanics and mediastinal torsions, then this might affect the back wall of the heart and the overall orientation of the pericardium. These factors may affect the mechanics of the back wall of the heart, and therefore dynamics of the ventricles and ultimately cardiac function.

As a result of all the above movement patterns, there are normal strain patterns within the myocardium[8] and it should be more active and dynamic in one section compared to another. But if there are adverse torsions acting upon the myocardium then this might cause an adaptation of the normal strain patterns. If the heart is mechanically malorientated and strained, this will decrease the heart's ability to regulate itself and so affect the way it reacts to changes in volume and pressure within the cardiovascular system. This may eventually manifest in cardiac disease.[9]

Another aspect of cardiac motion is that the back of the heart, where all the valves are located, will move in and out like a piston towards the left ventricle and away again. Without this elastic, longitudinally compliant movement acting evenly through the heart, the dynamics operating at the level of the heart valves may be affected and the leaflet actions become compromised. This may be a cause of (non-pathological) mitral valve shortening,[10] which is quite common.

This longitudinal expansion and contraction of the heart, coupled with ventricular rotations, may also be compromised if the AP diameter of the chest is reduced. During adolescent growth, the AP diameter of the chest naturally shortens and if this does not reexpand over time, cardiac dynamics may be altered in the long term, thereby affecting cardiac mechanics. The impact of left ventricular function and mechanics on the aortic valve and coronary vessels has already been noted, and osteopaths would consider that coronary vessel disease may be related in some way to altered physical tensions and movement dynamics of the chest, mediastinum and heart.

This movement of the posterior cardiac wall and its impact on flow dynamics gives rise to various interesting hypotheses. One is that the posterior wall of the heart needs to be correctly stabilized for appropriate valve function, and presumably efficient laminar flow through the major vessels entering and leaving the heart. Insufficient or altered posterior cardiac support could lead to valvular stress and incompetence, altered flow within the coronary arteries and reduced cardiac efficiency as a result. Not only this but the rest of the arterial tree also needs to be appropriately 'aligned' and positioned three-dimensionally in space, so that when blood flows through the vessel 'loops' that run through the body (Fig. 8.1), the flow has very little or no turbulence and so is more efficient and places less physical strain on the vessel walls (and causes hence less cardiovascular damage). This leads osteopaths to consider that overall posture, the dynamics of the mediastinum, thorax and pericardial relations, and the dynamics of blood vessels in the periphery (how they are affected by local

soft tissue tensions and torsions as they course through the trunk, head and limbs) and so on are all relevant to efficient and effective cardiovascular function. These concepts underpin some of the vascular techniques discussed below.

VENOUS ISSUES

Veins are capacitance vessels (blood reservoirs) that contain 65% of the blood supply. They have thinner walls than arteries but contain valves to prevent retrograde flow of blood. There can be some venoconstriction which is influenced by sympathetic nerves (venoconstriction increases cardiac preload). As previously stated, venous return is aided by muscular pumps and respiratory pressure changes between the thoracic and abdominal cavities.

In the erect posture, most blood and lymph vessels are oriented in a vertical plane, with the lower limb vessels, the abdominal vessels and the thoracic vessels all being directly superior or inferior to each other. Only the pelvic bowl is 'outside' this vertical pumping and fluid transport dynamic, being oriented on an oblique axis and posterior to the main fluid movement routes. The movements and pumping action of the pelvic floor thus become very important for venous (and other fluid) drainage from the pelvic bowl, a point which was raised in Chapter 7. General postural and somatic mechanical influences on fluid movements were introduced in Chapters 1 and 3.

LYMPHATIC ISSUES

Similar mechanical influences operate on the lymphatic system as for the portal system of veins. Virtually all abdominal lymph and lymph from the lower limbs and pelvis drains into the cysterna chyli before joining the thoracic duct and entering the systemic venous circulation via connections in the left thoracic inlet. Lymph nodes can be thought of as a meshwork of sinuses lined with tissue macrophages.

Lymphatics operate at a low pressure and small changes in pressure will close off the vessels quite easily. Hence lymphatic drainage is a light-touch technique as this is thought to promote flow,

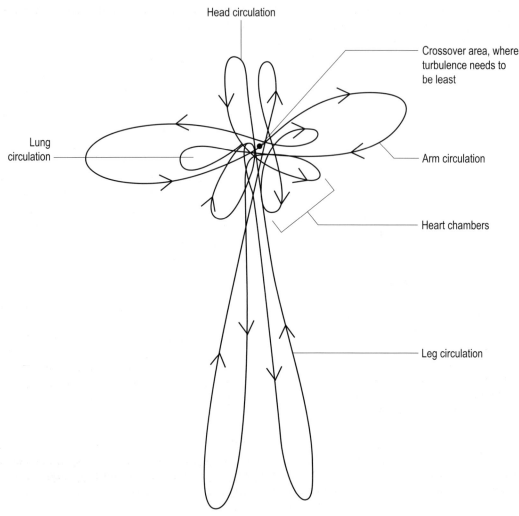

Head circulation

Crossover area, where
turbulence needs to
be least

Lung
circulation

Arm circulation

Heart chambers

Leg circulation

Figure 8.1   Spinal circulation through limb and body 'loops'.

whereas deep tissue massage would not in itself open lymphatic channels to promote flow. (Deep massage with higher levels of pressure may ultimately promote fluid movement through stretching of connective tissue, fascial and muscular tissues, thus improving their elasticity and compliance.)

No true lymphatic vessels are found in superficial portions of skin, central nervous system (CNS), endomysium of muscle or bone.

CNS – modified lymphatic function
- No true lymphatic vessels in CNS.
- Perivascular spaces contain CSF and communicate with subarachnoid space.

- Plasma filtrate and escaped substances in perivascular spaces return to the vascular system via the arachnoid villi which empty into the dural venous sinuses.
- Acts as a functional lymphatic system in CNS.

SOMATIC VASCULAR SYSTEMS

Issues relating to the somatic vessels were covered under the heading 'arterial issues' (see p. 217).

GUT CIRCULATORY ISSUES

As stated, altering blood flow in regional vascular beds can influence blood pressure. It has been found that periodic sympathetic modulation of mesenteric vascular resistance can initiate slightly higher frequency oscillations of arterial BP than can periodic sympathetic modulation of renal vasculature[11] and the impact of gastrointestinal vascular and mesenteric mechanics seems highly relevant to systemic blood pressure control mechanisms. Clinically, systemic circulatory issues cannot be addressed without first exploring the gut vascular beds and their reflex control.

Arterial issues

As mechanical torsion of the mesenteries affects local and general blood circulation and homeostatic regulation,[12] ensuring appropriate biomechanical function through the organs and mesenteries is important for whole-body control of blood flow as well as gut nutrition and drainage. The root of the mesentery is vitally important for the superior mesenteric artery, as is Toldt's fascia for the inferior mesenteric arteries, and the dorsolumbar junction and median arcuate ligament for the coeliac trunk. This latter can also be accessed from the front by passing 'through' the lesser omentum in the midline epigastric region.

Venous issues

Venous drainage is also important to gut function and is unusual insofar as the venous drainage is through the portal system to the liver and from there returning to the inferior vena cava and the systemic circulation. The liver is a vast filter for the gut's venous blood and if the filter gets 'clogged' in any way or the veins nearest the liver become compressed or torsioned, this can impede the flow of blood from the gut through to the inferior vena cava. There is a 'damming up' effect and varicosities through the gut tube can easily arise. These can manifest all along the length of the gut tube from the oesophagus to the rectum (where they are often visible as haemorrhoids). General venous drainage and portal circulation is also mechanically aided by the action of the thoracic diaphragm which gives a 'sucking effect' to abdominal and lower limb fluids as they pass towards the relatively negative pressure in the top of the abdomen and the thorax. Anything which impedes thoracic diaphragmatic actions could

interfere with global fluid drainage and impact on gut function.

ENDOCRINE ISSUES

Hypothalamus, pituitary and pineal

These are all cranial structures and are inaccessible to direct osteopathic palpation. As they are all situated in and around the third ventricle and the sella turcica, they are thought to be influenced by the mechanics of the sphenoid and temporal bones (as they sit close to the third ventricle). Osteopaths working with the primary respiratory mechanics would look at influencing these CNS structures via cerebrospinal fluid dynamics. Reflex relationships were listed above.

Thyroid and parathyroids

As these are embedded in the anterior throat and cervical fascias, the mechanics of the neck, throat, temporomandibular joint, tongue, thoracic inlet and upper mediastinum are all important. Techniques for these areas were discussed in Chapter 4. Reflex relationships were listed above.

Adrenals

The mechanics of the adrenals are intimately linked with those of the adjacent kidneys. Reflex relationships were listed above.

Pancreas

The pancreas is mechanically affected by the two kidneys and associated renal fascia, by the duodenum and the sphincter of Oddi, and the mesocolon for the transverse colon. It is also affected by the mechanics of the upper lumbar spine (over which it is draped). Techniques to influence these components have been included in Chapters 5 and 6. Reflex relationships were listed above.

Gonads

The testes are suspended from the pubis and inguinal region and are influenced by those mechanics, while the ovaries are suspended within the posterior layer of the broad ligament of the uterus and are located adjacent to the lateral pelvic walls. Reflex relationships were listed above.

EXAMINATION AND TREATMENT OF VASCULAR, ENDOCRINE AND IMMUNE SYSTEMS

FLUID (VASCULAR) SYSTEMS

Heart

Chapter 4 discusses the pericardial relations to the sternum, anterior ribcage, lungs, posterior mediastinal structures and dorsal spine. The top of the pericardium also links to the thoracic inlet structures and the cervical region, upwards to the cranial base via the pharyngeal muscles and fascia. This link is caused embryologically by the descent of the fetal heart to meet the developing diaphragm and through its enveloping in the intraembryonic coelum during the formation of the pleural and pericardial cavities.

The sliding surface techniques between the heart and the lungs which were described in Chapter 4 can, of course, be used to influence cardiac mechanics as well as those of the lungs. Releases through the chest, thoracic inlet and shoulder girdle and from the head through the neck to the chest can also indirectly affect the fascial continuum in which the heart and pericardium are embedded.

The techniques for the lobes of the lungs shown in Chapter 4 can be used to influence the pulmonary vessels, which are orientated along the same plane as (and are adjacent to) the bronchi. The vessels pass through the lung to the hilum and out to the posterosuperior wall of the heart to the right atrium. Releases utilizing a lung/lobar contact (via the rib) will indirectly unwind or release along both the bronchi and the pulmonary vessels.

Figure 8.2 shows a technique to balance and unwind the pericardial sac, which is aimed at releasing this structure close to the exit of the aorta, and hence indirectly influencing the coronary arteries.

Peripheral vasculature

Axillary and femoral triangle releases can be used to influence the mechanical dynamics of the vessels passing through those regions as they pass into

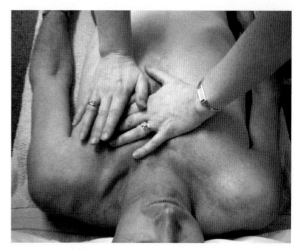

Figure 8.2 Coronary artery and pericardial sac balancing.

the limbs. The arteries can be worked on along their length by following the anatomical pathway of the vessels as they course through the body/limbs.

Gut circulation techniques

As many of the loops and arcades of the superior and inferior mesenteric arteries are located in the fascia embedded on the posterior abdominal wall by the flattened mesocolons (embryological remnants of dorsal mesentery), releases to these areas, by contacting into the paracolic gutters either side of the abdomen, can achieve a generalized release of the blood vessels passing in this region. Figure 8.3 shows a contact for the posterior abdominal wall

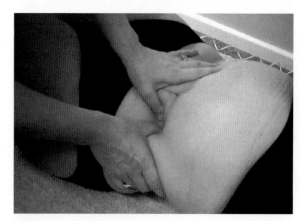

Figure 8.3 Mesenteric circulation contact via paracolic gutters.

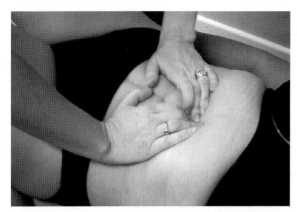

Figure 8.4 Coeliac trunk and portal vein contacts via the lesser omentum.

and paracolic gutter on the left. Direct inhibition and stretch to the peritoneum can be applied, or a functional/unwinding balancing technique can be utilized.

Figure 8.4 shows a similar contact but this time in the epigastric region, to influence the coeliac trunk. The coeliac trunk is located more deeply than the paracolic gutters and direct access to this vessel is limited as palpation is blocked by many intervening visceral structures. However, a generalized release of tissues at this epigastric point will influence the fascia in which the coeliac trunk is embedded. Both of these techniques are also influential for the neural plexi which surround the various blood vessels to the gut tube.

Figure 8.5 shows the contact for the root of the mesentery of the small intestine, to influence

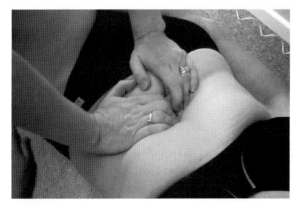

Figure 8.5 Superior mesenteric vascular release via root of mesentery.

the superior mesenteric artery. This is perhaps one of the most important abdominal vascular points to address. Pressure can be applied over the root of the mesentery, although care must be taken to avoid pressure onto the abdominal aorta. These vascular releases (and any deep work to the root of the mesentery) should be avoided in cases of abdominal aortic aneurysm (always remember to check pulses first, and to refer for investigation if in any doubt). When the technique is performed, gentle functional unwinding is usually the most effective.

Lymphatic techniques

There are numerous massage techniques to influence lymphatic flow. They are well reported and will not be discussed thoroughly here. Various techniques that should be employed or body areas that should be explored for their impacts on lymphatic circulation include:

- thoracic inlet release for thoracic duct entry into the venous system
- thoracic pumping (rhythmic pressure applied over the sternum)
- release of the cysterna chyli
- work on regional lymph nodes and associated tissues (especially the axillary and inguinal areas)
- general lymph massage
- organ lymph massage.

There are superficial and deep lymphatic systems, where the deep system drains everything *except* the skin. The superficial system drains into the axillary and inguinal nodes. Lymphoedema is almost exclusively a problem within the superficial lymphatic drainage system. Manual lymph drainage techniques attempt to encourage lymph flow towards open lymph channels and away from any blockage, on the presumption that many small anastomoses and accessory channels operate through the interstitium and some lymph can find a different drainage route. Manual lymph drainage is often accompanied by the use of compression bandages and management is for the long term, as lymphoedema will always progress if left unchecked.

The techniques used by osteopaths include stretch, soft tissue massage, articulation, general mobilization, functional unwinding or balancing techniques, and manipulation where necessary or advisable, in order to reduce tissue barriers to existing lymph channels and accessory lymph flow and to decongest swollen body parts. Osteopaths can also utilize the light-touch techniques often applied by physiotherapists in their treatment protocols for lymphoedema (manual lymph massage has a routine of pumping, scooping, stationary circles and rotatory movements applied to various parts). The additional techniques employed by osteopaths should work on the mechanical and soft tissue factors that are limiting the main and accessory lymph channels, beyond aiding fluid movements on a temporary basis during a manual lymph drainage massage.

The key to lymphatic drainage work is that it employs a light touch, so as to promote fluid flow without closing vessels through excess compression. Some osteopaths have begun to employ special light-touch/mobilization techniques onto the organs (or external body covering the organs), to promote local organ drainage. The movements must be applied in a specific alignment which matches the direction of lymph flow in that particular organ (each one having its own orientation). This can be a very useful adjunct for deep system lymphatic drainage techniques.

Some contraindications apply to lymphatic massage and mobilization, including cardiac oedema, acute infections, acute bronchitis and deep vein thrombosis. Care should be taken in patients with malignancies and bronchial asthma.

IMMUNE SYSTEM

Spleen

There are numerous techniques to influence the spleen and surrounding tissues, many of which involve working through the ribs and related soft tissues of the lower left thoracic cage. Figure 8.6 shows a sitting technique where the practitioner supports the external ribcage so that when external pressure or movements are applied, the inside of the upper abdomen is mobilized, thereby indirectly releasing the spleen.

Another general technique is the 'splenic pump' which involves rhythmic external bimanual compression of the left lower ribcage, to indirectly

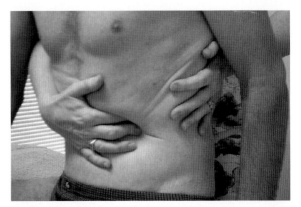

Figure 8.6 Sitting release of spleen and splenic ligaments.

'pump' or mobilize the spleen. This must be applied with caution. Pumping action which is too vigorous, too forceful or too quick only serves to irritate the local tissues. When the spleen is very active (such as with acute infection or allergic problems) then splenic pumping should be avoided and other, more gentle splenic releases performed.

Figure 8.7 shows a more direct route to approach the upper abdomen, in which the spleen is located. Note: the spleen cannot be directly palpated via the subcostal route, unless it is severely enlarged. The practitioner supports the lower ribs (8–10) so that they are slightly lifted off the couch and towards the midline of the patient. This will bring the spleen towards the abdominal contact (but not onto it). The abdominal hand creates some skin slack towards the subcostal region and eases through the visceral layers to feel as close to the splenic area as possible. Care should be taken not to have the fingers too stiff, as this will be uncomfortable for the patient and block the technique.

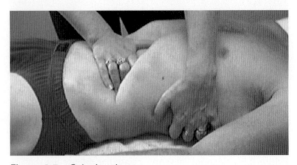

Figure 8.7 Splenic release.

Once the abdominal hand is somewhat subcostal, the two hands can then move slowly in concert, to affect a gentle mobilization through the posterior upper abdominal tissues, to affect the spleen and associated ligaments. A functional or unwinding/balancing technique can also be used.

Thymus

The thymus is linked with the mechanics of the transversus thoracis, the sternum and manubrium, the superior extensions of the pleural costomediastinal recesses and the superior extensions of the sternopericardial ligament, the heart and the lungs, the larynx, thoracic inlet and the thyroid cartilage, tongue and temporomandibular joint.

As well as working through the throat and related structures, releasing sternal and mediastinal torsions should ease movement restrictions around the thymus and improve local circulation and drainage. This is particularly useful in children presenting with any one of a number of inflammatory, allergic and infectious conditions that would benefit from support to the immune system. Note: this is not the same as directly mobilizing bacterially infected tissues, which would be contraindicated. The techniques would be designed to reduce any barrier to efficient function at the level of the thymus, so that the body's immune mechanisms can better operate to manage the infection in distant parts.

Bone marrow

To stimulate the nutrient arteries and veins, and hypothetically improve circulation and drainage to the bone marrow, any fascial and soft tissue tension and torsion operating around the nutrient foramen area of relevant bones could be worked on to reduce any constraints on the bone vascular supply. This would imply soft tissue and articulatory work as follows.

Humerus – release of soft tissues halfway down the medial border of the bone (inner aspect of upper arm).

Clavicle – release of thoracic inlet soft tissues attaching to the posterior (inner) surface of the clavicle facing the brachial nerves and scalenes.

Ilium – release of iliacus.

Scapula – release of infraspinatus, on the posterior surface of the scapula, close to the underneath of the spine of the scapula.

Ribs – soft tissue work to the erector spinae and articulation of the rib heads and costotransverse joints.

Femur – release of soft tissues on the medial border of the femur (inner aspect of the middle of the thigh), near vastus medialis.

This soft tissue work could constitute part of a general immune and lymphatic supportive treatment when required.

ENDOCRINE SYSTEM

Hypothalamus, pituitary and pineal

As these are all situated in and around the third ventricle and the sella turcica, they are thought to be influenced by the mechanics of the sphenoid and temporal bones (as they sit close to the third ventricle). Osteopaths working with the primary respiratory mechanics would look at influencing these CNS structures either directly or via cerebrospinal fluid dynamics. Otherwise, general 'gapping' work to the cranial sutures can be applied (utilizing small amounts of gentle direct pressure close to the suture sites around the sphenoid and temporals), as can articulatory techniques for the temporomandibular joint. This can be aided by general osteopathic work to the upper cervical spine, and soft tissues of the neck and throat.

The occiput (and the occipitoatlantoid articulation) can be very useful to consider specifically as it lies very close to the sphenobasilar synchondrosis. This junction is very closely related to the site of the pituitary and its mechanics are thought to influence those of the diaphragma sellae and the tentorium.

Thyroid and parathyroids

As these are embedded in the anterior throat and cervical fascias, the mechanics of the neck, throat, temporomandibular joint, tongue, thoracic inlet and upper mediastinum are all important. Techniques for these areas were discussed in Chapter 4.

Adrenals

The mechanics of the adrenals are intimately linked with those of the adjacent kidneys. Techniques to release the kidneys were described in Chapter 6.

Pancreas

The pancreas is mechanically affected by the two kidneys and associated renal fascia, by the duodenum and the sphincter of Oddi, and the mesocolon for the transverse colon. It is also affected by the mechanics of the upper lumbar spine (over which it is draped). Techniques to influence these components have been included in Chapters 5 and 6.

Gonads

The testes are suspended from the pubis and inguinal region and are influenced by those mechanics, while the ovaries are suspended within the posterior layer of the broad ligament of the uterus and are located adjacent to the lateral pelvic walls. Techniques to release the ovaries, testes and spermatic cord were described in Chapter 7.

References

1. Gayer G, Zissin R, Apter S, Atar E, Portnoy O, Itzchak Y. CT findings in congenital anomalies of the spleen. Br J Radiol 2001;74(884):767-2.
2. Ostermann PA, Schreiber HW, Lierse W. [The ligament system of the spleen and its significance for surgical interventions.] Langenbecks Arch Chir 1987;371(3):207-16.
3. Shadwick RE. Mechanical design in arteries. J Exp Biol 1999;202(Pt 23):3305-13.
4. Hoffman Sideman S, Beyar R (eds). Interactive phenomena in the cardiac system. New York: Plenum Press; 1993.
5. Pasipoularides A. Cardiac mechanics: basic and clinical contemporary research. Ann Biomed Engin 1992;20:3-17.
6. Toumanidis ST, Sideris DA, Papamichael CM, Moulopoulos SD. The role of mitral annulus motion in left ventricular function. Acta Cardiol 1992;47(4):331-48.
7. Moon MR, Ingels NB Jr, Daughters GT 2nd, Stinson EB, Hansen DE, Miller DC. Alterations in left ventricular twist mechanics with inotropic stimulation and volume loading in human subjects. Circulation 1994;89(1):142-50.
8. Azhari H, Weiss JL, Shapiro EP. Distribution of myocardial strains: an MRI study. Adv Exp Med Biol 1995;382:319-28.
9. Halperin HR, Tsitlik JE, Rayburn BK, Resar JR, Livingston JZ, Yin FC. Estimation of myocardial mechanical properties with dynamic transverse stiffness. Adv Exp Med Biol 1993;346:103-12.
10. Mishiro Y, Oki T, Iuchi A, et al. Echocardiographic characteristics and causal mechanism of physiologic mitral regurgitation in young normal subjects. Clin Cardiol 1997;20(10):850-5.
11. Grisk O, Stauss HM. Frequency modulation of mesenteric and renal vascular resistance. AJP – Regulatory, Integrative and Comparative Physiology 2002;282(5):R1468-76.
12. Holzer-Petsche U, Brodacz B. Traction on the mesentery as a model of visceral nociception. Pain 1999;80(1-2):319-28.

Chapter 9

Patient management in visceral osteopathy

GENERAL PATIENT MANAGEMENT

The essence of patient management is not to follow a set protocol that is predetermined for all cases but to appreciate which areas of the body may impact on the physiology, mechanics and vitality of the system or organ concerned and to explore what is uniquely required for that individual at that time. Any attempts to do otherwise will not result in the application of osteopathy.

In practice, this may mean something along the following lines. Some areas are more immediately relevant to explore than others (such as the ribs in asthma as opposed to the wrist, for example) but in order to resolve the ribcage problem to aid the asthma, the wrist may need to be addressed. This would be the case if in that patient, the wrist was part of a different pattern engaging the upper limb to the shoulder girdle and into the chest (thereby indirectly maintaining the rib and the lung/respiratory problem). In such a way, a seemingly unrelated structure or body area may ultimately be a major maintaining factor in the visceral condition and may be one of the key areas to work on to resolve the overall pattern limiting the self-healing and self-restoring mechanisms within that person. A different person will almost certainly have a completely different set of maintaining factors to their 'respiratory distress' pattern.

The key is to explore as much of the patient as possible, so that you are aware of the global pattern of restrictions within that person. At this stage, the presenting problem or symptoms are almost the least important thing to consider. The aim is to find out how the body as a whole is compromised or expressing adapted function. Then the body areas that are restricted or affected can be considered in the light of any mechanical or physiological relationships. A mechanical relationship is something like the wrist to chest analogy above: if the wrist is tight, the upper limb is used differently (at work, for example, typing) and if the arm is used differently, this engages the soft tissues of the shoulder girdle and the structures into the chest differently, which will impact on the respiratory activities of the chest.

If a global assessment is not made initially, treatment will not always be applied to the most appropriate places for that individual patient and focusing too much on local visceral factors gives limited results. Without that global assessment, neither practitioner nor patient can rationalize why treatment has not helped and may become disillusioned. Having a global evaluation means the patient can choose whether they wish to engage in the (usually more effective) global treatment or the (often less effective) local treatment.

COMPLEMENTARY, SUPPLEMENTARY OR ALTERNATIVE CARE?

There is debate about whether osteopaths provide complementary, supplementary or alternative care for patients, whether for musculoskeletal biomechanical problems or for various diseases, pathologies, postsurgical considerations, obstetrics or otherwise. The truth is that osteopathy can be all three, depending on the circumstances and presenting case.

SYMPTOM PATTERNS

The types of 'visceral problems' most often seen by osteopaths involve patients presenting with chronic, non-life threatening conditions, for which allopathic medicine can only provide symptom control or has limited impact. Such problems include chronic asthma (childhood or adult), recurrent ear infections, functional bowel disorders such as irritable bowel syndrome or chronic constipation, recurrent cystitis, organ prolapse and postoperative pain and scarring, for example. Osteopaths also become involved in the management of patients with complex medical problems such as cerebral palsy, Crohn's disease, autoimmune disorders, cancer, infertility and attention deficit disorders.

They also, of course, become involved in cases of visceral trauma (such as following a road traffic accident) where the organ has been damaged or removed and is now contributing to musculoskeletal dysfunction or adding to a preexisting visceral pathological presentation (such as a worsening of upper gastrointestinal tract reflux and irritation following lung trauma post whiplash, for example).

All the above will require general body treatment and local visceral treatment, coupled with an understanding of the presentation profile (and underlying pathology where present), so that any changes to the patient's presentation can be monitored, appropriately evaluated and management adapted accordingly. This involves the appreciation of the individual risk/benefit equation for that patient. The choice of which examination and treatment modes to utilize is also included in this equation, so as not to overstress damaged and weak structures or to compromise pathologically involved tissues.

The presentation profile is important, as many patients present with a variety of symptoms that all come and go in a 'regularly irregular pattern'. This effectively means that the patient finds it difficult to give an accurate daily pattern 'as it changes so much' and they find it difficult to analyse what triggers various episodes or makes them feel easier on any particular day. People with long-term problems become somewhat 'dissociated' from them and have a tendency only to recognize 'full resolution of symptoms' as the 'cure' or 'benefit' they are seeking. They initially find it difficult to appreciate that not all their symptoms may be relieved at once and that the pattern of their various symptom components may change first, before some start to ease, with other aspects gradually improving over time. This needs careful discussion with the patient so that they are properly informed of likely treatment outcomes and that they are not given false expectations.

It is also important for the osteopath to realize that managing various complex and long-standing visceral problems is more difficult than helping someone with a minor muscle strain or a joint restriction. A novice at visceral work (no matter how proficient with their existing osteopathic skills) will take longer to help someone than a practitioner well versed and practised in visceral patient management and techniques.

Often, practitioners who are highly proficient at dealing with a whole gamut of musculoskeletal disorders become disheartened when they first move into managing patients with visceral presentations, as they are used to patients that respond fully within only two or three treatments, for example. A couple of treatment sessions that include some organ stretching and mobilization and a bit of abdominal unwinding, for example, will not resolve chronic visceral dysfunction. The osteopathic care and management of patients with long-standing and complex visceral presentations requires a lot of clinical input, a lot of patient support, an ability to view the whole picture and not get lost in the minutiae of the case and an ability to remain vigilant and reflective over a long timespan, as positive changes are usually noted only over weeks or months, rather than days.

Patients are also likely to suffer relapses and they should be warned of this, as when they have gained relief from long-term suffering, they are much more emotionally shattered when a relapse occurs as they had begun to lower their defences and feel that they were 'over their problem'. Relapses occur for a variety of reasons but usually because tissues can only adapt so far, still fatigue easily and are still prone to the impact of the basic pathology or external factors such as emotions, diet or inhaled allergens, for example. If people are warned that relapses can occur, they are emotionally more prepared and can use that as part of their healing process rather than experience it as yet a further trauma in their lives. In most cases, subsequent recovery is usually quicker and easier than the timespan and effort that were required for the original relief of the presenting problem in the first place.

Getting an accurate picture of the various symptoms over time *before* treatment commences is very important, as both practitioner and patient need to be able to appreciate whether any changes that occur are part of the normal 'regular irregularity' or whether they represent actual positive change to the pattern of presenting symptoms.

OUTCOME MEASURES

One way to keep 'on track' with patient management and also to evaluate treatment efficacy and appropriateness is to use outcome measures as a regular aspect of clinical practice. This can be as simple as using a detailed symptoms diary or presentation profiles. Even a simple change to case history questioning methods usually provides much useful information. For instance, instead of asking 'How often do these symptoms recur?', ask 'How long is a good patch for you? If you have no or fewer symptoms for longer than 3 days or 3 weeks (or whatever is appropriate), is this good or would you normally expect to go that long on occasion with no symptoms or fewer symptoms?' Patients can often relate to this more easily and usually provide information such as 'Well, I never go for more than a week without some symptoms' or 'At least every 3 months I have a recurrence, reinfection or aggravation' (for example). These statements can then be much more easily reviewed for ongoing progress with osteopathic management.

ALTERED RESPONSES OVER TIME

Patients' problems often 'change' before they get better. Patients with chronic patterns of dysfunction can become quite psychologically used to their symptom patterns and find it quite distressing when these change, as they do not always interpret 'change' as 'improvement'. Rather, they view it negatively and become more depressed and distressed, which hampers their ongoing recovery. There are many challenges to managing patients over protracted periods of time, which are more involved than with the management of acute or short-term musculoskeletal biomechanical problems. Therefore practitioners wishing to move into visceral management will have to incorporate new time management and progression review strategies, in order to keep on track with treatment and to ensure appropriate care is always being given.

THE OSTEOPATHIC APPROACH

This chapter discusses how osteopaths may approach a variety of presenting problems and the aim is to stress the individualized application of treatment. Osteopaths do not treat 'conditions' – they treat 'patients with conditions' and osteopathy can only be applied by assessing the body and evaluating what in that individual is contributing to the problem and what is creating a barrier to homeostasis and healing within that patient. Although there may be common factors, each patient will have a unique combination of tissue tensions, irritations, restrictions and altered movement dynamics that should be worked on. This philosophical difference between osteopathic care and the allopathic application of manual techniques in various patients is fundamental.

Each chapter of this book provides information that is vital to understanding the osteopathic approach to various presenting problems and the reader should take care not to focus solely on the overview chapters as the techniques discussed within them will not provide a methodology for patient management without their being placed in a 'whole-body context'. For that reason, the information throughout the book is important in each patient scenario.

This chapter includes approaches to examination in various situations, from which the practitioner can identify factors that need to be treated or further explored. These examination and treatment approaches have all been included in one chapter rather than at the end of the separate systems in the overview chapters as it is extremely important to realize that osteopaths do not treat the systems separately, as does allopathic medicine. There is no osteopathic specialty that covers gynaecology or gastroenterology, for example, as this implies that only the organs or tissues within that system would be treated. This is absolutely not the osteopathic approach. Osteopaths can have special interests in the management of patients with gynaecological, respiratory or urinary problems, for example, but they would not treat only within that body system. They would explore and treat throughout the whole body (including adjacent organs in different body systems, global circulatory factors, mechanical and neural reflex links with the musculoskeletal system, emotional factors, sometimes diet and exercise routines and so on) to specifically address factors that are ultimately leading to compromise and lack of recovery within the symptomatic system. The various case management discussions reinforce this point. It is not possible here to discuss all the possible visceral presentations or conditions so those chosen are the ones more commonly presenting in practice.

The cases are not designed to show how osteopaths 'cure' various medical pathological problems. They illustrate approaches to exploration of a patient's presenting condition and provide examples of individual approaches to management (although they do not represent the only way to manage any particular patient with a similar problem). They will also show how patients often have many combined presentations and how varied torsions and tensions can combine to influence the overall presentation and progression. Remember that there will be a different combination of factors in each patient, culminating in compromised physiology that is impacting on the healing and resolution of their presenting problem, and that therefore the treatment of each patient will differ, even if they are presenting with the same condition. For that reason, not every minute or detailed restriction or tension has been noted for each case, only the most major components. Therefore the treatment discussions cover the more significant factors only.

For many visceral pathologies or problems, the aim of management (be it orthodox or osteopathic)

is often symptom support, maintaining quality of life, long-term reduction of medication and general patient support. In these circumstances, osteopathic care is complementary and supplementary to orthodox management. In some of the cases, though, the contribution of osteopathy as an alternative care regime may become clearer and it is hoped such cases will encourage further exploration and research into the overall scope of osteopathic practice. Sometimes the osteopathic approach will be the only one that brings further benefit to the patient, when other care protocols have nothing left to offer.

Only a very small insight into the management of patients with visceral problems using osteopathy has been illustrated here, as an introduction to the unique contribution of osteopathic medicine to patient care. Lay language is used in the case management discussions to allow a more philosophical (and practical) appreciation of the osteopathic principles used.

MANAGEMENT OF PATIENTS WITH RESPIRATORY PROBLEMS

CASES

Patient with chronic asthma and bronchitis

A 52-year-old lady presented for treatment for recurrent limb and back pain, associated with steroid medication for her chronic asthmatic condition. Whenever she had oral steroids for a period (required for acute episodes of asthma, bronchitis and/or chest infection), she had to suffer withdrawal symptoms as she halted the drug therapy. Periodically, then, she presented with the pain associated with the soft tissue reactions within her musculoskeletal system from this withdrawal.

This cycle of events had been established for a number of years and so she was a frequent visitor to various osteopathic clinics in an attempt to manage the withdrawal period. She would typically not manage more than 3 weeks with no antibiotic therapy or oral steroid use during the winter and in the summer months would not go for more than 3 months without them.

Until her recent presentation, the idea of treating her asthma osteopathically had not been aired by previous practitioners and it was thought interesting to see if any change could be initiated within her respiratory system, leading to a reduced frequency of asthma attacks and chronic bronchitis/chest infection. This would reduce the need for the oral steroid application and so would hopefully mean fewer musculoskeletal symptoms as she would have to withdraw from the steroids less often.

This lady had had asthma since 8 years of age and it was associated with house dust, tree and flower pollen and occasionally milk sensitivities. Her frequent chest infections had somewhat worsened over the 2–3 years prior to presentation. Her peak flow readings rarely got above 275 and usually hovered around the 250 mark. She had regular checks with an asthma clinic. A year or so prior to the current presentation, she had suffered a very bad bout of pneumonia, which made her overall chest condition worse for quite some time. Things were now beginning to stabilize again and had been helped by her husband retiring from work. The patient was an active person given her condition, liked walking and had a part-time job as a counsellor. Other history included hiatus hernia, chronic constipation and a previous cholecystectomy. She also had a hysterectomy for uterine fibroids and a mild problem with stress incontinence of urine due to pelvic floor weakness.

She was interested, if a little uncertain, about attempting to manage her asthma but was willing to try some treatments and review the results after a little time. This lady presented with a variety of findings, some of which are outlined in Figure 9.1.

She had a scoliotic pattern, with the right lumbar spine being a 'high side' (vertebral bodies rotating to the right) and the midthorax side shifted to the left and the left middorsals being a 'high side' (vertebral bodies rotating to the left). There was a counter-torsion pattern local to the upper dorsal and lower cervical spine areas, where the cervical spine was rotated right and the upper dorsals were rotated left.

The thoracic inlet was tight on both sides but more so on the left and the mechanics of the anterior chest on the left were particularly restricted due to the rib torsion and the effects of the costal margin tension induced from her history of gastrointestinal disorders. The left upper lobe of the lung was very tense and felt almost 'small/shrunken' and with respiration there

was not much movement or expansion in this region (this was also reflected in a lack of involuntary expansion at that level). The lower lobe was also bound down, with a strong torsion acting at the level of the oblique fissure (due to the opposing tensions from the thoracic scoliosis). The lower lobe expressed better respiration but it was still limited and the chest wall was generally inelastic. The sternal mechanics were limited. The diaphragm was tense throughout due to the variety of visceral tensions but was particularly so on the left, which meant the area of the spleen and left colic flexure was particularly immobile. The 11th and 12th ribs on the left were in an opposing torsion between the crurae of the diaphragm and the influence of the lumbar spine (being torsioned due to the action of the right psoas muscle).

The spinal torsion patterns were reflected down into the pelvis, where sacral torsion helped to compromise the action of piriformis and from that and the psoas restriction, the right hip was quite tense. Indeed, the lady was now beginning to suffer early degenerative change in the right hip which will further compromise the mechanics in this area. Other findings were noted but were not as prominent as those listed.

Treatment would follow several lines: to reduce the torsion between the upper and lower lobes of the lungs by working on the chest mechanics (particularly the sternum and costal margin areas), to improve the compliance of the lung, by working on the lateral chest wall and the diaphragm, to affect the lower lobe. This work would also be aided by subdiaphragmatic visceral mobilization (exploring her GIT problems). The compliance of the upper lobe would be explored by looking at the shoulder girdle mechanics and cervical spine relations, to help reduce the torsion at the level of the thoracic inlet. The action of the diaphragm, spleen and left lower lobe would also be helped by reducing crural tension, by releasing the 11th and 12th ribs on the left and working through the chain of torsion from the right hip, through piriformis and psoas, to the lumbar spine and the dorsolumbar region. Interestingly, through the attachments of the upper GIT organs to the front of the lumbar spine and diaphragmatic crurae and arcuate ligaments, tension in these areas will also affect the dorsolumbar mobility.

After some treatments to all the above, the pelvic floor and pelvic internal scarring was explored as

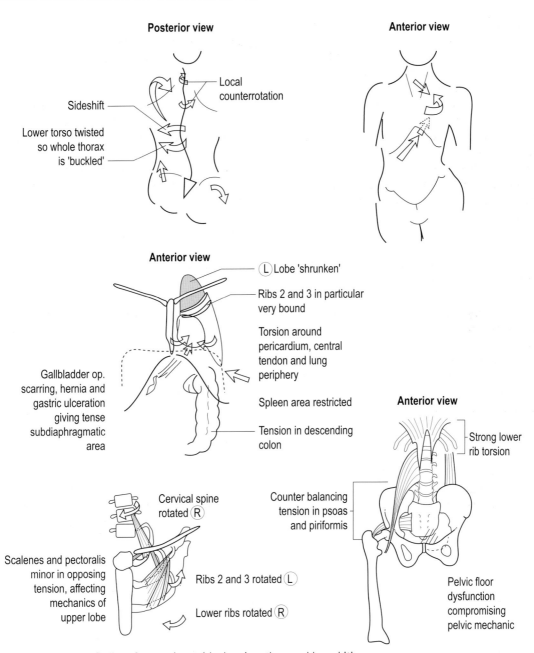

Posterior view

Sideshift

Local
counterrotation

Lower torso twisted
so whole thorax
is 'buckled'

Anterior view

Anterior view

(L) Lobe 'shrunken'

Ribs 2 and 3 in particular
very bound

Torsion around
pericardium, central
tendon and lung
periphery

Gallbladder op.
scarring, hernia and
gastric ulceration
giving tense
subdiaphragmatic
area

Spleen area restricted

Tension in descending
colon

Anterior view

Strong lower
rib torsion

Cervical spine
rotated (R)

Counter balancing
tension in psoas
and piriformis

Scalenes and pectoralis
minor in opposing
tension, affecting
mechanics of
upper lobe

Ribs 2 and 3 rotated (L)

Lower ribs rotated (R)

Pelvic floor
dysfunction
compromising
pelvic mechanic

Figure 9.1   Examination findings for a patient with chronic asthma and bronchitis.

this would help the whole abdomen respond better during respiration, which should have a beneficial action on overall lung function. It was also noted that there were a variety of cranial tension and torsion patterns but these, coupled with the influence of the very long-standing sacral torsion, were felt to be too established to be resolved before some release was provided to the core-link of fascia acting up through the mediastinum, anterior cervical spine to the cranial base (as well as dural membrane links from the pelvis) by the other work described. Once some expansion was available to the reciprocal tension membranes, then more locally applied work was carried out.

Techniques applied consisted of soft tissue massage to the spinal and chest wall muscles, local and specific articulation of the intervertebral and costovertebral articulations and general mobilization to the articulations of the anterior chest. Some vibratory and pumping techniques were applied to the thorax and some recoil techniques applied to the anterior ribs. General soft tissue massage and gentle visceral manipulation were applied to the abdomen and articulation and distraction techniques were applied to the right hip. Functional/balanced ligamentous techniques were applied to the lung areas, the lower left ribs and the sacrum.

This pattern was applied in a variation over a number of weeks and gradually the strong torsion patterns and overall posture of the patient began to 'soften', in preparation for beginning to change. Over the course of a few months, her peak flows began to improve after each treatment and her incidence of chest infection was reducing. It was interesting to note that over time, the very chronic facilitation (osteopathic lesion/somatic dysfunction pattern seen in the upper dorsal region, associated with the lung field) would flare up or down in concert with her respiratory distress or relief. This area would be worked on directly after a period of time but as a result of the strong torsion pattern around it from the ribcage mechanics, local work would have limited short-term effects, although articulation and soft issue techniques were always applied to the area to a degree.

Following treatment over the course of the last year, this lady has had a reduction of chest infection, managed to have many more weeks of the winter period free from the need to take oral steroids and had a much less troublesome time. Of course, her asthma is still present but the overall aims of the treatment programme seem to have been met and the patient is very keen to continue, to try to improve her respiratory function and reduce her overall aches and pains.

Patient with chest pain, breathlessness and sciatica

A 43-year-old woman presented with a 14-year history of recurrent chest infections, occurring 2–3 times each winter. In her early 20s she had had pericarditis and still had occasional ectopic beats if under stress. She was not currently medicated for

this problem. Around 1 year ago, she thought she had 'cracked a rib' while coughing during an episode of infection. This left her much more breathless for a while, with a girdle-like pain around the chest and a lingering sharp pain on the inferior right costal margin, which she had not had before.

Other factors included a 20-year history of low back pain, most likely associated with her nursing career (no specific trauma as aetiology). This had worsened in the preceding 10 years and in the last 7–8 years she had developed left leg symptoms of heaviness and aching into the lateral thigh and altered sensation (verging on numbness) into the dorsum of the foot. This had previously been attributed to sciatica and an MRI scan some years previously had diagnosed an L4–5 disc herniation. The leg symptoms had gradually been set off by spells of back packing, which had been quite arduous. After one occasion with her back/leg symptoms, she took to wearing a spinal support corset, which she kept on for 2 years. She had also sustained a local injury to her left knee (in the year preceding presentation) where she had split the knee open during a fall. An x-ray revealed osteophyte formation at the lower end of the femur, which had obviously preceded the fall but of which she had been unaware.

Other history included recurrent haematuria (21-year history), which had been extensively investigated with no conclusion. She had also had a bout of pericarditis after finishing her university course. She had felt tired for years and felt that her vitality was 'at a low ebb'. She had had a thyroidectomy in the last 5 years, for a benign swelling and was generally prone to breast lumps (more so in the right breast).

Her examination findings were complex and some of the main ones are illustrated in Figure 9.2. There were extensive and very chronic chest restrictions, due to the varied visceral pathologies. There was significant restriction in the bronchopericardial ligamentous complex and the right mid-ribcage was quite bound, including the liver and diaphragm. None of the dorsal spine articulations functioned very efficiently. Externally, the pectoral fascia of the right breast was particularly tight. There was restriction in the upper dorsal and cervicodorsal junction and the right cranial base, especially the temporal bone. There was a general torsion and restriction pattern throughout the body, particularly

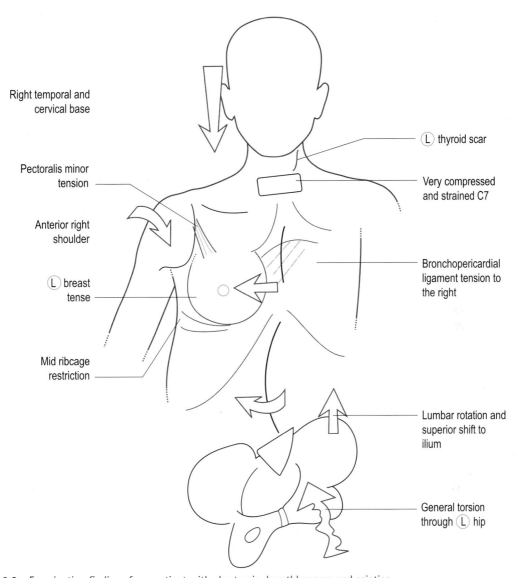

Right temporal and
cervical base

Pectoralis minor
tension

Anterior right
shoulder

Ⓛ breast
tense

Mid ribcage
restriction

Ⓛ thyroid scar

Very compressed
and strained C7

Bronchopericardial
ligament tension to
the right

Lumbar rotation and
superior shift to
ilium

General torsion
through Ⓛ hip

Figure 9.2   Examination findings for a patient with chest pain, breathlessness and sciatica.

engaging the left hip, ilium and the midlumbar spine.

Treatment started with the right side of the thorax and included sternal recoil techniques, functional unwinding to the anterior thoracic fascia to the liver and diaphragm and articulation and attempted manipulation to the upper dorsal spine and cervicodorsal junction. Some general unwinding to the cranium was done and some muscle energy techniques were applied to the accessory respiratory muscles (especially the scalenes). Work to the left

obturator internus and left hip was also included. This pattern of treatment was repeated over a few weeks and gradually some of the chest components began to loosen and the cervicodorsal spine was eventually released after much articulation, soft tissue and local stretching.

At this stage, her chest pain was less intense and less frequent but still present. On examination, it was only after quite a bit of treatment to the general chest and spinal restrictions that it was possible to feel 'down to the level of the lungs' with any accuracy.

Work could now be specifically addressed to the pericardium, lung tissue and bronchi and through the general mediastinal fascia. It was necessary to continually repeat work to the sternum and cervicodorsal area and to continue 'unwinding' through the head to the neck and also to the throat (for the thyroid scar) and its relations to the cervical fascia as it descended into the mediastinum. The cranial work also helped to release the left hip area (especially by addressing tension at the occipitomastoid suture area). General articulation was also repeated through the dorsal spine, to help with autonomic function and general postural/spinal mechanical balance and integration. The work through the cranium, pelvis and hip region improved lumbar spine mechanics (and therefore the sciatica) quite a lot.

After a few months of treatment, her chest function was definitely improving and she was suffering from less pain in all her main affected areas. However, she had developed a problem with headaches, which she had not suffered with before. This seemed to coincide with some changing mechanics in the spine, chest and shoulder girdle and with a particularly stressful time at home. These issues gradually improved and the headaches went away without requiring further investigation. Treatment continued by gradually working through the various findings previously noted, continuing to 'smooth over' local exacerbations as these recurred. The dorsal spine showed more specific (local) tensions, which did not spread through as much of the chest wall/pleura as they had once done, and it was possible to recognize the viscerosomatic changes to the related dorsal segments when her chest symptoms did temporarily return.

Over the course of nearly a year, her overall health improved, her chest symptoms eased and her sciatica was much reduced. She also acknowledged that there was quite an emotional trigger to her back symptoms and she also had much physical relief when she became engaged to be married.

These cases utilize various physiological relationships that can impact on respiratory function, which are further discussed below.

RESPIRATORY MECHANICS

As previously discussed, it is important to evaluate the movements of the musculoskeletal components of the thoracic cage in some detail, as many visceral restrictions and tensions will be indicated by altered, adapted or restricted movement patterns with the somatic thoracic cage. Pleural tensions and various ligament restrictions for the lungs will manifest as rib restrictions and somatic dysfunction at the level of the dorsal spine articulations, for example. The impact of these on whole-body mechanics as well as on respiratory function has been noted in earlier chapters. It is now interesting to consider just what type of impact these global, general and local chest restrictions may have on lung tissue, airflow and pleural circulation. With that type of understanding, an osteopathic approach to patient care can begin to be rationalized.

Thoracic wall movements take place in two compartments: the thoracic and the abdominal ribcage compartments. In patients with chronic airflow obstruction and in cases of respiratory muscle fatigue, there is notable thoracoabdominal discoordination.[1] This alteration to thoracic cage respiratory actions will impact on mechanical insufficiency and impairment of pulmonary function not unlike that often noted in scoliotic patients,[2] even in the absence of the physical skeletal distortion. Sagittal spinal curves change as a child grows and there is a statistically significant difference among different age groups, especially at cervicothoracic, thoracolumbar and lumbosacral junctions. The position of the sacrum (inclination and translation) and spatial orientation, as well as the global magnitude of thoracic kyphosis and lumbar lordosis, change with growth.[3] As a result, age-related changes in chest wall compliance must develop without hindrance in order not to impact on respiratory function.

The mechanical properties of the lung are important determinants of its efficiency as a gas-exchanging organ. Under normal circumstances the airways should offer very little mechanical impedance to airflow, allowing almost effortless and uniform distribution of fresh gas throughout the lung.[4] If there is efficient regional lung mobility as a result of efficient thoracic and abdominal ribcage motion patterns, then the lung tissue and internal airways (bronchioles) are kept compliant and there will be an even distribution of airflow within the airways. Under different mechanical loads and under different chemical influences, lung tissue will react and contract at different levels and so provide the lung with a reactive and active system for accommodating physical force and physiological needs to enable appropriate tissue function and gaseous exchange.[5] Gas travels within the airways much like a bolus of food does within the gut tube. There is a globular flow where the airway is stretched as the bolus of air passes. The airflow is always directed to the path of least resistance as this is where stretch is least obstructed. This enables good gaseous exchange (by allowing air to reach the periphery of as much lung tissue as possible), thus promoting effective homeostatic balance and normal respiratory function.[6]

Airflow is more limited in regions of the chest where movement is reduced and the more restricted some areas become, the more resistant that section is to regional airflow. This means some sections of the lung continue to 'contract' whilst others which are still receiving airflow, as a result of their local elasticity, will gradually 'overinflate'.[7] In the presence of general somatic ribcage restrictions, it is likely that the lobes/lung segments associated with those areas of the ribcage are also going to be slightly restricted and immobile. This means the person effectively 'breathes more in some areas of the lung than others'. This will create regional differences in airflow with regional changes to compliance developing throughout the lung, further adding to respiratory discoordination throughout the whole ribcage and associated structures. This can be complicated by the fact that there are regional differences in the viscoelastic properties of the pleura[8] and examination and treatment would need to ensure that these are not complicated by organ restrictions or somatic restrictions.

So, in terms of actual lung function, within the ribcage and within any general altered movement pattern acting on the respiratory system, any inhomogenous movement through the chest wall will create inhomogenous movement within the lung itself. As a result, the movement of the ribcage will actually affect lung pressures. This is not just the pressures between the parietal pleura and the visceral pleura; it is literally the gaseous interstitial and parenchymal pressures right within the lung tissue itself.[9] So, as the chest is mobilized (and during general body movements and respiration) dynamic changes are being created right within the depths of the lung tissue.[10] Lobar mechanics and the presence of fissures might allow extra degrees of freedom for the lung shape to conform to changes in thoracic shape during ventilation, which would reduce the non-uniformity of parenchymal stresses.[11]

Maintaining airflow is one thing but efficient fluid flow within the lungs is also necessary throughout the whole of the lung in order for it to function harmoniously and physiologically. Interstitial fluid movement and lung circulation are aided not only by chemical gradients but also by passive external mobilizing acting from the chest wall, through the connective tissue structures and through onto the lung tissue itself.[12,13] Regional differences in lung volume expansion result in regional differences in interstitial pressure within the lung parenchyma and thus affect regional fluid transport.[14]

Chest wall motion also aids pleural fluid flow.[15] Pleural fluid flows up around the outside/top of the lungs and also in between the lobes of the lungs and into the recesses and it drains centrally into the deep mediastinal nodes which are found around the bronchi and mediastinum. This means that all the fluid has to eventually drain from a dynamic situation (in and around the lungs) to a more static place deep within the mediastinum. The more efficient movement dynamics in the chest wall are maintained, the more the pleural fluid will be mobilized as a result of the shear forces acting between the two pleural layers that the somatic motion creates. Lobar mechanics, especially where these interact with the chest wall, may create a hydrostatic gradient in pleural pressure, facilitating the redistribution of pleural fluid.

Fluid flow really is important within respiratory disorders, because very many respiratory disorders are complicated by fluid effusion or oedema and fluid stasis.[16,17] Oedema and pleural effusion can also significantly affect the dynamic elasticity and resistance of the respiratory system.[18] When fluid stasis overcomes the normal chemical gradients, the passive mobilizing components within the respiratory system (i.e. somatic, pleural, connective tissue and lung tissue mobility and compliance) become quite important and these need to be kept dynamically flexible in order to improve deep lung fluid flow and help improve immunity and neural tissue reactivity, all of which can be compromised by the presence of the oedema.

As a result, it is evident that the mechanical components of the respiratory system are very relevant in the evaluation of lung function,[19] as they are vital for efficient lung physiology and healing and any change in them is a sure sign of impending problems.

General respiratory approach

- Whenever the chest wall is mobilized, especially when done in a three-dimensional manner and the more the pleura is stretched and engaged (during general articulations, somatic mobilization or whichever technique is being applied), the greater the benefit this will have on respiratory function.
- Make sure that examination and mobilization (where restrictions are noted) incorporates the whole of the body wall, so that the pleura (and underlying lung tissue) is being engaged right from the top to the bottom and all the way around.
- This examination and mobilization should also include ensuring that motion passes down into the pleural recesses and within and between all the lobes of the lung. The more homogenous the motion being passed into the lung tissue, the better the lungs will function.

BREATHING PATTERNS

This global emphasis on examination and mobilization is essential when the impact of airways function and regional restriction or change is appreciated. All the mechanical and physiological relationships discussed above will be affected when there is mechanical restriction in and around the respiratory system and alteration within breathing patterns. As a result, global musculoskeletal system restriction, torsions and tensions can have extensive physiological, emotional and respiratory consequences. Osteopathic care is directed at reducing or relieving those combinations of tensions found in the individual presenting, in order to alleviate physical stress and constraint on their individual breathing patterns and respiratory mechanisms.

Whatever the cause, breathing pattern disorders include changes in inspiration and expiration times and rhythms, predominance of upper chest or discoordinated chest breathing, mouth

breathing, shallow breathing, lack of or uneven diaphragmatic breathing, use of accessory respiratory muscles, changes in whole-body posture breathing patterns and palpable tissue changes, restrictions and torsions from head to toe. As a consequence, the patient's overall biomechanical balance will be affected, stress and strain will be present at various places throughout the musculoskeletal system and they will have additional regional differences in lung homogeneity, altered pleural compliance patterns and altered lung function tests.

Consequently, there is much that can be treated in these patients and many approaches to care that the osteopath can employ, including breathing exercises and pattern retraining, as well as the extensive manual approaches to the musculoskeletal, fascial, fluid and visceral systems that are standard within osteopathic care. The early chapters of this book indicate the approaches that osteopaths can use and the underlying philosophies that lead osteopaths to consider seemingly diverse tensions within the body when managing respiratory function. Chapter 4 on the respiratory and EENT systems gives specific visceral techniques that can be incorporated.

Some particular respiratory conditions are discussed below.

CHRONIC HYPERVENTILATION SYNDROME

One respiratory condition that is easily overlooked is hyperventilation syndrome. This is a complex disorder to diagnose in that it can present with a large variety of symptoms, none of which are pathognomic. Essentially, hyperventilation is a pattern of overbreathing where the depth and rate are in excess of the metabolic needs of the body at that time.[20] Exaggerated or excessive breathing can cause the respiratory centre's control of arterial CO_2 to fall, resulting in arterial hypocapnia. This affects the acid–base balance in the body, with pH rising to create respiratory alkalosis. Symptoms and signs can include the following.

- Headaches
- Numbness and tingling
- Ataxia and tremor
- Phobias

- Anxiety
- Depression
- Poor stamina
- Angina
- Tachycardia
- Breathlessness
- Wheezing
- Inability to breathe deeply
- Limb aching and stiffness
- Oesophageal reflux
- Heartburn
- Tendency to belching and bloating
- Sweating
- Muscular cramps
- Impaired concentration
- Sleep disturbance

As there are many differential diagnostic considerations with this type of list, the patient can often remain undiagnosed for years (or often have their symptoms confused with allergies) whilst other factors are ruled out.[21] The underlying physiology of many of the symptoms appears to include changes in vasomotor tone, metabolic changes in potassium, phosphate and calcium levels and changes in peristalsis (motility) and electrolyte handling.[22]

Breathing pattern disorders can also follow on from the presence of other disorders such as asthma, chronic obstructive pulmonary disease, conditions such as pleurisy and pneumonia and chronic interstitial lung diseases (such as sarcoidosis and asbestosis). Affected patients can demonstrate a range of breathing pattern changes, such as those described by Chaitow,[20] page 57.

Breathing patterns often provide clues as to the type of condition involved:

*Rapid shallow upper-chest breathing suggests loss of lung volume seen in restrictive diseases, where the work of breathing is increased to maintain ventilation.

*Prolonged exhalation time as witnessed in someone having an asthma attack indicates acute intrathoracic obstruction

*Prolonged exhalation (perhaps 'purse-lip' in severe cases) caused by chronic intrathoracic obstruction in patients with chronic obstructive airways disease

*Prolonged inspiratory time occurs in acute upper airways obstruction as in croup or globus (throat spasm).

Hyperventilation syndrome is something that can affect many patients and as it is related to chronic pain, it may be a complicating factor in someone presenting for help with a chronic low back pain condition (and not for their 'respiratory' problem at all). In these situations, recognition of the hyperventilation syndrome can be very useful not only for the practitioner, in that it helps to direct treatment to appropriate areas, but also for the patient, who will therefore receive more specific care that will be of long-term value to their pain presentation.

ASTHMA

Asthma is an increasingly common problem and has many causes. Although osteopaths can become involved in the management of patients with a variety of respiratory disorders, asthma is one of the more common ones. In order to appreciate the potential for osteopathic intervention with asthmatic patients, the following view may be helpful.

There is no peculiarity in the stimulus, the air breathed in is the same in the asthmatic and the non-asthmatic ... nor probably is there any peculiarity in the irritability of bronchial muscle: the peculiarity is in the link that connects these two – the nervous system – and consists of its perverse sensibility, in its receiving and transmitting on to the muscle ... it is clear that the vice in asthma consists not in the production of any special irritant but in the irritability of the part irritated.[23]

Diseases characterized by airway inflammation, excessive airway secretion and airway obstruction affect a large proportion of the population. These diseases include asthma, chronic bronchitis, bronchiectasis and cystic fibrosis. Airway production of chemokines, cytokines and growth factors in response to irritants, infectious agents and inflammatory mediators may play an important role in the modulation of acute and chronic inflammation. Several models exist to explain the processes by which airway inflammation is perpetuated in diseases such as asthma and chronic bronchitis. These include neurogenic inflammation, the perpetuation of the acute inflammatory response and cycles of airway epithelial cell-mediated and inflammatory cell-mediated recruitment and activation of inflammatory cells.[24]

An understanding of these mechanisms of airway inflammation may provide medicine with new therapeutic approaches to the treatment of these common and chronic diseases, in which osteopathy may be a major role-player.

Neurogenic inflammation is induced by conditions that stimulate small-diameter sensory nerves that end in the respiratory mucosa. When stimulated, sensory nerves in airways can mediate a complex set of local tissue changes in addition to their usual reflex responses. These local changes, which are collectively known as neurogenic inflammation, include alterations in mucosal blood flow, increased vascular permeability, leucocyte chemotaxis and changes in epithelial cell mucus secretion and ion transport.[25]

There are numerous reflexes operating within the lung tissue, including axonal reflexes which can be involved in a variety of functions including bronchodilation and constriction through the activation of pulmonary stretch receptors, for example.[26] The neural regulation of bronchial vasculature differs from that of the general systemic circulation in that vasodilator reflexes play a major part in determining blood flow. These reflexes originate in the upper and lower airways; those arising in the lower airways are the most potent and may increase bronchial blood flow severalfold and may cause swelling of the airway mucosa. Lower airways have afferent and efferent pathways in the vagus nerves, the former including sensory C-fibres and rapidly adapting receptors, the latter involving both cholinergic and non-cholinergic transmitters. In addition, neuropeptides released from the C-fibre terminals provide a local mechanism for vasodilation independent of central reflex control.[27] The vagal C-fibres in the trachea are found to be intimately related to the loose connective tissue within the lung, innervating it and providing a neural influence upon mast cells in the area, when stimulated.[28] It is the degranulation of the mast cells that induces a negative pressure of the interstitial fluid, so creating interstitial oedema by mechanisms mentioned above and others that are not fully understood.[29]

It has been suggested that local neural reflexes involving the release of these substances may contribute to airway inflammation and that axon reflexes may participate in the pathogenesis of bronchial asthma.[30] Continued stimulation of the axon reflex may lead to facilitation of this neural network, resulting in a lowered threshold for the triggering of local reflexes.[31]

Various factors may compound neurogenic inflammatory mechanisms. Neurogenic inflammation occurs (as stated) when substance P and other neuropeptides released from sensory neurones produce an inflammatory response, whereas immunogenic inflammation results from the binding of antigen to antibody or leucocyte receptors. There is a crossover (switching) mechanism between these two forms of inflammation. Neurogenic switching is proposed to result when a sensory impulse from a site of activation is rerouted via the CNS to a distant location to produce neurogenic inflammation at the second location. Food allergy inducing asthma is an example of neurogenic switching. Neurogenic switching provides a mechanism to explain how allergens, infectious agents, irritants and possibly emotional stress can exacerbate conditions such as migraine, asthma and arthritis. Thus neurogenic switching would also explain how the respiratory irritants lead to symptoms at other sites in these disorders.[32]

There may be another compounding factor for neurogenic switching, aggravating the phenomenon of neurogenic inflammation in the airways: the viscerosomatic and somatovisceral reflex concept discussed in earlier chapters. This key contribution to medical pathogenesis that originated within osteopathic philosophy may indicate another mechanism through which osteopaths can positively benefit patients suffering with asthma.

Although asthma has been considered as a condition of reversible airflow obstruction, many asthmatic patients, both children and adults, have evidence of irreversible residual airway obstruction in cases of persistent asthma (that may even be detected in some asymptomatic patients). This clinically demonstrable irreversible component of airways obstruction is also reflected by the presence of structural changes of the bronchi that contribute to geometric changes of the airways and to various degrees of functional impairment.[33] The airways become remodelled over time, with remodelling being a critical aspect of wound repair in all organs representing a dynamic process that associates matrix production and degradation in reaction to an inflammatory insult, leading to a normal reconstruction process or a pathological process.[34]

Chronic inflammation of the asthmatic airway leads to epithelial desquamation, goblet cell hyperplasia, mucosal and submucosal inflammation, prominent smooth muscle and collagen deposition below the basement membrane. The changes in the airway are attributed to chronic inflammation, the healing process and subsequent remodelling and contribute to three predominant mechanisms of increased airway resistance in asthma: decreased elasticity of airways; increased smooth muscle in the airway which may cause increased narrowing during bronchospasm; and collagen deposition beneath the basement membrane, resulting in airway wall thickening. Destruction and subsequent remodelling of the normal bronchial architecture are manifested by a progressive decline in lung function tests (notably FEV_1). Antiinflammatory medications, such as inhaled corticosteroids, have been shown to decrease this rate of decline in lung function, while the effect of bronchodilators is less conclusive. Beginning treatment with inhaled corticosteroids early produces a better clinical response compared to initiating treatment late, and early treatment may prevent airway remodelling and development of irreversible structural changes.[35] Osteopathic manipulation may also help to improve short-term forced expiratory volumes[36] and because of this potential for remodelling over time, the treatment of children with asthma may become very important, especially through the application of osteopathy which has the potential to maintain airway compliance and reduce airway inflammation through a variety of mechanisms as indicated.

The physical signs of asthma are manifest throughout the chest and include a retracted sternocleidomastoid (where the muscle is contracted and the clavicle is raised), which is more predominant than that found in COPD (see below). Signs for acute asthma attacks are more commonly noted than for the chronic (intervening) state and include increased respiratory rate above 30 breaths a minute, increased cardiac frequency above 120 beats per minute and (depending on age) pulsus paradoxus.[37]

CHRONIC OBSTRUCTIVE PULMONARY [AIRWAYS] SYNDROME (COPD)

COPD induces various changes in respiratory function that are somewhat different from those in asthma. In COPD, the adaptive changes include a relative expansion of ribcage or diaphragm/abdominal compartments, including changes in the diaphragmatic contour[38] which are not so noted with asthma. These changes in COPD are a result of hyperventilation of the lungs and particularly affect the diaphragm, which becomes chronically shortened, especially in its anterior fibres. The diaphragm is effectively in a full-inspiration position all the time. Although some sarcomere changes over time lead the diaphragm to adapt and maintain some of its contractile force, it gradually becomes unable to undergo changes in length. Its zone of apposition reduces and the fibres become more radial than axial, contributing to its reduced mechanical advantage.[39] The scalenes and intercostal muscles seem less affected. Tracheal mobility is also affected.

The physical signs of COPD include tracheal descent on inspiration, supraclavicular fossa recession, increased scalene and sternocleidomastoid activity and reduced palpation of the cardiac apex beat. The anteroposterior diameter of the chest increases to almost that of the transverse diameter, the rib angles become more horizontal and the diaphragm shortens anteriorly, as discussed.[37]

MANAGEMENT OF PATIENTS WITH GASTROINTESTINAL PROBLEMS

CASES

Patient with Crohn's disease

A 30-year-old woman suffering from spinal pain and Crohn's disease presented with a 17-year history of lower dorsal pain and discomfort and a 16-year history of Crohn's disease. Her current symptoms were generalized abdominal discomfort and irregular bowel habits associated with the Crohn's disease and severe spasmodic episodes in the epigastric and left upper abdominal quadrant. These started immediately after the second resection operation she had for the Crohn's. These episodes had been increasing in intensity in the first year postoperatively. She was also prone to more episodes of diarrhoea following this second operation. She was hospialized for a short while to try to stabilize her condition, with limited success. She had been having general osteopathic treatment elsewhere for her back pain (with partial relief) for a year prior to her current presentation, which was 3 years post-operatively. The first Crohn's operation had been 15 years ago and the second 5 years ago. On both occasions, to resolve the pathology in the terminal ileum, about a foot of intestine was removed. The first operation gave good relief for some years but the second did not have such a successful outcome.

Other history included some riding falls as a teenager, which may have contributed to her back pain, and a fall onto her coccyx. The patient is not sure but she does suffer from intermittent coccygeal pain and the area is sometimes swollen and tender. These latter symptoms can be associated with an exacerbation of her Crohn's symptoms. She had glandular fever at 8 years of age.

Her back pain was thought to be a combination of old trauma and referred irritation from the Crohn's and the more recent abdominal spasms were attributed to adhesions following the second bowel resection.

On examination, the following findings were elicited.

- Generalized abdominal tenderness, with a tendency to cramp on slightly deeper palpation of the organs.
- Significant fascial pulls to the sites of greatest scarring/adhesions within the abdomen. These centred around the small intestine and the duodenojejunal junction and into the descending colon/splenic flexure area. These pulls within the organs and the scar tissue associated with them fed through to the upper lumbar spine, and the left L1–2 area was particularly fibrotic and bound down.
- A slightly swayback posture, with a very rigid and fibrotic dorsal spine. There was no one area that seemed to display a particular viscerosomatic lesion pattern on presentation as all the spine seemed equally restricted/affected along its length.
- Marked restrictions at the suboccipital area and through the cranial base (implicating the vagus). The right temporal was particularly involved.
- A general fascial pull of the thorax down onto/into the abdomen, such that the patient felt she could not quite stand as upright as she ought to be able to. This pull seemed to be directed towards the liver and diaphragm and also to the small intestine restrictions mentioned above.

These findings are illustrated in Figure 9.3.

Initial treatments were to the thoracic-abdominal pull, which was considered the most 'active' component. Releasing this should lessen the strain on all other structures and begin to clarify the picture. Initially, the abdomen did not have a sufficiently 'resilient' feel to it to make much use of direct/local work at this point.

Her first treatments then were fascial unwinding and functional work to the mediastinal fascia and the diaphragm and sternum. This released the pull through to the cranial base (and the upper cervicals/vagus) somewhat. It also altered her posture slightly over a period of time so that her dorsal spine was not so kyphotic. After a few sessions of treatment, her abdomen became slightly less reactive and direct work (using the functional technique) was utilized. There would still be occasional reactions to this but, overall, her symptoms were beginning to settle.

After a few months the nature of her symptoms changed, in that she developed a slightly different pattern of pain and the timing of her periodic abdominal contractions/cramps would be slightly different and be differently relieved by her anti-spasmodic medication. Her medical practitioners felt that no changing pathology was occurring and it was possible that this alteration was in relation to the changing function of her tissues.

At this stage of her osteopathic management, the external constriction on the remaining intestines had reduced, allowing better local peristalsis and better fluid dynamics (of blood, lymph and peritoneal fluid); the smooth muscle of the gut also seemed less irritated. There seemed to be, though, a different type of change occurring at the spinal level. The nervous system (the sympathetic and the parasympathetic) seemed not to be controlling the gut more efficiently; rather, these nerves seemed to be exerting a control that was slightly more erratic than before. Concurrently, the palpatory findings of her spine had also 'come into focus' more. The dorsal spine now exhibited a 'classic' viscerosomatic reflex pattern for the small intestine area and the vagus was palpably more active. The nervous system appeared to be trying to 'function differently' but was still not sufficiently improved to influence gut function more efficiently. Thus, it had moved out of its 'diseased pattern' but had not yet moved fully into a more physiological pattern. Therefore, at this stage, work was directed more to the spine using

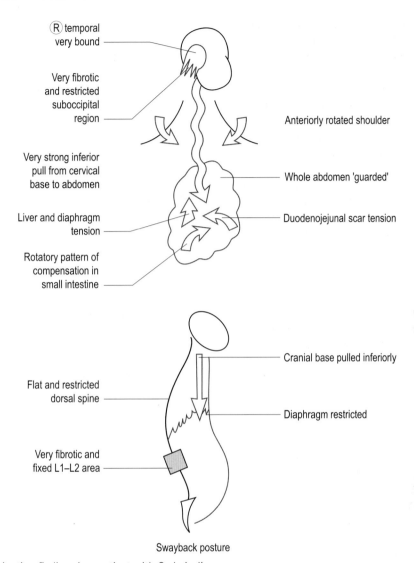

R temporal
very bound

Very fibrotic
and restricted
suboccipital
region

Anteriorly rotated shoulder

Very strong inferior
pull from cervical
base to abdomen

Whole abdomen 'guarded'

Liver and diaphragm
tension

Duodenojejunal scar tension

Rotatory pattern of
compensation in
small intestine

Flat and restricted
dorsal spine

Cranial base pulled inferiorly

Diaphragm restricted

Very fibrotic and
fixed L1–L2 area

Swayback posture

Figure 9.3   Examination findings in a patient with Crohn's disease.

neuromuscular techniques, articulation and high-velocity thrust techniques. Very quickly, the abdomen altered its habit for the better, although it was not yet fully stabilized. Note: before this, the spinal work seemed very ineffective and had not brought the changes noted latterly. Also, the abdominal work now did not seem to be as responsive as before.

It appeared that there was a phased/staged response to treatment as the physiology of the organ and its controlling nervous structures adapted to the changes induced through treatment. As spinal work continued, her overall pattern of spinal pain, general abdominal discomfort, irregular bowel

habits and episodes of gut spasms stabilized and improved and were gradually maintained through a long-term combination of global (visceral and musculoskeletal) approaches. This overall plan should continue over time, being adapted in the short term when there are any aggravations or alterations to her condition.

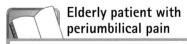

Elderly patient with periumbilical pain

An 81-year-old lady presented with a history of periumbilical pain which was fairly constant.

This was worse after eating and when walking. She also felt that she simply couldn't stand upright, as this caused too much 'stretching' discomfort in the abdomen, and that her back seemed to 'collapse' over her abdomen all the time.

These problems had started quite suddenly, 2 years previously. She had been walking along when out of the blue she had a pain in the abdomen and she had to stop walking immediately. This was not concurrent with any sharp increase in kyphosis or acute alteration in any spinal posture. She consulted her GP, who referred her for various tests, CT scan and x-ray, ultrasound scans and a barium enema. All were negative. The consultant felt he could not help her and she was discharged (which she found distressing). Eventually she presented for osteopathic treatment, as this had helped for other pains in the past and she was keen to try it for her current symptoms.

On examination, this lady seemed to be in good health for her age and her previous history had revealed nothing serious or significant. She was of slight build and was now quite kypholordotic and probably had a degree of osteoporosis.

Her overall posture was certainly not helping the general function of any of her visceral cavities and would probably be maintaining compression onto or congestion around the abdominal organs. Her posture and other examination findings are illustrated in Figure 9.4. She had spent the past 2 years walking around doubled up because of her symptoms and this would have had dramatic effects upon an underexercised osteoporotic/degenerative skeleton. It seemed unlikely that she would ever stand up straight again.

Local examination of the abdomen revealed a very compressed state in the subdiaphragmatic region and the lower abdomen had undergone a degree of ptosis as a result. The tissues of the upper GIT were very tight and the surrounding peritoneum was very bound down. The liver and kidneys (especially the right) seemed very immobile and the aorta appeared to be kinked/buckled and was pulsating quite strongly. She had had extensive tests and a diagnosis of aneurysm had been ruled out. The root of the mesentery of the small intestine (which contains the superior mesenteric artery) was particularly tense. It seemed possible that this posture alone was probably causing poor circulation in the gut, leading to pain and discomfort, and that if the mobility and

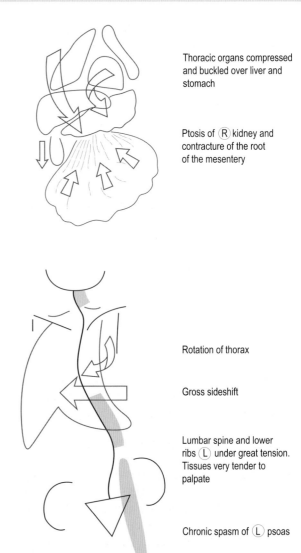

Thoracic organs compressed and buckled over liver and stomach

Ptosis of (R) kidney and contracture of the root of the mesentery

Rotation of thorax

Gross sideshift

Lumbar spine and lower ribs (L) under great tension. Tissues very tender to palpate

Chronic spasm of (L) psoas

Figure 9.4   Examination findings of a patient with periumbilical pain.

alignment of the tissues and organs could be improved then she might gain some relief.

After a few sessions of treatment, which was directed at her spinal posture (and general biomechanics) as well as her viscera, there was some slight improvement in her short-term ability to stand and in the extent/duration of her symptoms.

The spinal work was limited due to the degenerative state of the spine and the longevity of the tension, and the abdominal treatment, which consisted of local direct functional work and some mobilization, was guided by tissue reaction and local comfort/pain levels. Gradually, less of the abdomen was tender and more of the organs had a degree of mobility. However, she continued to have symptoms and relief after treatment was only short term.

She was reluctant to give up on the treatment, as some change had occurred, plus she was not confident that a return to a consultant would yield further answers. However, after a few more sessions with slight improvement, it seemed impractical to continue without another attempt at investigation and her GP was contacted requesting copies of all the tests (which confirmed a hiatus hernia which had been suspected during osteopathic examination). A second opinion with a different consultant was eventually organized. In the end, a diagnosis of midgut ischaemia following infarction of the mesenteric circulation was made. She has resumed an orthodox course of treatment, with hopefully a greater degree of success.

The osteopathic intervention was not wasted in this case. If anything, it helped this lady's confidence, gave her some rationale to consider her symptoms against and lead to an ongoing osteopathic appreciation of her tissues over time, allowing a better evaluation of any changes. This latter point is quite important, as it provided further evidence that the GP and consultant could reflect upon as part of the orthodox management protocol and decision-making process.

Some of the relief gained by this lady after treatment was because of the emotional supportive nature of the treatment situation but there may have been a short-term improvement in tissue blood flow through non-infarcted gut tissue, which was being compromised by the mechanical distortion, giving temporary relief.

Elderly patient with bowel incontinence

A 70-year-old lady presented with bowel incontinence and altered bowel sensation. She had periodic bouts when her stools were looser than at other times, although not quite like diarrhoea. She had faecal urgency during these times and would lose motions quite frequently. This had all started gradually around 15 years previously and the problem was thought to have been diverticulitis. It started with just discomfort in the abdomen and over the years she

became incontinent. She had various investigations and long spells with no treatment but eventually had two bowel operations, which did not relieve her problem. Her only other suggested management plan at that stage was a colostomy.

Other history included a long-standing back problem which was related to years of dancing, needing ongoing osteopathic care over the years. She had a bad fall onto her coccyx 50 years previously (for which she received osteopathic treatment) and a road traffic accident at 7 years of age, which was not apparently serious. She had had two children around 40 years ago, with no apparently obstetric complications.

Initial examination was fairly localized as it was felt that working on distal factors first would not bring sufficient change locally, due to age-related changes in her tissues (meaning they would not unwind globally with ease). The sacrococcygeal joint was very loose but the coccyx was pulled to the right side and had marked intraosseous strain within it. The rectum had very poor tone but was also being somewhat compressed by the uterus, which was slightly pressing against it. The sacrum had very poor movement and the lumbosacral articulation was very restricted. The upper lumbar spine was very tender and had chronic facilitated soft tissue changes, which may have been related to the bowel autonomics. Her right hip was a little tight, which was partly related to tension in the pelvic floor muscles and piriformis. The sigmoid colon was a little tight and irritated. These findings are illustrated in Figure 9.5.

Initial treatment was per rectal adjustment of the coccyx, with some initial attempts to release the uterus through the anterior wall of the rectum. General functional release was applied externally through the pelvis and soft tissue work and articulation were given to the upper lumbar region. Initial response to treatment was good, with fewer bowel symptoms in that week, although there was a little sensitivity in the bladder, as a reaction. Treatment continued with general functional release through the sacrum and pelvis and to the sigmoid colon, using gently rhythmic stretches and releases. Uterine balancing and functional work through the general pelvic connective tissues from there to the pubis was also performed and the right ilium was found to be in less torsion. As this patient's symptoms were cyclic in nature, she could indicate when her

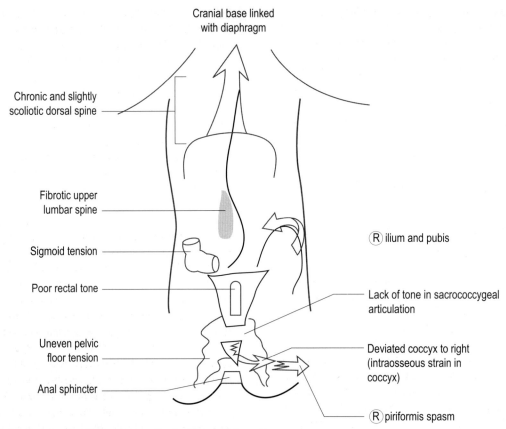

Figure 9.5 Examination findings in a patient with bowel incontinence.

next exacerbation was likely to be and although this did occur, it was not as bad as usual.

Work continued as above with occasional per rectal work, with the rectum beginning to have more tone and the coccyx not being so loose. Overall, the pelvic torsion was reducing. After a few treatments, it was decided to work on some of the more general tensions, which included problems within the right foot and lower limb and work through the abdominal tissues as a whole. At her next scheduled hospital appointment, they decided to delay any further surgery, as she was beginning to maintain some improvement. The medical team would 'watch and wait'.

Treatment was continued over some months, with intermittent per rectal adjustments to the coccyx and surrounding tissues, work through the pelvic, lower limb and cranial base and, after one occasion of relapse, to the coeliac and mesenteric plexi via the lumbar region and the liver, to help the overall tone of the gut tube. Her overall progress was that each treatment would help to relive her symptoms and lead to a reduction in faecal incontinence, although it would always build up again over time. She was suffering fewer bouts overall, though, since treatment was initiated. Intraosseous release of the coccyx did always seem to improve bowel/sphincter tone in this patient and the spinal changes were better maintained if right leg and dorsal spine/diaphragm treatment was performed (which had been gradually introduced into the treatment regimen, as other factors had started to change).

In terms of long-term management, osteopathic care could be continued, with the patient suffering incontinence albeit less frequently, or she could go ahead and have further surgery. At this point, the patient felt she would consult with her medical team and consider what she wanted (or could manage with) in the longer term.

Patient with rectal prolapse and somatic pelvic pain

A 54-year-old lady presented with a history of pelvic symptoms, both visceral and somatic. She had intermittent general low back pain and buttock aches and her rectum 'felt like a concertina', with the feeling that the 'whole thing has come down'. She also had occasional stress incontinence of urine. These (rectal and bladder) symptoms were especially prevalent when coughing or playing squash. She felt that occasionally faecal matter would get lodged in the rectum and she would perform manual evacuation on herself via the vagina to ease this. Maintaining a good diet seemed to have mostly addressed a previous problem with constipation. Her left hip was worse than the right and she had intermittent left femoral neuralgia symptoms. She was also prone to some cervical spine aching and stiffness on occasion, if she had been 'overdoing things'.

Previous obstetric history was of two children, both uncomplicated pregnancies and vaginal deliveries. She had stitches with the first but possibly not with the second (no forceps or other intervention occurred). She saw a gynaecologist about 2 years prior to her current presentation as she thought there may be a prolapse. No major prolapse was found, although an operation was offered, which the patient declined. She does try to do pelvic floor exercises but is not sure of progress. Her general health is good and she tries to exercise regularly (golf and walking).

On digital vaginal palpation, there was a slackness to the posterior wall of the vagina, through which small pockets/bulges of the rectum could be felt and occasionally there are faeces present in these 'spaces' which can be dislodged with the finger.

On examination, there were several factors, local and general, which were of interest. There was a generalized pelvic torsion with quite a degree of unevenness throughout the pelvic organs. The tone in the pelvic floor was not too bad but there was certainly tension in parts of the levator ani and through to the (left > right) obturator membrane/muscles. Some of the pelvic torque and the organ tensions were contributing to a left piriformis problem. The uterus was tense through the uterosacral ligament to the left sacroiliac joint, especially its lower pole. The adnexa was tense and this radiated up through the rectum. There was also restriction within the descending colon. These findings are indicated in Figure 9.6.

In general, there was poor motility to the sacrum and this was related to tension in the cranium and through the cervical spine to the thoracic inlet. These upper spinal patterns were not unrelated to the patient's job as a hairdresser. Within the cranium, there was a right-sided tension, especially through the right wing of the sphenoid and the temporal bone. These areas of tension were accompanied by a sideshifting pattern through the cervical spine to the thoracic inlet.

Treatment was directed at releasing the cranium and thus the sacrum and also working directly with the soft tissues of the pelvis. The obturator tension and that within the levator were of prime importance to the pelvic/hip pain and were also related to the support of the organs. Unless the pelvic floor unevenness was resolved, any work on the uterus and rectum would not be fully maintained. However, there were (as stated) significant local uterine and rectal tensions which needed to be 'kept at bay' for the whole pattern to resolve. This required local treatment which consisted of functional work to the organs and fascia, inhibition and gentle massage to the pelvic floor muscles, functional work to the sacrum and occasional general articulation of the pelvis and low back. Treatment was both internal (per vaginam) and external. Globally, the cranial and thoracic inlet problems needed closer attention so that their influence on the sacrum could be reduced and repeat treatment to the pelvic soft tissues would allow the central nervous system to gradually readapt and the fascia of the pelvis to gradually remould/strengthen itself.

Her symptoms gradually improved over time until she had considerably longer periods with no symptoms and when they did return, they were more quickly relieved. She was also given guidance (during the per vaginam examinations) on how she was performing her pelvic floor exercises, so that she could more successfully manage her symptoms 'at home'.

Patient with hiatus hernia

A 45-year-old patient presented with hiatus hernia, 'trapped wind and heartburn'. This had gradually built up over the last 10 years or so and coincided with coming off antidepressants which she had been

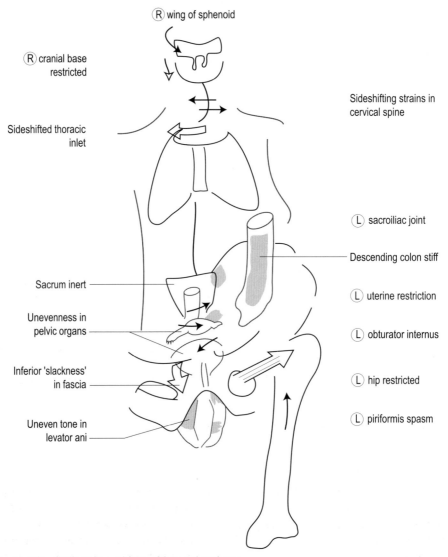

R wing of sphenoid

R cranial base restricted

Sideshifting strains in cervical spine

Sideshifted thoracic inlet

L sacroiliac joint

Descending colon stiff

Sacrum inert

L uterine restriction

Unevenness in pelvic organs

L obturator internus

Inferior 'slackness' in fascia

L hip restricted

Uneven tone in levator ani

L piriformis spasm

Figure 9.6 Examination findings in a patient with rectal prolapse.

taking for the preceding 5–10 years (following some family tragedies). A gastroscopy and barium meal revealed the hernia but showed no evidence of ulceration. There was some food-related exacerbation of symptoms and also an occasional aggravation coinciding with her menstrual cycle, which was now beginning to be a little erratic as she was menopausal.

Previous history revealed a long pattern of irritable bowel syndrome which had been triggered by a very stressful divorce. The IBS was not as bad as it used to be. Her father had had various stress-related

digestive problems and she herself was trying to manage the stresses in her life a bit more effectively.

On examination, there were various findings, which are indicated in Figure 9.7. There was a general hardness and tension throughout the stomach. Some tension was present in the diaphragm muscle but the ribs themselves were not too bad. The overall pulls in the abdomen were towards the diaphragm and the general peritoneal movements and organ tensions were not too bad, considering the long history of IBS. There were some quite chronic mid to lower dorsal spine restrictions but the upper

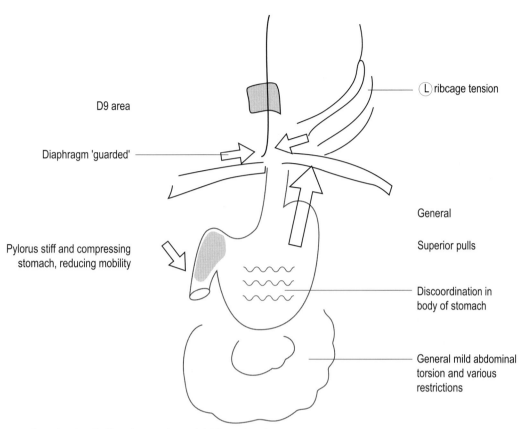

D9 area

Diaphragm 'guarded'

Pylorus stiff and compressing
stomach, reducing mobility

(L) ribcage tension

General

Superior pulls

Discoordination in
body of stomach

General mild abdominal
torsion and various
restrictions

Figure 9.7 Examination findings in a patient with hiatus hernia.

cervical spine was functioning reasonably (again, this was quite good, considering her tendency to stress). After this initial treatment, she felt quite sickly and had a bit of general abdominal discomfort although she had had less reflux.

On subsequent examination, the pylorus was softer, although the body of the stomach was still tight (indicating a temporary increase in distortion between functioning parts, which is not uncommon during an ongoing visceral treatment plan). A lot of soft tissue work and inhibition was given to the dorsal spine and functional work and articulation to the ribs, to help ease the autonomics. Work to the stomach ligaments in general and to the coeliac plexus in particular was given and specific mobilization ('very local articulation') to the D9 vertebra was applied.

Following this treatment, she was much improved and her stomach was palpably looser. Treatment continued to be directed at the stomach

and the diaphragm/dorsal spine. Tensions in the greater curvature area lingered a little but gradually the whole upper abdomen became more integrated. The patient gradually eased off her medication for the hiatus hernia symptoms and she remained reasonably symptom free. It should be possible to maintain this situation with general 'top-up treatments' every few months, providing no other new stressors develop.

This case is quite interesting in that the patient recovered very quickly, which is unusual for this type of problem. In many cases much more local work needs to be done in the chest and general abdomen, for example, as well as whatever else is individually relevant to that particular patient. It is always good to remember that it is only necessary to treat what is actually present in the patient and not to work on 'factors that are theoretically related' regardless of whether they are restricted or poorly functioning in that patient or not.

Patient with long-standing constipation

A 30-year-old patient presented with a recent aggravation (in the preceding 6–8 months) of a long-standing problem with constipation. The constipation had been ongoing since he was a child but was stable and he tended to pass a motion every 3–7 days. The presenting symptoms consisted of terrible bloating (from lunchtime onwards), 'terrible wind' and lots of 'noise/gurgling', especially in the rectal area. These symptoms had been present to some degree in the last 5–6 years but had been much worse in the last 6–8 months. Around 8–9 years ago he had had a mild nervous breakdown, had lost a lot of weight, split with his fiancée and become quite depressed. In the last 3 years he had been tolerating his depression less well. He found he was continually tired and found the problem was very limiting to his social life.

Other history included an operation for tonsils and adenoid removal as a child and correction for a right inguinal hernia at 10 years of age. In the preceding 2 years he had had some generalized low back pain (for no apparent reason) and a 'trapped nerve in his neck', for which he had received previous osteopathic treatment.

On examination, there was a very strong restriction with the atlas and the cranial base and there was a general torsion through the lower thorax/upper abdomen, which focused around the splenic flexure of the colon, on the left. There was marked tension through the descending colon and sigmoid, both of which were quite full. There was tension in the transverse colon and the duodenojejunal junction. Chronic restriction was also apparent at the dorsolumbar junction, with torsion at the right ilium, sacroiliac joint and inguinal region (Fig. 9.8).

Initial treatment was directed at soft tissue massage to the colon and general unwinding through the abdomen. Functional work to the cranial base was applied, which was very compressed. Articulation was given to the atlas joints. Over a few weeks, work was continued in a similar vein, with stretching and mobilization work through the lower thorax, to release the rotatory torsions around that region. Local work to the viscera was still a little difficult (especially access to the left subcostal region, which could only be worked on indirectly, initially). Symptoms gradually became more infrequent and

the patient was finding things generally less noticeable and embarrassing at work. Treatment at this stage had to be adjusted to accommodate a left thoracic inlet and lower cervical sprain (resulting in some mild neuralgia in the left arm) which arose following a strain during an exercise class.

After a few months of treatment to the various abdominal, thoracic, diaphragmatic and upper cervical strains, the symptom picture was more controlled and there were generally fewer exacerbations. The pelvic restrictions were proving a little complex, as the torsion pattern kept 'swapping' from side to side, engaging one ilium and then the other. This seemed to indicate that some factors were not being addressed and that the pelvic torsion was 'reacting' to some lingering tension pattern which had not yet been adequately resolved. As more tension was gradually released on the left side of the abdomen (with the descending colon and sigmoid), the chronicity of the left psoas was more apparent and with more direct work to this, the pelvis further stabilized. This also required further work to the cranial structures but did settle over time. The abdomen as a whole was beginning to soften and the junctional areas of the spine were more integrated.

The treatments were gradually spread out until a balance was found between lifestyle and monetary factors and the degree of retightening that occurred (in other words, the patient could only attend so often and this was done just frequently enough to keep that current improvement at a stable level). Occasional exacerbations would occur but these were addressed. The patient settled into a comfortable 'maintenance' treatment programme, with which he was quite happy.

These cases utilize various physiological relationships that can impact on gastrointestinal function, which are further discussed below.

GASTROINTESTINAL MECHANICS

The omentum

The omentum is worthy of first mention as it has a regulatory role for overall gut (and abdominal) function. The omentum has various biochemical and immunological functions which are unique and can be related to specific anatomical structures,

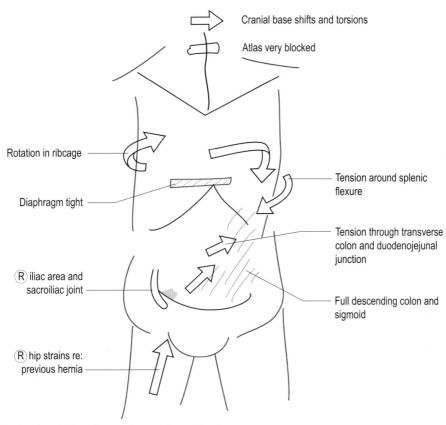

Cranial base shifts and torsions

Atlas very blocked

Rotation in ribcage

Diaphragm tight

Tension around splenic flexure

Tension through transverse colon and duodenojejunal junction

(R) iliac area and sacroiliac joint

Full descending colon and sigmoid

(R) hip strains re: previous hernia

Figure 9.8   Examination findings in a patient with constipation.

some of which may be traced back to its embryological sources. The omentum's actions of absorption and adhesion formation, neovascularization and infection defence protect against irradiation damage, accelerate healing of dead space and improve the complication rate and quality of life after application to a wound bed, for example, following injury or surgery.[40] It effectively 'patrols' the abdominal cavity and the various organs contained within it, helping to combat irritation, infection and damage to tissues. Regardless of which organ is involved, general omental function will improve abdominal function and aid overall tissue health and organ vitality. It therefore makes a very good starting point for a general 'visceral' approach to the abdomen. It is also interesting to realize that small excised sections of omentum have uses throughout the body, to help tissue repair and healing after various surgical procedures, such as complex cardiothoracic procedures[41] and

within neurosurgery.[42] Omental mobilization coupled with general gastrointestinal 'articulation' may also aid peritoneal fluid flow and therefore tissue health.

Mechanical gut sensation

The gut (or intestinal tract) is a long tube which has various muscular layers used to propel food at different rates along its length. It has a mucosal lining, with various glands and other structures either in its walls or entering into its lumen, to help lubricate the passage of food and to break it down and digest it. Each section of the gut has a special function (digestion of different types of foodstuff or water reabsorption, for example) and between each section is a muscular junction or 'sphincter', which controls the passage of food from one part to the next. The food is passed along by a series of peristaltic waves (contractions and relaxations in the muscular tube of the gut). Mechanical gut sensation is very important in the optimum functioning of the gut and is normally a subconscious phenomenon.

Gastrointestinal 'motility' really encompasses a number of events[43] which include:

- myogenic events in the smooth muscle cell (myocyte) leading to contractions
- neurogenic events, which coordinate smooth muscle activity by both intrinsic and extrinsic nerves
- coordinated smooth muscle contractions, which lead to increased luminal pressure
- propulsion, which is the net result of the above.

Neural control of peristalsis and sphincter function, all of which must work in concert for normal gut transit and digestion to be achieved, involves parasympathetic, sympathetic and enteric nervous modulation.[44] As a result, there are numerous reflexes operating between different sections of the gut tube, such as the gastrocolic reflex, the duodeno-oesophageal reflex and so on. Each section of the gut tube also seems to have its own pacemaker and rhythmicity generator, which functions in accordance with a global gut transit pattern.

There are numerous receptors within the gut tube and several that can act as mechanoreceptors. For example, the vagus nerve supplies stretch receptors as well as tension receptors to the wall of the gastrointestinal tract.[45] Many of these vagal mechanoreceptors appear embedded in connective tissue elements that would be exposed to shearing forces during stretch muscle contraction and, coupled with spinal afferent receptors, can monitor peristalsis and distension.[46] It is also apparent that mechanical stimuli from the mesenteries are important and can even influence other visceral functions and homeostatic regulation.[47]

So, the various peristaltic waves, global intestinal movement and mesenteric torsion, gastrocolic (and other) reflexes, pacemakers in the gut, rhythmicity generators and so on, which are controlled by various neural feedback loops, all integrate to influence gut function and transit.[45,48,49]

Osteopathic theory proposes that local neural control can be influenced by viscerosomatic and somatovisceral spinal reflexes; through reflex loops operating within the pre-aortic ganglia (e.g. coeliac and superior mesenteric); and through reflexes operating between sections of the enteric nervous system. Any spinal or associated soft tissue restriction or tension in relevant areas could compromise neural integration, while local soft tissue tension and torsion, inflammation and scarring within (and around) the gut tube could lead to altered reflex control of peristalsis and gut transit and may impact on normal mechanical gut sensation. It also seems that the normal general intestinal mobility movements could be important for its self-monitoring mechanisms, such that poor or altered gut mobility will impact on function via neural feedback loops.

If one section of the gut tube is expressing symptoms, the maintaining factor(s) which are mediated via the various feedback loops and reflexes may be within quite distant parts of the gut. Hence oesophageal reflux could be maintained by duodenal, ileocaecal valve or lower colon restrictions. If one sphincter is dysfunctional, the others will reflexly adapt their rate and rhythm of function (which may override chemical and other signals that would normally regulate these factors) and as a result they might then begin to express dysfunction in their own right. Hence the relationships between the following become quite interesting within osteopathic examination and treatment.

- Sphincters
- Fixed sections of gut tube
- Suspended sections of gut tube
- 'Hinges and corners'
- Fascial supports
- Mechanical links to the musculoskeletal system
- Peritoneal tensions
- Adjacent visceral restrictions

Many gut disorders and pathology have altered gut sensation and altered gut peristaltic activity (either hyperperistalsis, discoordinated peristalsis, or weak or absent peristalsis), which can manifest as a separate clinical entity or be part of a wider clinical presentation, as a corollary to inflammatory problems, ulcerations or other disease processes. Osteopaths are able to address the secondary 'adaptive' changes in gut transit, sensation, contracture and rhythmicity disorders that accompany such problems as gastric ulcer, colitis, diverticulitis and Crohn's, for example. Osteopaths also seem able to address these problems where they present without accompanying pathology in ways that are perhaps as successful as medication and other treatments, in some cases (although not all patients will respond to a manual approach, depending on what maintaining factors are involved, such as emotional, allergic or other environmental or traumatic considerations).

Osteopaths may well impact positively through their ability to interact with the autonomic and enteric nervous systems (either through reflex relationships or by direct mobilization and engagement with the gut tube locally), as discussed in earlier chapters. The neurological impact on gut function cannot be overstated. In fact, some refer to the gut as 'a neurological organ'[50] and suggest that many functional gut disorders (see below) seem to be related to dysfunction within the enteric nervous system and other components of the gastrointestinal innervation, making these prime targets for therapeutic intervention in these disorders.

Mesenteric and peritoneal circulation

The role of the control of mesenteric circulation as part of regional blood flow distribution has already been mentioned, as has the influence that local torsion and tension within the mesenteries can have on local mesenteric blood flow. Active digestive function requires an increase in mesenteric mucosal blood flow, without which intestinal absorption of nutrients cannot proceed. This requires a very complex level of communication between the mucosa to relevant resistance vessels, which is much more involved than for any other organ.[51] Microvascular regulation in the gut, then, is critically important to function and any factor that impedes it will create splanchnic dysfunction that could manifest with many symptoms. Although most studies into the effects of reduced splanchnic circulation focus on the critically ill patient, small changes in regional blood flow within the splanchnic circulation may have clinical relevance. One example of this is 'abdominal migraine' which is further discussed below.

Osteopaths would hypothesize that many functional gut disorders may also involve some small disruption to regional gut perfusion, mediated through the sympathetic nervous system perhaps, and that this may be under the influence of viscerosomatic and somatovisceral spinal reflexes, for example, thus making the problem potentially amenable to osteopathic care.

Similarly, peritoneal fluid flow is considered vital to gastrointestinal function and organ health and osteopaths would consider that they could influence fluid dynamics within the abdominal cavity (mediated this time more through the physical relations and tensions in the peritoneal ligaments and mesenteries and the mobility of the organs rather than via neural reflexes). Peritoneal fluid flow dynamics are further discussed below, under the topic of 'adhesions and postoperative scarring complications'.

Neuroendocrine immune components

Enteric neuroendocrine communication is complex. There are many links between the central nervous system, the immune system and the gut through the lymphatics embedded within the intestines and through complex hormonal and neurological feedback loops. Any work with the patient's overall health, vitality and whole-body biomechanics can be aimed at improving neuroendocrine-immune communication, with the goal of reducing the overall burden on homeostatic and healing mechanisms and reducing (in this instance) gastrointestinal tract dysfunction and symptoms.

Some particular gastrointestinal conditions are discussed below.

GASTRO-OESOPHAGEAL REFLUX DISEASE, HIATUS HERNIA AND GASTRIC ULCERS

Gastro-oesophageal reflux disease (GORD), hernias and ulcers are all common upper digestive tract problems. There can be many compounding variables which contribute to a patient's presentation and (in the case of ulcers), despite the presence of bacterial infection in many cases, there is a contribution that osteopathy can make. Much of orthodox medicine's approach with these problems is manifested in symptom control, with the use of antacids, barrier medications, acid reducers and so on. These clearly are easy for the patient to take and give short-term symptom relief and the patient can easily self-administer 'top-ups'.

Osteopathic management is designed to aid recovery from inflammatory processes (when present), to normalize gastric emptying (where possible), to influence the general motility and peristaltic pacemaker regions of the stomach and upper gastrointestinal tract (including the pyloric and cardiac sphincters and the sphincter of Oddi) and to improve diaphragmatic, oesophageal hiatus and cardia functions in general.

Much of the treatment can revolve around spinal reflexes with the sympathetics and parasympathetics and local mediastinal and chest releases to ease the lower oesophagus and the diaphragm. Much work should be done to the diaphragmatic insertions along the arcuate ligaments and the lumbar spine, as well as considering the impact of the adjacent thoracic organs such as the heart and lungs to the lower oesophagus. Subdiaphragmatically, the liver needs examination and treatment, where necessary, and work to the lesser omentum is usually required (especially where ulceration is present, as the majority of ulcers are located along the lesser curvature of the stomach and the duodenal cap). Particular care should be taken with subdiaphragmatic examination and treatment, due to the likely presence of oesophageal varices which can be ruptured, causing extremely serious gastric bleeds. Another caution which should be considered is the potential presence of food within the lower oesophagus, which is blocking the return of the stomach from the thorax in cases of hiatus hernia. Any sudden jerking techniques (such as those historically described for the manual reduction of hiatus hernia) should be avoided. An alternative is discussed in Chapter 5.

The above suggestions are not the full extent of possible treatment regimes. Associated factors found within each individual patient will determine whether cranial base work or pelvic work is required, or something with the lower limbs needs to be addressed, so that ultimately the physical environment of the stomach is eased.

'FUNCTIONAL' GUT DISORDERS

There are many gastrointestinal problems where there is no demonstrable pathology but the patient presents with a range of symptoms relating to altered gut transit, peristalsis and mobility, depending on which level of the gut is affected. These disorders are collectively called 'functional' gut disorders and, as mentioned above, they seem related to dysfunction within the enteric nervous system and related autonomic nervous system components. The symptoms associated with these disorders often arise from the changes to mechanical gut sensation and the discoordination of reflexes operating throughout the gut tube. Such problems can be initiated by several routes.

- Emotional factors.
- Short-term problems such as parasitic gut infection (which irritates the gut and creates inflammation, contracture and pain, for example) which will distort overall gut function, often persisting after the infestation is resolved.
- Sensitivity to various environmental or food substances (but no true allergic response is noted).
- Scarring from other procedures, such as caesarean section, gynaecological operations, appendectomy and so on.
- Mechanical tensions and injuries in adjacent or related musculoskeletal and fascial structures, that lead to physical or reflex compromise in local gut physiology and function.

The modulating effect of all these types of external stimuli to the gastrointestinal tract has long been recognized, as has the fact that the gastrointestinal tract is capable of carrying on all its major functions after all extrinsic nerves have been cut.[52]

This 'automatic function' of the gut is due to the local nervous mechanisms in the walls of the gastrointestinal tract and the inherent properties of the smooth muscles in its walls and from the actions of gastrointestinal hormones. The external stimuli via the neurohypophysis, various CNS centres and the parasympathetic and sympathetic nervous systems act to guide and influence the motility of the GIT (with the guiding signals arising from information received from visceral, cranial and somatic afferents, as well as intracerebral or psychic inputs). Under normal circumstances, they only influence gastrointestinal activity which would promote optimal automatic functioning for the body's best performance and efficiency.

Current evidence indicates that functional gut disorders are consistent with an alteration in the peripheral functioning of visceral afferents and/or in the central processing of afferent information in the aetiology of their associated altered somatovisceral sensation and motor function.[53]

> Osteopathic treatment hypotheses include work to the related neural reflex centres, as previously discussed. They also include work to the organs and smooth muscle components of all of the gut tube (including the bile duct) that engages the myogenic properties of smooth muscle. As this is stretched 'in series' (usually in a longitudinal direction), this will help 'reset' normal reflex activity in that structure, leading to a more normal smooth muscle 'resting tone' and a more coordinated peristaltic response during normal gut transit. Stretching and general mobilizing of the gut tube sections is a key component to normalizing enteric reflex control of gut function and any tissue tension, scarring, inflammation, torsion or contracture will impact on mechanoreceptor activity and contribute to discoordinated reflexes. Work is also directed to surrounding and adjacent soft tissues, including musculoskeletal structures, where indicated.

'Functional' gut disorders include biliary dyskinesis, dyspepsia, globus (the sensation of something stuck in the throat), dysphagia, aerophagia (repetitive air swallowing or ingesting air and belching), sphincter of Oddi dysfunction, gastroparesis (overlong emptying of the stomach) and pelvic floor dyssynergia (obstructing rectal outlet).

Functional gut disorders are also aided by stress management, the use of symptom diaries and cognitive behavioural therapy, to help change thoughts, perceptions and behaviours to control symptoms.

IRRITABLE BOWEL SYNDROME

Irritable bowel syndrome (IBS) is a very common disorder, which merits separate discussion. It is a mixed bag of symptoms and complaints, which are quite variable in their presentation in any one individual. It is usually a diagnosis of exclusion, i.e. it is made in the absence of any other identifiable pathology.

The syndrome consists of:

- bloating
- early satiety
- nausea
- heartburn
- feeling of incomplete emptying on defaecation
- borborygmi
- flatulence.

Other symptoms that are consistent with IBS include:

- constipation
- pain on passing a motion
- diarrhoea
- altered stool consistency
- loss of appetite
- scant stools
- weight gain.

Symptoms or signs that are generally inconsistent with IBS include:

- arthralgia
- fever
- gastrointestinal bleeding
- night sweats
- steatorrhoea
- weight loss
- vomiting.

Other important factors:

- LACK OF ANY OTHER DIAGNOSIS.

Things not included in the irritable bowel syndrome:

- chronic, non-painful constipation
- chronic, non-painful diarrhoea.

The site of the pain that people with IBS complain of can be in a number of different areas of the abdomen, illustrated in Figure 9.9.

There are many different factors which have been identified as having a relation to the onset of IBS. These include dietary, emotional and other types of stress, postoperative complications (such as adhesions) or in association with another abdominopelvic condition such as endometriosis or prostatitis and hormonal factors, for example.

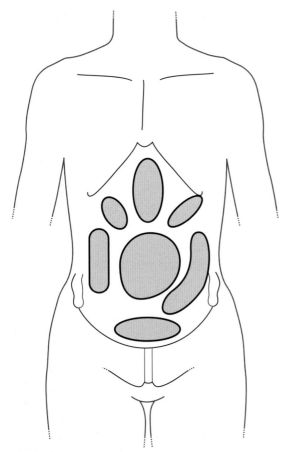

Figure 9.9 Sites of pain associated with irritable bowel syndrome.

It may also follow some sort of reflex irritation of the nervous system.

When gut transit is impaired for any reason, the lining of the gut will become irritated and normal function begins to be disturbed. Peristaltic reflexes accommodate and gradually the motility of the whole gut tube becomes dysfunctional, compromising local function with a gradually emergence of the symptoms of IBS.

The osteopathic hypotheses underlying irritable bowel syndrome are similar to those for 'functional' gut disorders in that reflex activity, local tensions, torsions and restrictions in the gut and surrounding tissues and general abdominal mechanical and postural efficiency are important. The findings in irritable bowel syndrome sufferers are often much more widespread than for most functional gut disorders (which can be locally focused to the organ expressing the symptoms).

Management is also along similar lines (given the caveats below) and should always be individually applied, according to the examination findings in each particular patient. Remember that change is slow and so many aspects of the treatment may need continual repetition over many months. This requires a long-term care strategy and IBS is definitely not responsive to 'quick-fix' concepts.

IBS can seem complicated and confusing but with a little patience, time and careful assessment, the syndrome can often be improved and in many cases much reduced with a combination of treatments, both physical and dietary. Given a little time, the gut will 'relearn' a better habit and settle into a less troublesome pattern of function. IBS symptoms will return if emotional, dietary or other 'stressors' are not (or cannot be) removed or reduced. Osteopathic care can help manage and contain the problem but will not resolve it in all cases without additional input from the patient and maybe other healthcare professions.

In terms of osteopathic treatment, it is important not to be 'diverted' to the section of the gut or abdomen that is 'symptomatic that day'. This type of short-term management is misguided and does not address underlying gut reflex and habit problems, which can only be helped by working on *all* the tensions and torsions in that patient, rather than just those that seem active on the day of any particular treatment. Don't forget that in treating the gut, habit retraining is vital, for example through the use of cognitive behavioural therapy. This includes retraining the mental components of a patient's 'relationship' with their IBS. They will have a tendency to focus on the known factors and familiar habits (thus negatively reinforcing them). It is the practitioner's job, through focusing on the underlying factors and relevant sensations, to help 'steer' the patient to a different mental picture of their gut function, so that they can then positively reinforce changed bowel habits rather than recreate them.

INTESTINAL/INFANTILE COLIC

The causes are not understood but infantile colic is a very common disorder, defined as distress or crying in an infant which lasts for more than 3 hours a day, for more than 3 days a week, for at least 3 weeks, in an otherwise healthy infant. It is considered that most infants will 'grow out of' infantile colic by 4 months and have no further problems. Many cases can be associated with lactose intolerance, reflux oesophagitis (immature sphincter development), inexperience of parents and maternal postnatal depression. Osteopaths would also consider several other aetiological factors and treat accordingly.

Osteopathic hypotheses focus around the role of visceral afferents within the vagus and the potential of birth strain for creating cranial and upper cervical compression and tension onto the vagal nerves in and around the jugular foramen in the skull. They also include local thoracic, diaphragmatic and intestinal tension and irritation, which can again result from intrauterine or birth strains (including caesarean births, which don't give the infant the advantage of normal 'elastic recoil' following a vaginal delivery to 'unlock' the cranial bones, which can be somewhat moulded even without an actual vaginal birth having been attempted).

Osteopathic work focuses on gently easing any strain patterns within the cranial bones, soft tissues and surrounding upper cervical spine structures, as well as working through related dorsal spine segments (for neural reflexes) and through the diaphragm, chest and abdomen. Other general treatment may be required throughout the infant's body in order to help the important head and chest compressions and torsions to unwind and fully release.

Many parents and lay people have become accustomed to the term 'cranial osteopathy' and have for many years consulted osteopaths as a way of relieving infantile colic. The name itself creates some tension within the profession, as many osteopaths who utilize the technique consider the name an anathema, as it incorrectly describes their approach and (through the growth of 'craniosacral therapy') associates osteopathic techniques with therapists who may not have sufficient medical and clinical scientific training to safely and effectively work in this field. Osteopathy in the cranial field (which is the preferred term) was developed by Sutherland[54] who considered, amongst other factors, that inherent motion occurred within the CNS,

which was related to embryological movements and vital forces within the person. His work established concepts of how to work with this motion and the reciprocal tensions operating throughout the dural, membranous and fascial systems of the body (which are based on the principles of tensegrity). The techniques employed by osteopaths working in the cranial field are very subtle and as a result, there is debate concerning the validity of the approach. However, many practitioners use it almost exclusively in their work and consider that, empirically, there is great benefit to its application, especially in infants and children.

However, it is not the case that osteopaths who work in the cranial field using Sutherland's techniques or similar approaches have the only way of relieving infantile colic through the application of osteopathic principles. Any gentle and general unwinding and releasing techniques applied to the head, torso and cervical spine can be employed, as can gentle soft tissue techniques to the chest, spinal muscles and whole body of the infant, for example. The approach is much the same as for adults with functional gut disorders, except that the forces and techniques applied are adapted to the infant body. These can therefore be applied by osteopaths without any training in Sutherland's work. However, in complex cases, the experience that osteopaths working in the cranial field have developed in infant palpation and interpretation of soft tissue findings may bring something extra to the management of these infants, which should not be overlooked.

Whatever the osteopath's own views of Sutherland's work, the concept of reciprocal tension and the primary respiratory mechanism, any work with the mechanics of the cranial bones (both cartilaginous and membranous), their soft tissue relations (such as the dura and other membranes), the fluid systems within the skull (the circulation of cerebrospinal fluid and venous drainage through the sinuses, for example), and so on, is a complex approach. Understanding the way the cranial bones articulate with each other and the cervical spine and the interplay of muscular, ligamentous and fascial connections between these bones requires much study, without which general osteopathic treatment cannot be attempted with any specificity or efficacy. As a result, these techniques will not be described in detail here.

FAECAL INCONTINENCE AND RECTAL SPASM

Most osteopaths would not view themselves as budding proctologists but there is much that can be done through the application of osteopathic principles for those patients suffering from rectal dysfunction (be it spasm or incontinence following pelvic floor or anal sphincter damage). This focuses on general lower gastrointestinal tract mobilization, work through local neural reflex pathways and particular attention to the levator ani component of the pelvic floor, coccygeal mechanics and the pudendal nerve. Patients respond differently and variably, depending on the extent of the damage and amount of prolapse.

CONSTIPATION

Constipation is another common problem that is resistant to general medical intervention. As it is multifactorial, it can be difficult to isolate the primary cause or causes within any particular patient and as a result, therapy is often applied on a 'try it and see' basis.

Constipation is an endpoint diagnosis defined by a constellation of symptoms, including infrequent passage of stool, difficulty passing stool, faeces that are either large and hard (or in small pieces), abdominal pain, palpable stools in the abdomen, stools in the rectal vault or faecal soiling.[55] Whether the underlying problem is one of stool consistency, poor cognition, motivation or fear on the part of the sufferer, or whether it is related to gut motility, altered rectal sensation, stool retention or disordered emptying mechanics, orthodox management begins with rectal emptying of impacted stool followed by maintenance of regular soft stools to eliminate fear of pain with defaecation.

Constipation may be related to discoordinated gastrointestinal (enteric) reflexes[56] and also to pelvic floor weakness and dysfunction, for example.[57] Both of these components may be amenable to osteopathic treatment. The osteopathic approaches

to neural irritation and enteric discoordination have already been discussed (and relate to general and local organ mobilization and restoration of normal compliance and myogenic activity) and the osteopathic approaches to pelvic floor dysfunction are mentioned below and have been discussed with reference to techniques in Chapter 7 (where pelvic floor dysfunction in general is reviewed). General abdominal massage seems of value and may help with stool consistency as well as enteric reflex activity. Stimulating fluid dynamics by mobilization may improve local tissue health and thus promote more effective gut peristalsis. Vagal function is particularly important and so much work should be addressed to any mechanical factor (where present) that can impact on vagal function (such as the mechanics of the upper cervical spine and cranial base).

INTESTINAL CIRCULATORY PROBLEMS

Various problems can affect the circulation of the intestines. On the arterial side, these include 'abdominal migraine', intestinal ischaemia and 'abdominal angina'. Relative gut ischaemia as a result of long-term sympathetic nervous system stimulation could be a precursor to these types of problems, which may arise through various viscerosomatic and somatovisceral reflexes and which could give an imbalance in the regional distribution of blood throughout the body, according to osteopathic hypotheses introduced in previous chapters. On the venous side, these include gastrointestinal varicosities, usually as a result of portal venous congestion.

Whatever the underlying mechanism, efficient intestinal circulation is essential for normal gut function. Various techniques have been described in previous chapters to explore the neural or physical tensions and torsions that can impact on intestinal circulation.

Intestinal ischaemia and 'abdominal migraine'

The mesenteric vessels can be exposed to atherosclerotic damage and occlusion, much as with other vessels. Gut necrosis accompanies acute infarction and requires urgent medical intervention. However, not all gut ischaemia may be so marked and there may be various situations in which there is a type of gastrointestinal 'angina' or a sympathetic neural disturbance leading to a relative ischaemia in gut tissue which would compromise local function and induce various symptoms and discomforts. Although the impact of atherosclerotic vessel disease is beyond osteopathic intervention, one variation of altered gut blood flow may be amenable to manual intervention. This is the condition of 'abdominal migraine'.

There is evidence to suggest that, in children, episodic abdominal pain occurring in the absence of headache may be a migrainous phenomenon.[58] There are four separate strands of evidence for this:

- the common coexistence of abdominal pain and migraine headaches
- the similarity between children with episodic abdominal pain and children with migraine headaches, with respect to social and demographic factors, precipitating and relieving factors and accompanying gastrointestinal, neurological and vasomotor features
- the effectiveness of non-analgesic migraine therapy in abdominal migraine
- the finding of similar neurophysiological features in both migraine headache and abdominal migraine.

Abdominal migraine is one of the variants of migraine headache. It is also known by other terms, including 'periodic syndrome'. This variant most typically occurs in children. They usually have a family history of migraine and go on to develop typical migraine later in life. The attacks are characterized by periodic bouts of abdominal pain lasting for about 2 hours. Along with the abdominal pain, they may have other symptoms such as nausea and vomiting, flushing or pallor. Tests fail to reveal a cause for the pain. Occasionally there may be EEG findings suggestive of epilepsy but this is rarely related to seizures. Medications that are useful for treating migraine control these attacks in most children. There are various criteria for the diagnosis of abdominal migraine which have been outlined by Dignan.[59]

Osteopathically, the management would be to focus on any restriction present that related to the autonomic (particularly) sympathetic innervation to the gut. Consideration would also be given to the root of the mesentery and the posterior abdominal wall mechanics, as both of these impact on the superior mesenteric artery and plexus. Local general abdominal work may also be of value.

MANAGEMENT OF PATIENTS WITH GENITOURINARY PROBLEMS

CASES

 Patient with recurrent renal infection

A 50-year-old patient presented complaining of recurrent renal infection. She was retired from her job through ill health and stress.

Past history revealed that she had had one episode of undiagnosed abdominal pain at age 12–13 years. She had then been of good health until just after she gave birth to her first child. She had her first bout of diagnosed pyelitis 6 months after the baby was born. Then, during her third pregnancy, she had some sensations of 'collapsing' (her middle 'giving way') and renal pain. Since the birth of her children, she had had a 20-year history of recurrent renal infection, which had eventually depleted her health and energy so much that her quality of life was markedly affected.

She had had various tests and investigations over the years and was diagnosed with clubbing of the calyces. This was predominantly on the right side and causing some kinking of that ureter, giving pain and causing disruption to the flow of urine, thus aggravating the pyelitis. For some years, things were not too bad and she was having 1–2 episodes of infection per year and could cope. Then, in 1993, things took a turn for the worse and the antibiotics didn't help as much as before. She had further investigations and one urologist inserted a stent into the right ureter to see if that relieved matters. However, this had to be removed 3 weeks later, due to pain. He suggested pyeloplasty, which the patient declined. She eventually had another stent fitted, where part of the ureter was deliberately disrupted so that any newly formed scar tissue would 'realign' things. This did help for 7 months, then the infections started again.

So, on her osteopathic presentation, she was suffering from chronic loin pain, a 'collapsing' sensation through her right side, as though there was nothing in there to 'hold her upright', and discomfort and some pain around the right costal margin.

On examination at the first session, the tissues were too irritated to do any direct work (in fact, it was to be five sessions before direct work on the kidney was possible, due to tissue 'sensitivity') and a functional/balanced ligamentous tension approach was applied to the 12th rib area and posterior abdominal wall. The aim was to diffuse tension around the kidney and begin to reduce 'facilitation' within the tissues. Some gentle release was done with the lower dorsal spine and also around the liver (again using functional techniques only), as these areas were also very immobile and sensitive. She had slight pain the day after treatment, was then OK and then had an infection 1 week after treatment.

Subsequent treatment continued as before, focusing on the 12th rib and liver. There was also some slight work on the renal fascia, via the other GIT organs that attach to it. She was slightly eased with this second treatment – not quite as bad overall, although she did have local pain on the day of the treatment. At the third session her tissues were less sensitive to touch and were more elastic. It was to be expected that she would continue to get infections but the aim was to reduce their frequency and their intensity (or at least the intensity of the associated symptoms).

At the third treatment, some work via the cranial base was added and by the fourth treatment (8 weeks after presentation) she was definitely feeling a bit better. The collapsing sensation had certainly changed and it was now 6 weeks since she had had an infection, which was very good for her. She still had right loin pain. On this treatment some work was applied to the psoas, lumbar spine (soft tissue massage and inhibition and articulation) and general work to the abdominal/peritoneal tissues and surrounding gastrointestinal organs around the kidney. The general pattern of her restrictions is illustrated in Figure 9.10.

After that treatment, she did have an infection but not as long lasting, nor as severe. The tissues themselves were a little more sensitive than at the preceding session but this would have been due to the after-effects of the infection. They were not as sensitive as on the first visit, though.

On this treatment, more work was applied to the cranial base, some to the cervicodorsal area and to

the right lung in general. A direct contact onto the right kidney was achieved for the first time and some balancing work was applied to the ureter area. The mobilizations performed were still very gentle, barely more than functional with a bit of exaggeration at some points to create a very slight stretch. Thereafter she continued to ease and treatment continued to be on the areas already identified (e.g. 12th rib, lung, cervicodorsal area, psoas and hip). Her pain levels were gradually decreasing, although she did have the occasional 'flare-up'. However, she was more mobile, less tired, less depressed about her long-term prospects and generally making good progress.

She was also continuing to have general osteopathic treatment for her neck and upper back from an osteopathic colleague, for intermittent aches and pains (a history of a few years' duration). This shared-care approach seemed reasonable for her situation, as that way the visceral components could be focused on by the practitioner more experienced in that field and the other could concentrate on the general musculoskeletal components (all of which would help all symptoms over time, anyway).

 ## Patient with undescended testicles

This case involved a 6-year-old boy who had bilateral undescended testicles, the right being worse than the left, in that the left testis was more frequently in the scrotum than the right. The parents had been advised that an operation was necessary but they were wary of this if it could be avoided.

As explained below, there may have been something impeding the descent of the testes, either by blocking their path (such as a tight inguinal area) or something holding them back, as in some form of embryological remnant, which may impact on the overall progression of the case. It was explained to the parents that treatment would be very much on a 'trial basis' and if no change was apparent after 3–4 treatments, then medical advice should be sought again.

General history revealed a Venteuse birth and eczema from 18 months old. Some slight asthma was present and the child's posture and general movements were a little stiff and awkward (there was no neurological or other pathological cause for these latter symptoms).

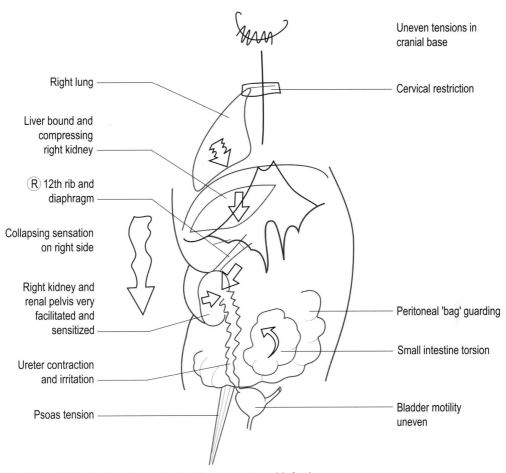

Uneven tensions in
cranial base

Cervical restriction

Right lung

Liver bound and
compressing
right kidney

(R) 12th rib and
diaphragm

Collapsing sensation
on right side

Right kidney and
renal pelvis very
facilitated and
sensitized

Ureter contraction
and irritation

Psoas tension

Peritoneal 'bag' guarding

Small intestine torsion

Bladder motility
uneven

Figure 9.10   Examination findings in a patient with recurrent renal infection.

On examination, there was a complex pattern of tensions around the right ilium, which was bound in all directions. These tensions are shown in Figure 9.11. There was a marked tension in the right hip joint, which accompanied the right ilial torsion. The right inguinal region was therefore quite compromised, with the tissues around the superficial inguinal ring, inguinal canal and symphysis pubis all quite swollen, irritated and sensitive to touch. There was a general fascial torsion pattern throughout the whole right leg to the foot, which was related to the overall postural imbalance and awkward gait pattern. The mid to lower dorsal spine, right ribcage and right abdominal wall were all quite bound and inelastic. Some of this tension was present on the left but not nearly so noticeably as on the right.

Initial work was directed to the right hip and inguinal region, with gentle traction and some soft

tissue unwinding through the area. Work then continued with soft tissue massage and stretching to the right abdominal wall, to the lower ribcage bilaterally and to the upper lumbar and lower dorsal spines. Some work was given to the cranial base and to the sacrum. The right foot was also articulated and mobilized.

After a couple of treatments the testes were both more frequently in the scrotum and the boy's general posture and walking were not so awkward. Treatment continued with the general work to the abdomen, inguinal region, hip and ilium, with secondary work to the cranial base and right foot/lower leg. Once these areas became more stabilized and the right ilium was consistently more mobile, the testes were definitely more frequently in place, with the left being present in the scrotum almost always. The pubic swelling had reduced and there was much less local swelling.

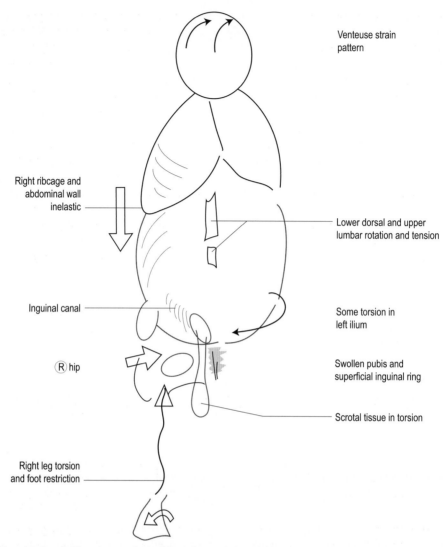

Venteuse strain
pattern

Right ribcage and
abdominal wall
inelastic

Lower dorsal and upper
lumbar rotation and tension

Inguinal canal

Some torsion in
left ilium

®hip

Swollen pubis and
superficial inguinal ring

Scrotal tissue in torsion

Right leg torsion
and foot restriction

Figure 9.11   Examination findings in a patient with undescended testicles.

At this point, the boy was reexamined by the consultant and it was agreed that surgery may not be required after all and a watching brief was undertaken. Now, work was also directed to some other components in the patient's overall pattern, which included the thoracic inlet, first rib, lungs and further (more extensive) cranial work. After some 6–8 months of treatment, the testes were almost permanently in the scrotum and the patient had some maintenance work over the next few months to maintain the situation, which remained resolved.

Patient with pain on urination

A 25-year-old male patient presented with penile pain on urination and some occasional pelvic pain during intercourse. This had been ongoing for the last 4 years or so, with an intermittent pattern, sometimes as many as 3–4 episodes of painful urination a week. No actual lower urinary tract cause had been identified for this problem over the years. He also had some generalized abdominal discomfort, 'indigestion' and 'bowel sensitivity' which he considered a 'side issue'; again, this was chronic in nature.

Past history included a diagnosis of non-Hodgkin's lymphoma 3 years previously (which had taken a little while to finally diagnose). He received chemotherapy and steroid therapy and had surgery to remove nodules in the intestine, during which some of the small intestine was resected. He eventually got the 'all clear' from that but around a year ago developed right hip problems and had to have a hip replacement (performed around 6 months prior to the current presentation). Since the hip replacement, the right hip pain had been quite severe and his gait was altered, leaving him with a sensation that the legs were different lengths, which he found quite troublesome. Other history included asthma, which was exercise-related but now well managed and not giving him any noticeable concerns.

On examination, there were problems almost everywhere one looked. The major components are indicated in Figure 9.12. The hip pain seemed a straightforward mechanical problem but the penile pain would require repeated analysis of the pelvic and associated factors, before being able to understand if it was a referred pain or related to the pelvic floor, prostate or some of the abdominal components, for example. It is also likely that the problem may have been partly provoked by a history of triathlon competition (including bicycle riding, which is known to aggravate the pudendal artery and nerve), although the patient had not complained of the problem during that period.

Findings included generalized abdominal tension, a strong torsion through the longitudinal midline

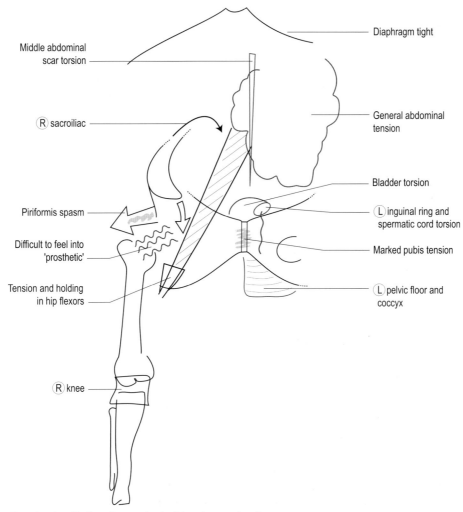

Middle abdominal scar torsion

Diaphragm tight

(R) sacroiliac

General abdominal tension

Bladder torsion

Piriformis spasm

(L) inguinal ring and spermatic cord torsion

Difficult to feel into 'prosthetic'

Marked pubis tension

Tension and holding in hip flexors

(L) pelvic floor and coccyx

(R) knee

Figure 9.12   Examination findings in a patient with pain on urination.

abdominal scar and tensions into the pubis. The left vas deferens and spermatic cord were under torsion and the right hip was quite compromised, given the operation. There was still considerable piriformis, right pelvic floor, right psoas and general hip musculature irritation, spasm and tension. The right sacroiliac joint was very compressed and the patient had poor spinal curves throughout, these being very flattened. There was chronic and marked restriction at the upper lumbar, D6–8 region, D2 and the upper cervicals. All these areas had small rotatory (and opposing) torsion problems, so the spinal mechanics were very distorted as a whole.

This patient required a lot of care over the course of a year, during which time there were several changes to his overall mechanical pattern, which in the short term gave some symptoms into the neck, left leg and dorsal region, as tissues that had been chronically bound for years gradually adapted to a new biomechanical balance. This sort of 'two steps forwards, one step back' progression is not at all uncommon with chronic rehabilitation. Effectively, posture and gait have to be relearned and all the relevant muscles have to be re-coordinated over time.

Initial treatment was directed at the sacrum but this was very dense and it was difficult to feel 'into' it. It was also very difficult to feel through the tissues of the right hip region as the hip replacement was (naturally) blocking normal tissue responses. However, with some treatment it was felt that a better physical sense of the local tissue would emerge, giving a more detailed analysis with respect to the urinary symptoms. Work continued with intraosseous strain work across the pubis to the sacrum and through the length of the spine (with general soft tissues, articulation and some manipulation where required). As the tissues around the right hip region released a little, it was possible to do more with the perineal region, through the prostate and lower pelvic fascia and through the inguinal canals and rings (for the vas deferens torsions).

During this time there was some difference through the right hip symptoms and occasional relief from the penile pain and urinary symptoms. So, there was some overall benefit but progress was slow. General work was continued through the spine, cranium, pelvis and lower limbs, with the global work on each area gradually benefiting the other dysfunctioning parts. General abdominal visceral releases were required to ease out the scar

tensions, and local bladder unwinding (particularly in relation to the pubis tensions) was performed. As required, some other work was necessary through the left leg, through the midcervicals and shoulder girdle and into the feet.

After the course of a year, the hip pain was much more free, the overall postural mechanics were changed for the better and the pattern of pain on urination and on sexual intercourse was reduced in frequency and intensity. It is anticipated that this patient will require ongoing maintenance treatment to keep the progress stabilized.

Patient with urinary frequency

A 65-year-old woman presented with urinary frequency, urgency and some occasional incontinence. The incontinence was not related to pelvic weakness but followed on from an extreme episode of urgency where she couldn't get to a toilet quickly enough. This had been ongoing for the last 5 years, gradually progressing. Over the years, the pattern had been variable and not consistent, although the patient now had the frequency problems every morning and the urgency problems at least once a week. There had been no treatment from her GP to date (apart from putting her on hormone replacement treatment, which she felt had not really changed the symptoms). The GP was going to refer her for possible surgery if she wished at some point.

Previous history revealed a fall onto her bottom many years ago, with no long-lasting symptoms. She had intermittent low back pain and hip stiffness and an x-ray had revealed age-related degenerative changes to the lumbar spine and right hip. Her other history was unremarkable except that she had had four children. The smallest baby was 8.5 lb and the largest just over 10 lb. She had stitches each time and forceps with the first. The pregnancies and deliveries were otherwise unremarkable and she had had no associated symptoms (until possibly the more recent urinary problems in the last 5 years).

On examination, her general mechanics were not too bad and included some expected tensions within the lumbar spine, pelvis and hip related to the degenerative problems. The pelvic floor was generally uneven and the whole pelvis had a reasonably strong torsion pattern oriented around the right hip and ilial area. On per vaginal examination she had a urethral torsion, with the lower urethra being quite scarred and kinked. The bladder neck was a bit tight in relation to the arcus tendineus but the trigone area still had reasonable tone (as did the general vaginal vault). There was a very slight uterine ptosis, which was more of a slight 'sagging' onto the top of the bladder rather than anything more significant. This would be causing some bladder irritation, though. These pelvic findings are illustrated in Figure 9.13.

Initial treatment was given to the right hip and pelvis, with a general mechanical approach. Some internal release of the pelvic floor and urethra was given. After a couple of sessions, the patient also required some work through the right ascending colon, the lower lumbar spine and the general peritoneal relations, as the pelvic mechanics started to alter. She began to have quite good relief from her urinary frequency, although she could still have some urgency and the occasional wet episode.

Internal release of the bladder, vagina, uterus, urethra and pelvic floor was continued and externally, supportive release was still being given to the lumbar region, throughout the dorsal spine and into the right hip and leg. Some work was also given to the thoracic inlet, cervical region and head as she had been having a sinus problem for the last year and it was felt that the local mechanical tensions in the head region were adversely affecting the release and changes within the sacrum and pelvic region as a whole. After some further treatment, she also required some balancing work to the right kidney and 12th rib regions and through the left leg, which initially was not comfortable with the changing gait mechanics.

After a couple of months of treatment, the pelvic floor was much more integrated and the pubic and hip mechanics had all released. She still had some right hip and lumbar restrictions but these were not affecting the pelvis in the same way and her urinary

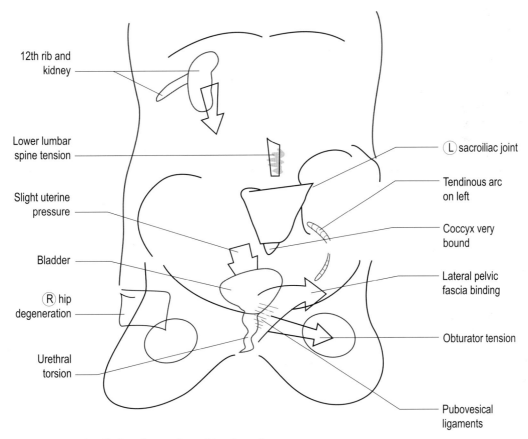

Figure 9.13 Examination findings in a patient with urinary frequency.

symptoms had practically disappeared. She elected to 'see how it goes' and to return for further treatment on an 'as needed' basis. This patient illustrates the point that it is not necessary to release 'everything' in order to achieve the desired patient outcomes.

Patient wanting conception assistance

A 36-year-old woman presented with pelvic pain and fertility problems, wanting some assistance with conception. She had had pelvic pain for the preceding 3 years, which was initially just 1 week premenstrual but then increased to the whole of the second half of each cycle.

Her gynaecological history had started 15 years before with a burst ovarian cyst, followed by a small fibroid removal the following year. She then had 8–10 years of no gynaecological problems or symptoms. About 5–6 years ago she had stopped taking the pill and was trying to conceive, so was 'paying more attention to her cycle'. She wondered if this interest helped her to focus more on the pain but she started to experience pelvic discomfort, which developed into some pain (although not as severe as currently). She had an hysterosalpingogram which indicated that the right tube was blocked and a laparoscopy was performed, which identified that both fallopian tubes were twisted and bound down through numerous adhesions, which were partly addressed during the procedure.

She continued to try to conceive and did have one naturally conceived pregnancy but this was miscarried at 9 weeks, apparently due to low progesterone levels. She then had an unsuccessful attempt at IVF. Following this, her current consultant performed a second laparoscopy which revealed the presence of polycystic ovaries and endometriosis. These were assumed to have been 'masked' in the first laparoscopy by the previous adhesions. There was some more local surgery to address these recently revealed problems. Her consultant then said she probably had '6 months of better ovarian function before things became dysfunctional again' so she felt she had quite a constrained 'window of opportunity' to try to conceive. Hence her decision to try osteopathic care.

Other history revealed back pain for the preceding year, following a skiing accident and an ongoing

(but very intermittent) problem with irritable bowel type symptoms, which she attributed to stress levels.

On examination, there were some marked local torsions and scarring tensions through the right lower abdomen and pelvis. The right leg was generally less 'elastic' but the sacrum was very unstable when a 'listening' technique was used, indicating that it was trying to balance many conflicting tensions through the pelvic region. Most of these tensions were within the right deep pelvic region, relating to the uterine and fallopian tube/ovary problems. The abdomen as a whole was a bit 'inert' and the tissue were a little difficult to feel through. There was marked tension in the root of the mesentery, some small intestine irritation and 'dragging' into the right iliac fossa and some tension from the mesentery into the midlumbar spine (which was locally adding to autonomic nervous irritation). These findings are indicated in Figure 9.14. Other findings included a kyphotic upper dorsal spine and a congested feel to the adjacent tissues.

Initial treatment was directed to the abdomen, where a generalized functional release was given. After that treatment she had some low back pain but this eased off within a few days. Her premenstrual symptoms were not as marked and she felt generally better. Work was then addressed to her spinal restrictions, throughout the abdomen and into the right iliac fossa and psoas area. At this stage the releases were fairly non-specific, as the tissues as a whole had to become more 'engaged' in global movements and not be so generally restricted. As tensions dissipated, it was possible to work more closely through the abdominal wall into the tubal tension patterns and local ovary torsions.

Her next menstrual cycle was more comfortable and although there was still some midcycle pain, the strong 'premenstrual' element had significantly reduced. Treatment was again addressed to her more global pelvic and spinal restrictions and it was decided to perform an internal per vaginal examination on the next treatment, to work more closely on the uterine and tubal tensions. However, this was not performed, as the patient cancelled because she was 6 weeks pregnant by then. The pregnancy was successful and she finally gained her longed-for child.

This case is interesting in that it gives some insight into gynaecological 'assistance' for conception and indicates that not all osteopathic gynaecological work needs to be done internally. It is not possible

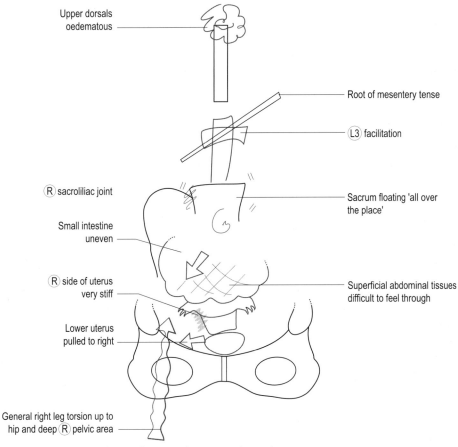

Figure 9.14   Examination findings in a patient wanting conception assistance.

to state definitively that the osteopathic care had been the 'missing part of the picture' which enabled her to conceive (as conception is a multifactorial issue) but it certainly did not hinder her success.

Note: many patients with fertility problems do require considerably more osteopathic care and often deeper tensions cannot be successfully released without internal work. However, this is always the choice of the patient and even if the practitioner feels it would benefit them, some patients only want to pursue an 'external' approach to gynaecological care.

 Patient wanting support for fibroid problem

A 46-year-old woman presented with a 2-year history of fibroids, for which she wanted some support. The patient didn't want a hysterectomy if at all possible. She had abdominal 'bloating' and 'swelling' and an accompanying tendency to urinary frequency and constipation due to pressure from the fibroids. In the preceding 6–8 months her condition had been worsening and she was having occasional vaginal bleeds.

With this patient, it was decided to attempt treatment to give her relief and to keep in contact with her medical team and for her to have repeated scans as indicated, to monitor her overall condition (so that further pathology was not overlooked, for example). She had had one child, who was now 10 years of age, and she felt very good with that pregnancy, as she had (obviously) no 'period pain' at all, which was 'very nice for a while'. The delivery was uncomplicated and she had a few stitches, which had healed with no problems. Otherwise her medical history had been uncomplicated; she had had only one episode of back pain, on a holiday when she had 'slipped a disc', and had low back aches and some posterior left leg aches/'sciatica' for a year or two, some years previously.

The fibroids had started to bother her around 2 years ago, as stated, when she was having quite a stressful time with family illness. Her most recent scan revealed that she had multiple fibroids, with the largest measuring 9.5 cm across and two other smaller ones at 6 cm across. She also had a right ovarian cyst which measured 5 cm. On abdominal palpation, these were quite noticeable, as were surrounding abdominal and pelvic restrictions and tensions. These are indicated in Figure 9.15.

The right side of the pelvis/uterus was more bound than the left inferiorly but the left side of the uterus seemed more bound superiorly. The uterus as a whole was not too much 'in spasm' but there was quite marked sidebending through the uterine body, with the top of the fundus being quite bent to the left (as a result of the fibroid masses).

The movements of the uterus were strongly reflected within the sacrum and there was quite a strong lumbosacral and upper lumbar torsion pattern that would need addressing. There were also conflicting torsion patterns between the different fibroids themselves, each seemingly 'vying' for position. The dorsal spine was a little restricted generally and there was some diaphragm/lower ribcage tension, which could be stress related. The cranial base had a strong pull down into the pelvis and the upper cervical spine was quite tight.

Treatment was first given to the lower abdomen in general, trying to balance the tissue around the uterus as a whole. Some local articulatory work to the spine and related soft tissues was given. There was some initial relief of abdominal 'cramping' post treatment and the patient felt able to sit more comfortably upright. Over a few months, work was directed to the upper lumbar region, with articulation and manipulation and some stretching and articulation

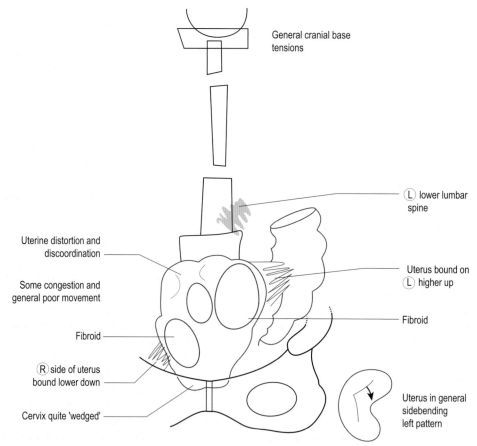

General cranial base tensions

L lower lumbar spine

Uterine distortion and discoordination

Uterus bound on L higher up

Some congestion and general poor movement

Fibroid

Fibroid

R side of uterus bound lower down

Cervix quite 'wedged'

Uterus in general sidebending left pattern

Figure 9.15   Examination findings in a patient wanting support for a fibroid problem.

to the upper cervical spine and functional work to the cranial base and sacrum. Local gently balancing work was applied through the abdomen to the uterus, to try to ease the overall balance within the uterus. No direct articulation or strong treatment was directed at the uterus. Surrounding work was also applied to the abdomen and to the chest/lower ribcage and diaphragm.

Gradually her bleeding episodes calmed down and a scan revealed no further enlargement of her fibroids. The uterine consistency was improved and she was generally more comfortable within her abdomen. She continued to have some treatment intermittently for a while, to help monitor the situation.

These cases utilize various physiological relationships that can impact on genitourinary function, which are further discussed below.

UPPER URINARY TRACT MECHANICS

There are many conditions affecting the kidneys and osteopaths often deal with the consequences of these, rather than becoming involved in the primary care of those conditions themselves. The two most common conditions that osteopaths deal with are the consequences of renal infection (and the chronic pain that can develop in some cases) and renal colic, which can present as atypical low back pain. Renal mobility can be impaired post infection, due to the consequences of muscular 'guarding' and also the connective tissue changes that occur during the inflammatory/infective process. Similarly, renal calculi can also lead to irritation of the tissues and leave associated structures in an altered state.

In practical terms, patients will not present at an osteopathic clinic with acute renal pathology but will present either with a 'confused presentation' of early renal infection/colic and associated musculoskeletal symptoms, or the long-term consequences of renal colic or repeated renal infection such as chronic loin-groin pain and chronic dorsolumbar pain, for example.

Pyeloureteral motility and ureteric peristalsis

The kidney has very complex functions and the range of its physiological actions will not be discussed here. The elements of renal function that

interest osteopaths combine physiology with the mechanical and neurological influences in and around the kidney.

Renorenal reflexes (operating between the two kidneys) have been identified, although their exact function is not clear. However, they are stimulated by mechanoreceptors within the corticomedullary region and the wall of the renal pelvis. From the tubules within the kidney, the transport of urine to the urinary bladder is under pyeloureteral control, which is not a 'passive drain' but an active transport mechanism under the control of myogenic and neurogenic factors.[60] There seem to be locally operating pyeloureteral reflexes controlling the flow of urine. Spontaneously acting myogenic pacemakers in the renal pelvis initiate ureteric peristalsis and promote the flow of urine to the bladder. The control must remain efficient, as urine flow must be maintained in many body positions (including many hours of being horizontal at night) and during general locomotion and other activities during the day. It seems that factors such as the degree of filling of a particular calyx or local stretch may determine the initiation of the pacemaker activity at a given site.[61] However, the neurogenic influence (which may be as strong, or more so, than the mechanical stimulus) is also important in the control of activity and peristalsis throughout the whole ureter.[62]

This combination of neurogenic and myogenic reflexes may be influenced by changes in local soft tissue dynamics operating with the kidney, renal pelvis and ureter (all embedded in the renal fascia). Osteopathic hypotheses would indicate that mechanical torsion and irritation (or slight renal ptosis, for example) in and around the renal and dorsolumbar region/posterior abdominal wall may influence the physical properties of the renal pelvis and ureter sufficiently to negatively impact on the efficiency of the above reflexes. 'External factors' such as tension or adhesions in the peritoneum or surrounding organs, for example from gall bladder surgery, duodenal irritation or various colon problems, may impact on the renal fascia and hence onto kidney and ureteric tissue. Similarly, as discussed above, problems in the arcuate ligaments, diaphragm, 12th rib mechanics and particularly the actions of psoas are thought by osteopaths to contribute to renal mobility problems (and therefore distortion in the operation of the pyeloureteral reflexes). Even such factors as the use of stents (which are quite routinely employed to keep the ureter patent in various pathological situations) can lead to renal and ureteric complications,[63] which can leave residual mechanical and palpatory impact long after their use or removal.

Renal colic

There is extensive sensory innervation of the ureter, which is self-evident from the suffering caused by renal colic (from the passage of a stone in the ureter) which is one of the most severe forms of visceral pain. The sensory innervation of the ureter and renal pelvis plays a role in local changes in pyeloureteral motility/peristalsis and in producing neurogenic inflammation. Any irritant on the lining of the ureter (from the passage of a rough/sharp stone, for example) will create local inflammation and contracture of the ureter. This will only serve to 'clamp' the ureter even more tightly around the damaging stone, creating a vicious cycle of contraction, irritation, inflammation, oedema and more spasm. This can leave the ureter quite scarred, stiff, less elastic and compliant and with possible altered response to the neurogenic and myogenic stimuli for peristalsis and the flow of urine.

Although osteopaths may be unable to significantly influence the aetiology of renal calculi production or change the fact that bacteria create renal infection, they can at least help manage the after-effects of these debilitating conditions, particularly for those who suffer regularly. They aim to do this by gently stretching and mobilizing the kidney (when the patient is not suffering acutely) as well as the ureter, with the aim of reducing local smooth muscle spasm, increasing compliance of the renal pelvis and ureter, and improving circulation and drainage to the renal tissues in general. Mobilizing the renal fascia encourages renal and ureteric mobility, which should help manage the above factors and aid the physiological reflexes operating within the kidney and ureters, all of which can promote the restoration of more normal renal functioning.

Vesicoureteric reflux

This may be a cause of recurrent urinary tract infection, with the reflux causing 'back-damming' of urine, incomplete emptying of the renal pelvis,

urethral dilation and consequent renal irritation and compromise. The problem can be congenital or following some sort of ureteric constriction, for example, and often presents in childhood.[64,65]

The mechanics of the vesicourethral junction are of interest to osteopaths, who consider that mechanical distortion of the lower ureter, bladder and associated tissues may compromise the reflex activity of the vesicoureteric junction, contributing to reflex and its attendant complications. Various techniques to evaluate and treat the vesicoureteric junction have been described in Chapter 6. It is not suggested that osteopaths can manage the consequences of primary reflux or severe outlet obstruction, which is not the case. However, in some mild cases, there may be some functional improvement that can be maintained through the application of manual techniques.

Enuresis

Enuresis (reflex incontinence) is a troubling condition, which has a variety of causes. One issue may be a relationship with bladder hyperreflexivity and vesicoureteric dyssynergia.[66] The osteopathic hypothesis is that unstable or inappropriately inhibited bladder wall (detrusor) reflexes may 'confuse' sphincter mechanics and actions, leading to enuresis. This instability may be related to physical tensions and torsion in the bladder and surrounding tissues. Note: this concept is further discussed below. Osteopathic management would be to treat any tissues or tensions that may be contributing to adverse bladder, urethral and renal mechanics, which may be disrupting urinary tract mechanoreceptors and sensory feedback loops. This can even include links via the urachus and the umbilicus to the liver and diaphragm, via the bladder and pelvic floor to the coccyx and via the dural membranes to various cranial torsions and tensions, for example (as well as work to spinal reflex centres and other neural components). The umbilical link can be very influential in children consequent upon a variety of intrauterine and birth-related issues.

LOWER URINARY TRACT MECHANICS – FEMALE

During micturition, the pelvic floor has to relax and to change from being like a horizontal platform into being something shaped like a hammock (bulging inferiorly). As the pelvic floor drops, so the bladder can descend. It also rotates backwards and the bladder neck must be mobile away from the internal surface of the pubis, to prevent awkward kinking or torsion at the top of the urethra. After micturition, with pelvic floor contraction, the bladder has to rebound and come back up again.[67] Various pelvic tensions, problems with scars, altered symphysis pubis mechanics, pelvic floor spasms or weakness will alter the lower urinary tract mechanics and irritate or 'confuse' the various mechanosensitive reflexes controlling and guiding the whole process of micturition and thus preventing incontinence and a whole host of urinary disorders (such as urgency and frequency).

The muscular coat of the bladder is called the detrusor. During the filling stage, the detrusor has to stretch with adequate compliance to avoid the pressures in the bladder building up.[68] The bladder needs to be compliant, meaning that as the bladder fills, there has to be the same internal pressure when it contains 50 ml of urine as when it contains 700ml of urine, for example. The bladder needs to be nicely 'elastic, spreadable and *compliant*' so that it does not trigger sensations of being full too early. Tension and contracture within the detrusor muscle, or a lot of tension/scarring/mechanical problems in the connective tissue ligaments around the outside of the bladder and the surrounding peritoneum or pelvic floor, may affect the compliance of the bladder and therefore affect bladder function.[69-71] This mechanical distortion can disturb not only filling sensation reflexes but also the interplay of reflexes that would normally prevent voiding activation until the bladder is sufficiently full and the person is in a socially acceptable and comfortable place to void. As a result, the bladder can become hyperirritable and unstable, leading to urethral dyssynergia, or contribute to vesicoureteric dyssynergia and possible reflux. The tension causes irritability in the detrusor because it 'confuses' the mechanoreceptors that inform the central nervous system (at cord level S2–4) of bladder fullness.

The mechanics of the symphysis pubis, obturator muscles, general pelvic connective tissues, pelvic floor and other pelvic organs are all particularly important for lower urinary tract function, as mechanoreceptors running *throughout* the pelvic

bowl can influence micturition and voiding control. Pelvic floor problems are particularly troublesome, especially if the muscle cannot relax and therefore presents some sort of outlet obstruction to the bladder. In this case, voiding is harder and the person has to strain more to pass urine. This makes the bladder wall thicker (hypertrophy) and more irritable.[72] In this way, problems start small with a few local mechanical torsions and tensions, which accumulate and gradually increasingly disturb the voiding and micturition reflexes, leading to symptoms in both men and women.

Orthodox literature also describes the need for a normal stable, functioning sacral cord in order for micturition and continence to be properly coordinated.[73,74] And, coming back to the osteopathic idea of facilitation and irritation within the spinal cord, many somatic and visceral nerves converge on that section of the cord so if there is irritation in any of those areas, bladder function becomes distorted.[75-77] Therefore, even if local visceral treatment is not considered, work done to somatic structures which send fibres through to S2–4 (where these are irritated or compromised) will influence that neural reflex arc (note: this includes anything that can be done to address problems in the feet (S1–2) or posterior thigh, for example). So even if the patient's foot is the only part treated, there may be an effect onto the bladder, strange as it may seem!

Urgency, frequency and incontinence

As a result of all this tension, altered mobility and reflex activity, urgency, frequency and incontinence can result from the accompanying detrusor instability and urethral dyssynergia. Osteopaths can work on bladder compliance, on suppleness in supportive ligaments and surrounding organs and tissues, and work with the pelvic floor, general pelvic mechanics and hips and low back, for example, to reduce reflex discoordination.

Chronic recurrent cystitis and lower urinary tract infection

Osteopathic hypotheses also consider that recurrent bladder infection and cystitis may be related to pelvic congestion, bladder irritability and contraction, contributing to incomplete bladder emptying and retention of urine. Coupled with irritation to neural pathways, this may well compromise local mucosal tissue health and immunity and contribute to an increased tendency to infection or inflammation and an impaired ability to recover from the same.

Bladder prolapse

Bladder prolapse and pelvic floor weakness are major causes of urinary incontinence and may be influenced (if the prolapse is not too severe) through osteopathic management. Urinary prolapse is discussed below with genital prolapse.

Pelvic floor considerations in urinary tract mechanics

As introduced above, the pelvic floor itself is quite important for urinary tract mechanics as it has to relax and move in order to allow the bladder to move and empty. Also, if the pelvic floor does not work appropriately, it does not send the right neural messages back through to the sacral spinal cord and this 'confuses the way the bladder is told to act', as part of the sacral cord integration of bladder reflexes.

Most people are familiar with the concept that a weak or partially paralysed pelvic floor causes urinary incontinence through prolapse (with or without genital and/or rectal prolapse and anal sphincter dysfunction). However, many more problems are associated with a pelvic floor that has too high a resting tone; in other words, one that is too tight, in spasm, shortened and poorly mobile and responsive as a result. Many painful perineal and urogenital conditions are associated with a hypertonic pelvic floor[78] which are definitely amenable to manual techniques and osteopathic management. Internal per vaginal, per rectal and external perineal work to the pelvic floor and perineum is valuable in many cases of vaginismus, vulvadynia, dyspareunia and so on, as well as for lower urinary tract problems associated with pelvic floor dysfunction.

Treatment would include trigger point therapy to the hypertonic and painful muscles. Mobilization of surrounding connective tissue structures and work through the pelvis and low back/hip areas to improve abdominal, pelvic and symphysis mechanics can also be beneficial.[79] Inhibition and

unwinding/balancing to the pudendal nerve (via a perineal contact, for example) can also be very useful in 'diffusing' adverse pelvic reflexes and their painful sequelae.

LOWER UROGENITAL TRACT MECHANICS – MALE

The mechanics of the male bladder are influenced strongly by the prostate and any prostate restriction can not only affect sexual and reproductive function but can also impact on urinary flow and bladder wall activity and compliance.

The prostate and seminal vesicles should move up and down with the natural mobility of the pelvic floor[80] but often this movement is reduced when infection, inflammation or some type of pathology is present, when pelvic bony/articular dysfunction occurs or the mechanics of the pelvic floor are disturbed. The actions of the pelvic floor and pelvic bones help to indirectly mobilize the lower urinary tract in the male as well as the female.

The osteopathic management in a variety of male urogenital problems consists of general pelvic mobilization and perineal work coupled with work through the pelvis, hips and low back and (in many cases) through the lower limbs (as injury to the legs is a common accompaniment to pelvic biomechanical problems). Prostatic massage is also a very useful tool which osteopaths can apply. Note: prostatic massage can be done externally as well as internally, via a perineal contact which, whilst not as effective as per rectal mobilization and drainage, is certainly of value and can be repeated frequently with less emotional and physical discomfort for the patient.

Prostatitis and prostadynia

The conditions of prostatitis, prostadynia and prostatic hypertrophy are all very common and management can be challenging as many of these conditions are quite chronic.[81]

As stated above, there is a lot that osteopaths can do for these types of pelvic pain problems. Manual medicine techniques can be utilized (perhaps with the exception of cases of acute infection and carcinoma). Many cases of prostatitis and prostadynia are resistant to standard medical approaches and one of the reasons for this is that bacterial infection is often commonly misdiagnosed.

In fact, non-bacterial prostatitis is far more common than bacterial prostatitis[82] and if someone has not responded to antibiotic therapy, this often indicates that they are suffering from a non-bacterial prostatitis. In such cases general mobilization can be very effective as it helps reduce general pelvic congestion, improves local compliance in the prostate and with work to reduce spasm and shortening of the pelvic floor, overall urogenital health can be fairly easily improved.

Testicular disorders

Left testicular varicosities are very common and result mainly from the difference in venous anatomy from left to right. On the right side, both the ovarian and testicular veins have a (relatively) short oblique route, draining up to the inferior vena cava, so there are not too many problems draining the right ovary and right testicle. On the left, however, the left ovarian vein and the left testicular vein actually take a different route which is more vertical, going up the length of psoas, up the side of the lumbar spine and actually joining to the left renal vein. So whereas the right vein drains obliquely, the left vein is longer, more tortuous and has a harder job draining.[83] Poor drainage can give problems with varicosities in relation to the ovary or testicle on the left. Left testicular varicosities are the single most common cause of painful swelling in the testes but are often amenable to osteopathic treatment (if the varicosities are not too severe). Whether for ovarian or testicular function, the mechanics of the left kidney and renal fascia and torsions of the left renal vein are of interest. The mobility of the left arcuate ligaments, 12th ribs and diaphragm/posterior abdominal wall is also important, as are the inguinal canal mechanics for the testes.

Testicular descent is closely related to and depends on the development and reorganization of various ligaments within the embryo and in early childhood. The functions of the gubernaculum are particularly relevant.[84] This structure runs on the inside of the abdominal wall, from near the underneath of the 12th ribs to the inguinal region, where it passes through the inguinal canal and into the scrotum. It forms a 'track' along which the testes descend (using many chemical signals as a guide). Descent can be incomplete and, if left

unresolved, this can impact on long-term fertility issues for the individual concerned. Most unresolved cases are surgically managed but osteopaths may have an input in some situations (where the abdominal location is periodic and the testis occasionally appears in the scrotum, or where local inguinal mechanics, swelling, irritation and tensions may be blocking the descent, for example).

Osteopaths also have another hypothesis, which concerns the gubernaculum directly. This is a very unscientific description but in essence, the gubernaculum can be considered as a tether to testicular descent, and abdominal wall, renal fascia and gubernaculum tension could act as a sort of 'bungee rope' constantly pulling back on the testis and disturbing its normal pattern of descent. Thus osteopathic management may also take into account any abdominal wall tensions, problems with the kidneys, renal fascia, 12th ribs, psoas and quadratus lumborum, for example, which would also need to incorporate lower limb, hip and pubic mechanics (as these would be inter-related with the above).

Also, embryological formation and signalling are thought to be related to/affected by mechanical factors in the tissues concerned. If the abdominal muscles and associated joints/skeletal structures were tense, this may be interfering chemically with the descent signals, complicating the process further (this hypothesis is also not proven).

Delayed resolution of the undescended testicles results in them remaining within the too warm abdominal cavity longer than is natural and this has consequences for fertility, with the sperm count being reduced once the testicles are descended and an increased susceptibility to torsion is likely. Some authors feel there is also a link with testicular cancer in later life. Ninety-seven percent of newborns have both testes within the scrotum and most of the remainder gradually descend over the next 9 months. As stated, it is generally considered essential that the condition is resolved before puberty and surgery is the preferred treatment (hormone therapy is rarely considered).

Pelvic floor ischaemia and perineal biomechanical problems

The pelvic floor is also important for prostate and pelvic floor function and has a role in sexual function and particularly ejaculation and pain on ejaculation.[85] The pelvic floor is very important for the stabilization of the base of the penis and a lot of men who have prostate problems also end up with pain on ejaculation, which can create many psychological problems in relation to the sexual act. Relieving tension in the pelvic floor may have the added benefit of improving their emotional balance and therefore indirectly improving sexual function. Even without considering its role in sexual function, the pelvic floor itself can literally be the cause of a patient's pelvic pain, even without any involvement of the prostate or other pelvic organs. Perineal spasm in males is very common and often accompanies 'ordinary' biomechanical problems of the pelvis, low back and hips.

Pelvic floor disorders may also be related to pudendal artery syndrome, which can lead to ischaemia of the local tissues and be related to erectile dysfunction.[86] It is often accompanied by pudendal nerve compression and is usually managed surgically by pudendal canal decompression. However, general osteopathic work to the pelvis and pelvic floor may be of value, especially if the condition is not too established. It is also interesting to note that many men suffer from urogenital problems as a result of the mechanical stresses and strains caused by bicycle riding.[87] The most common expression of this is genital numbness, coupled with haematuria, torsion of the spermatic cord, infertility and erectile dysfunction, as well as general perineal pain and discomfort. Osteopathically, the general mechanics of the pelvic bowl and pelvic floor would be considered, to improve overall 'bicycling mechanics', as well as advice on the types of bicycle seat that may be less compromising.

GYNAECOLOGICAL MECHANICS

As discussed in previous chapters, any movement from one pelvic organ (or the pelvic floor) is immediately transferred through to the others and any gross somatic/bony pelvic movement is going to affect that dynamic relationship.

The mechanics of the uterus and fallopian tubes are extensively discussed in Chapters 7 and 10. In particular, the link between the uterus, the sacrum and the symphysis pubis should be emphasized, as it relates to many complex urogenital tract movements. The uterosacral ligament is one of the most influential for uterine mechanics and it has extensive attachments with the sacrum, piriformis, ischial spine, coccygeus and sacrospinous ligament and can attach to the cervix, vagina and/or lower uterine body.[88] Hence, local diagnosis of its tension really depends on careful physical examination, as there is quite a degree of anatomical variation. Osteopathic management in a whole variety of gynaecological disorders is not possible without a very detailed and three-dimensional understanding of genital tract mechanics and an appreciation of the interrelatedness of general pelvic mechanics.

As previously mentioned, some of the connective tissue ligaments of the uterus contain smooth muscle fibres themselves, so they are not just inert fascial supports. The uterosacral ligament can also be the site of much pelvic pain, whether in relation to its own tension and stress or as a common site for endometrial lesion implantation, for example.[89,90] The uterosacral ligaments contain smooth muscle and hormone receptors[91] so they are capable of contraction, which means that they can tip the uterus in one direction or another. If the sacrum moves, then that elastic momentum is going to be passed onto the uterus and vice versa. Where the uterosacral ligaments have hormone receptors in them, at different times of the menstrual cycle (in relation to the different hormone levels) the consistency, strength and ability to support and guide uterine movement will vary. So, movement of the uterus may differ from one part of the menstrual cycle to another.

Pelvic pain

There are a variety of causes of pelvic pain and some of these arise from the organs and some from the musculoskeletal system. Causes include musculoskeletal, gynaecological, urological, gastrointestinal, postsurgical and psychological factors.[92-97]

Apart from the many pathological conditions affecting the pelvic organs, other mechanisms are involved, which may be amenable to osteopathic intervention (even if also accompanied by various pathological states or disorders). Referred pain and nociceptive reflexes are thought to operate through the autonomic nerves (from the spinal cord at the upper lumbar level). Through this neural reflex pathway, many aspects of musculoskeletal dysfunction or irritation can 'summate' and lead to pain being interpreted as being visceral in origin. Chronic pelvic pain is particularly debilitating and pain control can be difficult where central sensitization and altered pain behaviour mechanisms have developed.

The musculoskeletal system can also contribute to pelvic pain because of its relationship to support of the pelvic organs and its influence on the fluid dynamics of the pelvis. Additionally, many of the pelvic floor muscles themselves can become tense, contracted and in spasm, giving a variety of pain syndromes within the male and female pelvis.

Other causes of pelvic pain include gastrointestinal tract problems such as irritable bowel syndrome, sigmoid problems such as polyps and haemorrhoids. In males, rectal spasm can be associated with sacroiliac lesions, coccyx problems and sacral biomechanical problems, which can impact on prostatic and bladder function.

It must not be forgotten that there are a variety of psychological associations with pelvic pain. There is a huge unresolved debate about which came first, the depression or the pain, and in years gone by a diagnosis of 'hysteria' or malingering was quite common. However, now, there is better appreciation of the complexity of the situation and people are willing to believe that chronic pain is deeply debilitating and will adversely affect a patient's life, with very long-term consequences. Thus the depression can come after the pain rather than before. As understanding grows, a sort of balance is being struck in relation to the psychology of pain and how it affects people, and how this relates to their diagnosis. This point is very important in practice, as many patients cannot fully progress without the additional input of cognitive behavioural therapy, stress management or other psychological support, which the osteopath may not be able to manage alone.

Fluid dynamics

Problems with fluid dynamics (such as venous congestion and varicosities) can be the cause of many cases of chronic pelvic pain.[98,99] 'Pelvic varicosities' may commonly be discussed in relation to haemorrhoids, for example, but venous congestion affects all the organs. Internal pelvic varicosities cannot be seen but they are a recognized cause of pelvic pain and the osteopathic approach is quite

interesting, as we can look at all sorts of factors to encourage general venous return and help prevent the whole pelvis being congested, swollen, 'heavy' and irritable. This is done through thoracic diaphragm and pelvic floor mechanics, thoracic 'pump' mechanics, general abdominal mechanics and peritoneal cavity integrity, for example. Interestingly, different gynaecological conditions present with differing amounts of general pelvic congestion. For example, endometriosis often presents with widespread swelling and oedema throughout the pelvis, whereas fibroids are not associated with the same widespread congestion.

One anatomical consideration is very important for ovarian and testicular venous drainage: for the ovarian and testicular veins, the anatomy is different left to right, a point which was introduced above. Ovarian varicosities and general pelvic varicosities are 'difficult to see' but as modern imaging techniques improve, so the diagnosis of pelvic varicosities is more easily and commonly made.

Uterine peristalsis

In this train of thought, the term 'uterine hyperperistalsis' has been coined to describe adverse, uneven or excessive uterine contraction. This is thought to be related to endometriosis and it might even be a causative factor.[100] There are natural, small movements and contractions within the uterus which, if they happen in an aphasic or slightly hyperactive state, seem to contribute to endometrial shedding through the fallopian tubes into the abdominopelvic cavity during menstrual flow. It is thought that this is perhaps a more likely cause of endometriosis than simply retrograde 'leakage' during menstruation. However, there is incomplete understanding about what causes the hyperperistalsis and a potential link to neural irritation (via some sort of somatovisceral or viscerovisceral reflex, or local tension in the uterine wall and peritoneal relations) is an interesting hypothesis.

Fibroids

Fibroids are a (generally) benign condition affecting many women. They can be responsible for general pelvic pain and can disrupt fertility in some cases. They are often associated with abdominal discomfort and bloating, both of which can be distressing to the woman concerned. If surgical removal is not advisable or unwanted, then osteopaths may have a limited role in some aspects of symptom management in some cases.

The prime consideration is to explain to the patient that the aim is not to 'treat the fibroid', in the sense that a few manipulations are going to cause the fibroid itself to shrink or disappear. Instead, the aim is to improve uterine compliance, reduce general uterine stiffness and congestion and effectively allow the uterus to be softer and more elastic so that it can accommodate the physical presence of the fibroid(s) more subtly, and for the remaining 'normal uterine tissue' to be as uncompromised as possible. In lay terms, it is as though a stiff and thickened uterus is trying to accommodate one too many billiard balls and relaxing the tissues and promoting drainage and general mobility will allow the uterus to soften and allow the balls to stack more comfortably.

Endometriosis

Endometriosis is related to many cases of pelvic pain. It can cause adhesions within the abdomino-pelvic cavity which can then cause altered position and altered mobility of the organs.[101-103] The effects of this on those other organs can give rise to additional symptomatology, such that endometriosis is a 'big problem' whichever way it is considered. Interestingly, though, the amount of pain is not actually related to the size or extent of the endometrial lesion, nor, in fact, to the site of the adhesion.[104] Surgical intervention can be of limited use and instead, inducing amenorrhoea through medication often reduces the pain[105] and can be a therapeutic option.

> *i* Note: adhesions are not simply 'tissues stuck together'; there is not simply a bland inert scar which has just grown and become established. Adhesions are living tissues; they are often innervated,[106] they have their own vasculature and they are literally part of the body and can contribute to symptoms in their own right, apart from the tethering that they cause to other structures. The osteopathic approach to adhesions is discussed below.

Endometriosis itself, regardless of what it can cause in terms of adhesions, is often present in fertile women with no pain whatsoever, which makes it a prime component in many cases of infertility, as women do not seek early treatment as there are no prompting symptoms. The general impact of endometriosis on fertility and conception (whether there was pain present or not) is discussed below. There are many theories as to the causes of endometriosis and some even now consider that it may be a paraphysiological condition,[107] such that it is something that occurs naturally. The currently unanswered question has to be why the natural phenomenon of endometrial tissue found in the abdominopelvic cavity causes a problem for some people and not for others.

Whatever its cause, it induces marked changes in local urogenital mechanics and often involves the small intestine, sigmoid and rectal mechanics as tension spreads through all adjacent tissues and adhesions can be present between gastrointestinal and genitourinary organs. Pain patterns can be intense and patients can be difficult to manage in that their tissues are often hypersensitive and sometimes they can tolerate only very small amounts of input. Also, as gynaecological work is best done in the first half of the menstrual cycle (which is less uncomfortable for patients and avoids possible very early pregnancies, even if these are rare in these women), only one or two treatments may be possible per menstrual cycle and so any treatment plan is necessarily conducted over a protracted period of time, making monitoring of progress difficult in the short term. Practitioners are best advised to treat accordingly for, say, three cycles and then to compare overall symptom levels and pain patterns, rather than focus on day-to-day changes.

Pelvic prolapse

The functions of the pelvic floor in relation to pelvic organ support have been discussed in Chapter 7 and the development of pelvic organ prolapse as a unitary concept in pelvic biomechanics (all tissues and structures, including the pelvic floor and pelvic bowl, being interrelated and multi-aetiological to prolapse) has been introduced. So, whether through obstetric trauma, congenital connective tissue weakness, pelvic floor injury (for example, after coccygeal trauma), any disruption to the pelvic floor and pelvic tissue continuity will contribute to pelvic organ prolapse. Added to this are other biomechanical factors such as organ prolapse being related to impact sports and to foot arch stiffness and lack of shock absorbency,[108] and thus the area of whole-body biomechanics that are important for pelvic organ support becomes quite broad.

Ovarian conditions

Polycystic ovarian syndrome is a complex disorder that requires particular medical intervention. However, some general osteopathic support can be given to the patient, which may help to offset some of the hormonal imbalances and address some of the local pelvic effects of the syndrome. Ovarian cysts often require surgical intervention but some aspects of the pain may be amenable to osteopathic intervention and postsurgical support is certainly possible. Given current understanding of the underlying mechanisms, any possible connection between reflex mechanisms and general pelvic biomechanics to the aetiology of ovarian cysts would be conjecture only.

Perineal conditions, vaginismus and vulvadynia

See above discussions on pelvic floor considerations in urinary tract mechanics, as the same factors within the pelvic floor (for example, shortening, spasm and poor mobility) can affect genital and vaginal function as well as urinary function. Conditions such as vaginismus and vulvadynia are linked to various pelvic floor dysfunctions and tensions. In particular, vulvadynia is being increasingly linked to pudendal neuralgia and osteopaths have potentially many options for assessing pudendal nerve function. For example, this can be achieved by evaluating the S2–4 foramina and the mechanics of the cauda equina, by looking at piriformis, coccygeus and perineal tissues, and by sacroiliac and hip biomechanical links.

In conclusion, the osteopathic profession, with its high degree of palpatory awareness and experience and anatomical analysis, is uniquely placed to help many patients suffering from pelvic pain. No other profession utilizing manual approaches has the same degree of skill or similar hypotheses that enable them to consider the mechanics of the urogenital tract and the impact on pelvic physiology and function.

CONCEPTION AND INFERTILITY

Conception and fertility are clearly related to many hormone patterns and cycles and no exploration of a patient is complete without this type of analysis. However, there are also many mechanical factors relevant to conception which, if compromised, in some people seem to reduce fertility and limit the ability to conceive or maintain an early pregnancy.

As already discussed, uterine peristalsis is a cyclically occurring natural phenomenon that changes throughout the menstrual cycle. Physiologically, to aid reproductive function, the uterus needs to be active, contracting rhythmically to move both ovum and sperm together within the tube and so on. So, reproduction is not just about sex; it includes the action of the whole genital tract, which is compromised if it is irritated and torsioned or has adapted mobility.

Following intercourse (during which the vagina, cervix and uterus have to sustain and comfortably accommodate various strong mechanical movements), rapid and sustained sperm transport from the cervical canal to the isthmical part of the fallopian tube is provided by cervicofundal uterine peristaltic contractions that can be visualized by vaginal sonography. Peristaltic contractions normally increase in frequency (and presumably also in intensity) as the proliferative phase of the menstrual cycle progresses. However, in women with infertility and endometriosis, for example, uterine hyperperistalsis will nearly double the frequency of contractions during the early and midluteal phases in comparison to fertile and healthy controls and this appears to be a common finding.[109] During midcycle, these women display a considerable uterine dysperistalsis (in that the normally long and regular cervicofundal contractions during this phase of the cycle become more or less undirected and convulsive in character). This can severely hamper sperm transport and therefore conception.[100] Hyperperistalsis may also constitute the mechanical cause for the development of endometriosis in that it transports detached endometrial cells and tissue fragments via the tubes into the peritoneal cavity.

Endometriosis and other conditions that cause abdominopelvic adhesions can cause many problems and pain and are generally related to difficulties with fertility and conception.[110-111] The adhesions can affect the contractions and peristalsis which occur naturally within the uterus (and fallopian tubes), at different stages of the menstrual cycle and which are related to conception, as discussed above.[100,109] The adhesions can also affect the ovary. Tubal torsion or adhesion/spasm could affect the ability of the ovum to pass through the fallopian tube, for example (which is hindered when the tube is a bit kinked or tethered). The endometriosis/adhesions seem to irritate from the outside of the uterus, to 'confuse' the mechanoreceptors of the visceral peritoneum and hence the musculature of the uterus, thereby distorting uterine peristalsis.

Osteopathic mobilization and release of the pelvic tissues and work through the genital tract, including the local and internal mechanics of the cervix, uterocervical and uterotubal junctions and within the tubes themselves, can all play a role in normalizing uterine peristalsis and rhythmicity. Osteopaths can also consider the vaginal mechanics and the way the uterus can move and orient itself and the cervix for optimal sperm collection.[112] The biological valve operating at the cervix is also important for conception. There are various cervical changes during the cycle, where there is increased mucus production around ovulation and a softening and opening of the cervix just after it. This opening (or not) can permit (or block) sperm penetration, which will ultimately impact on conception. Osteopaths consider that uterine torsion or tension and poor cervical mechanics can distort the cervical valve or cause neural/circulatory irritation that may compromise its cyclical function, thus inhibiting its role in conception.

Additionally, any reflex irritation through the autonomic nerves can be addressed, as can global pelvic and other related biomechanical problems that are impacting on pelvic circulation, drainage, immunity and function in general. Even if the osteopath only addresses the painful and inhibiting components of vaginismus, painful penetration and intercourse (dyspareunia), the patient will often relax more during the sexual act, thereby aiding conception through reduction of stress. Osteopaths can often help to 'calm down' tissues which have

been 'traumatized' by hormone stimulation, egg retrieval, implantation and general examination, which helps the women feel that they are getting a chance to recover as much as possible in between attempts (which lessens some of the emotional burden for them). It is extremely important not to give false hope to patients with conception difficulties, as there are no guarantees that osteopathic intervention will benefit them and there is currently no supportive evidence in this field. These patients are particularly emotionally vulnerable to suggestions and possibilities, which the practitioner must bear in mind.

Osteopathic work with patients following a programme of assisted conception (whether that be intrauterine fertilization or some other procedure) can also be rewarding. Work can often be oriented to help them prepare for the procedures, by 'making the most of what they have got' in the sense that maintaining efficient circulation, reducing irritating neural signals and reducing pain and congestion by alleviating organ stiffness and immobility can all help prepare the genital tract for implantation and pregnancy. It is common that once implantation has occurred, patients will not consent to any osteopathic work, let alone local pelvic work, and practitioners will end up playing the same waiting game as the patient in order to see if conception has occurred or, if not, what the next process for that patient may be. Patients with infertility can often try many complementary or alternative therapies at once and it is easy for them to become 'overloaded', which must be borne in mind. However, they are not always agreeable to the idea of doing one thing first, then another, as time is usually a severe issue for these women and their partners and most do not want to try a few cycles of each thing separately, 'just to see'.

Osteopaths have an active role in issues of conception and infertility but because of all the above, it is often difficult to assess their exact impact.

Male infertility

Very little work has been done on the osteopathic input into male infertility. However, the most plausible approach would be to consider testicular, seminal vesicle and prostatic function, with the aim of improving local mechanics, neural reflexes and circulation/fluid drainage components and reducing any pain and discomfort within the pelvic and perineal region associated with coitus. General work to the biomechanics of the bony and articular pelvis, hips and low back would also be implicated, as would other work throughout the body designed to aid the pelvic biomechanics or reflex areas of the spinal cord/higher centres. All the considerations that relate to the osteopathic management of pelvic floor spasm, perineal ischaemia, prostatitis and prostadynia and so on are relevant for male infertility problems that have their origin within the pelvic organs. Attention may also be given to the hypothalamic-pituitary axis and the global influences of sperm production and male reproductive function.

MANAGEMENT OF PATIENTS WITH POSTOPERATIVE PAIN AND ADHESIONS

CASES

Several of the above cases have included work through scarred and adhesed tissues but the following two are interesting, one for the fact that the treatment was carried out quite soon postoperatively and the other because, although simple, it is an unusual presentation.

Patient with abdominal scar haematoma

A 58-year-old woman had been presenting for ongoing treatment for a sore knee and hip since a 'bunion' operation a year ago. She had also been suffering from diverticulitis for some years and was scheduled for a bowel resection, to ease some of those symptoms. Just prior to her bowel operation, a scan revealed a tumour on her left kidney, which would be explored during her resection operation. This was performed and the tumour was not removed at that time. However, she developed strong abdominal pain and midline discomfort around the scar site and further testing revealed the presence of a blood clot/haematoma just deep to the incision. Aspiration was not carried out immediately and the medical team were monitoring progress. She was booked for a further operation to resolve the renal tumour problem, in a few months time.

Her presentation for help with the abdominal problems was 6 weeks postoperatively and there were a lot of conflicting tensions through the abdomen, which are indicated in Figure 9.16. Note: the patient had also previously had a hysterectomy and ovarian removal (on two separate occasions) and prior to that, an appendectomy. It was decided to perform symptomatic relief only, by working locally and very gently around the scar site, along the abdominal wall around the incision and on some of the major 'visceral' tensions. Very gentle fascial balancing and unwinding was applied, with no direct pressure onto the scar site. The haematoma (which was apparently 6–8 inches long and 2–3 inches wide) was not directly 'engaged', but only the surrounding tissues, in order to give 'space' and relief to the other abdominal wall tissues. This treatment was repeated for a couple of sessions, whilst she awaited her further operation (for the kidney problem). No further medical treatment for the haematoma was given and the problem and symptoms gradually eased over the treatment sessions, following which she proceeded with the renal operation.

Although the osteopathic care in this case for the postoperative complications was shortlived, it demonstrates the general support that can be given to patients in these situations, when there may be few other avenues for short-term relief. It is always important to remember that further complications can always occur postoperatively and the practitioner must be acutely aware of any factors requiring the patient to re-present to their medical team as necessary, if the patient is not already arranging to do so themselves.

Patient with vaginal pain and abdominal discomfort, post caesarean

A woman presented for treatment for an unusual complication following a caesarean delivery, where little vaginal trauma had been possible, as the patient had not dilated further than 2 cm and the baby had not descended very far at all into the pelvic birth canal. The problem was perineal and vaginal pain, at the side of the entrance to the vagina and just inside the labia. This would occur on penetration, with intercourse. There was also some right-sided lower abdominal discomfort at one

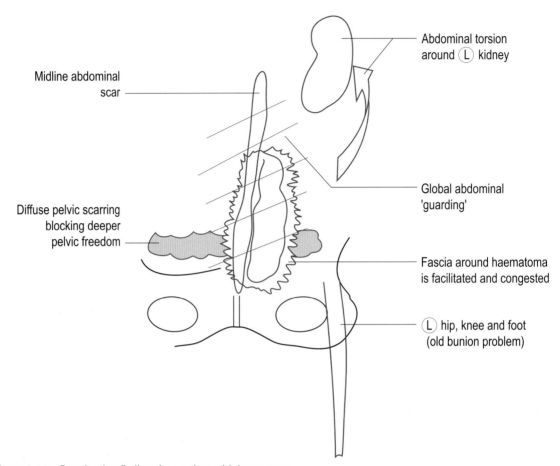

Midline abdominal scar

Diffuse pelvic scarring blocking deeper pelvic freedom

Abdominal torsion around (L) kidney

Global abdominal 'guarding'

Fascia around haematoma is facilitated and congested

(L) hip, knee and foot (old bunion problem)

Figure 9.16   Examination findings in a patient with haematoma.

end of the caesarean scar. The patient presented 7–8 weeks post delivery.

The case was unusual in that there are generally no vaginal complications following a non-vaginal birth and the patient had some palpable tight bands of tissue just inside the right side of the vaginal entrance, which her midwife had not seen before in any similar situations. The caesarean scar itself was healing well and there were no other significant pelvic, low back or abdominal problems. There was no previous abdominal surgery and nothing that would have set up the pelvic and perineal tissues to express the presenting problem.

On examination, there was general tension along the caesarean scar, with some stronger focus to the right side, where the abdominal wall muscles were a little more tense and irritable than the left. On the left side, the inguinal region as a whole was a little tense but only from the inguinal canal downwards, and the left round ligament was a little tense. After some other general exploration, it was determined that the problem lay with the round ligament tension, which was pulling on the vagina, after it had passed over the face of the pubis and onto its insertion into the labia/side of the vagina and perineal region. This tension is indicated in Figure 9.17. Some local caesarean scar unwinding was performed and some releases over the face of the pubis and with the round ligament were performed. A local inhibition was applied to the labial insertion of round ligament and to the tight vaginal bands which were present on the left side. After a couple of treatments the problem had resolved and the patient could have intercourse free of pain.

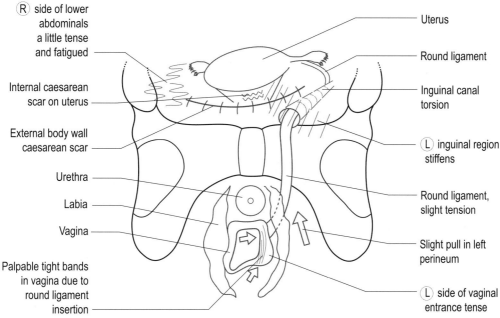

R side of lower abdominals a little tense and fatigued

Internal caesarean scar on uterus

External body wall caesarean scar

Urethra

Labia

Vagina

Palpable tight bands in vagina due to round ligament insertion

Uterus

Round ligament

Inguinal canal torsion

L inguinal region stiffens

Round ligament, slight tension

Slight pull in left perineum

L side of vaginal entrance tense

Figure 9.17 Examination findings in a patient with vaginal pain post caesarean.

ADHESIONS AND POSTOPERATIVE SCARRING

The way that adhesions form is a complex subject and it is surprising how little is known about the function of the peritoneum and its own physiology and why it sticks together on some occasions.[113] However they are produced, postoperative and postinfective adhesions can give rise to many painful syndromes, which osteopaths are well placed to help manage. Adhesions often produce strong tensions and torsions within the abdominopelvic cavities and can often contribute to a variety of musculoskeletal mechanical problems even in the absence of visceral symptoms or pain. Many of the techniques for their examination and treatment are relatively simple and should be part of every osteopath's repertoire.

The osteopathic profession's interest in the management of adhesions is long-standing. Early osteopathic texts refer to examples of treatment for adhesions, especially within the field of gynaecology.[114] These early approaches included organ mobilization through the abdominal wall and via per rectal and per vaginal internal approaches. There was also an interest in 'stretching' and

'releasing' various fascial and connective tissue structures as part of the established core to many osteopathic approaches.[115] All these approaches are still current today.

Whether induced by infection, inflammation, ischaemia and/or surgical injury, peritoneal adhesions are the leading cause of abdominopelvic pain, bowel obstruction and infertility. The treatment of pelvic adhesions and their associated morbidity contributes to a significant portion of healthcare expenditure.[116,117] While postsurgical peritoneal wounds heal without adhesions in some patients, others develop severe scarring from what seemed the same operation. Also, in one patient, adhesions can develop at one surgical site and not another. The predisposition to form adhesions is not fully understood[118] which makes management protocols challenging.

Adhesions occur in more than 90% of patients following major abdominal surgery and in 55–100% of women undergoing pelvic surgery. Small bowel obstruction, infertility, chronic abdominal and pelvic pain and difficult reoperative surgery are the most common consequences of peritoneal adhesions.[119]

Adhesions are not necessarily formed by foreign bodies in the peritoneal cavity, such as fragments of gauze swab left behind from an operation or powder from surgical gloves. It is thought more likely that the actions of cutting tissue and causing minor abrasions all combine to produce mesothelial trauma. This is the stimulus for an inflammatory response, followed by adherence of adjacent involved peritoneal surfaces. Interestingly, adhesion formation does not tend to occur between the abraded peritoneal surfaces of mobile intraabdominal viscera, which suggests that maintaining intestinal motility (peristalsis) in the early postoperative period is important in the prevention of adhesions.[120] Maintaining general organ mobility is a way of aiding this. Patients can be examined and treated within hours or days of surgery; at which stage gentle non-invasive functional or 'listening' techniques are applied to defuse general tissue torsions and relax superficial tension.

Peritoneal fluid flow may also be important to adhesion formation. The fluid can drain or be absorbed throughout the peritoneal surfaces, entering the lymphatics of the abdomen from a variety of directions (as shown in Fig. 9.18). Adhesions may also occur through the surgical practice of non-closure of the peritoneal layers, following a variety of operative procedures (such as caesarean section), although this point is quite contentious.[121]

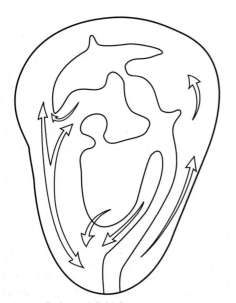

Figure 9.18   Peritoneal fluid flow.

Once staples or stitches are removed from the external wound (or laparoscopic site incision) then gentle mobilization of the organs and abdominopelvic cavity can commence. This is usually within 4–8 weeks after surgery. Osteopathic palpation is applied only within tissue response barriers and within any pain or discomfort tolerances for the patient. Note: 'mobilization' does not mean vigorous stretching. It consists of carefully applied small movements that would not stress the healing tissues. Functional, balancing and unwinding techniques can be used within hours or days of surgery, as these place no significant range of motion through the scar or incision sites.

Adhesions are highly cellular, vascularized and innervated structures, making them living tissue that is capable of regeneration,[122] and causing pain in their own right,[123] as stated above. Some may even contain smooth muscle cells and therefore be capable of reacting dynamically and causing tension and tissue tightening.[124]

Osteopaths do not aim to 'get rid of' adhesions and do not claim to separate adhesed structures; doing so would require ripping of tissue and rupture of vessels and nerve fibres. Osteopaths will work to reduce the influence that the adhesion is having on adjacent structures, reducing adverse mechanoreceptor stimulus, improving circulation and tissue health at the cellular level and allowing more peritoneal areas to slide over each other, where possible. This is achieved through gentle movements to organs and tissues, to 'unwind' without causing tissue distress and injury. Some aspects of the pain that may arise as a result of the adhesion do so through creating an alteration in mobility in affected organs and tissues. The torsion of the organ causes, amongst other things, an irritability of the muscular components within that organ (be it uterus, intestine or some other organ).

Visceral osteopathy involves the use of mobilization applied directly to the organs through the body wall, or indirectly through movements applied to body sections that are attached/physically related to the organs within the body cavities. It also involves the per vaginal or per rectal mobilization of tissues such as the pelvic floor, uterus or coccygeal articulation, to improve movement consequent to adhesions and other traumas/tensions.

The osteopath can use 'listening' techniques and also direct mobilization to explore either mobility or motility. Gentle stretching and articulation can be applied, as well as indirect, functional, involuntary mechanisms or other gentle release-type techniques. As adhesions create tensions between organs, and between them and sections of the body cavities, tensions can appear throughout the peritoneal 'bag' in which the organs are sited. This can be treated by working through the peritoneal layers as a 'whole' and viewing the organs as a united system.

Visceral tissues respond best to gentle rhythmic techniques and often a small release can have large effects. It is often easy to overtreat the viscera and supportive tissues, so once a degree of change has been achieved, that area should be left to rest until the next treatment session. Practitioners often underestimate the amount of time it takes to unwind chronic adhesion patterns and techniques often need to be repeated several times, in order to maintain changes to tissue pliability and elasticity and to help reduce any CNS sensitization that is invariably present.

Adhesion management may be necessary for many different patients and could be required consequent to upper gastrointestinal tract surgery, renal or other abdominal procedures, following laparoscopic work or general trauma (in the pelvis, abdomen or thorax). It is a very satisfying aspect of osteopathic work.

CONCLUSION

This chapter is a very small introduction to the highly complex and skilful application of osteopathic management in a variety of visceral (and musculoskeletal) problems and within the care of pregnant and labouring women. It is hoped that it gives the reader some insight into the concepts and hypotheses that osteopaths utilize in the application of their principles in these situations and some introduction to the techniques used. It marks the beginning of a long and very satisfying journey into the broader scope of osteopathic practice and osteopaths' contributions to modern healthcare.

References

1. Fitting JW, Grassino A. [Technics for the functional evaluation of the thoracic cage]. Rev Mal Respir 1986;3(4):173-86.
2. Leong JC, Lu WW, Luk KD, Karlberg EM. Kinematics of the chest cage and spine during breathing in healthy individuals and in patients with adolescent idiopathic scoliosis. Spine 1999;24(13):1310-5.
3. Cil A, Yazici M, Uzumcugil A, et al. The evolution of sagittal segmental alignment of the spine during childhood. Spine 2005;30(1):93-100.
4. Bates JH. Lung mechanics – the inverse problem. Australasian Phys Engin Sci Med 1991;14(4):197-203.
5. Fredberg JJ, Bunk D, Ingenito E, Shore SA. Tissue resistance and the contractile state of lung parenchyma. J Appl Physiol 1993;74(3):1387-97.
6. Similowski T, Bates JH. Two-compartment modelling of respiratory system mechanics at low frequencies: gas redistribution or tissue rheology? Eur Respir J 1991;4(3):353-8.
7. Kamm RD. Shear-augmented dispersion in the respiratory system. Symp Soc Exp Biol 1995;49:277-95.
8. Suki B, Hantos Z. Viscoelastic properties of the visceral pleura and its contribution to lung impedance. Respir Physiol 1992;90(3):271-87.
9. Chihara K, Kenyon CM, Macklem PT. Human rib cage distortability. J Appl Physiol 1996;81:437-47.
10. Stamenovic D, Glass GM, Barnas GM, Fredberg JJ. Viscoplasticity of respiratory tissues. J Appl Physiol 1990;69(3):973-88.
11. Lai-Fook SJ, Rodarte JR. Pleural pressure distribution and its relationship to lung volume and interstitial pressure. J Appl Physiol 1991;70(3):967-78.
12. Negrini D, Ballard ST, Benoit JN. Contribution of lymphatic myogenic activity and respiratory movements to pleural lymph flow. J Appl Physiol 1994;76(6):2267-74.
13. Serikov VB. Porous phase model of the lung interstitial fluid motion. Microvasc Res 1991; 42(1):1-16.
14. Serikov VB. Porous phase model of the lung interstitial fluid motion. Microvasc Res 1991; 42(1):1-16.
15. Lai-Fook SJ. Mechanics of the pleural space: fundamental concepts. Lung 1987;165(5):249-67.
16. Ingram RH Jr. Physiological assessment of inflammation in the peripheral lung of asthmatic patients. Lung 1990;168(5):237-47.
17. Sahn SA. The pathophysiology of pleural effusions. Annu Rev Med 1990;41:7-13.

18. Dechman G, Sato J, Bates JH. Effect of pleural effusion on respiratory mechanics, and the influence of deep inflation, in dogs. Eur Respir J 1993;6(2):219-24.
19. Avanzolini G, Barbini P, Cappello A, Cevenini G. Influence of flow pattern on the parameter estimates of a simple breathing mechanics model. IEEE Trans Biomed Engin 1995;42(4):394-402.
20. Chaitow L, Bradley D, Gilbert C. Multidisciplinary approaches to breathing pattern disorders. Edinburgh: Churchill Livingstone; 2002.
21. Niggemann B. Functional symptoms confused with allergic disorders in children and adolescents. Pediatr Allergy Immunol 2002;13(5):312-18.
22. Foster GT, Vaziri ND, Sassoon CS. Respiratory alkalosis. Respir Care 2001;46(4):384-91.
23. Barnes PJ. Neural control of human airways in health and disease. Am Rev Respir Dis 1986;134:1289-314.
24. Shelhamer JH, Levine SJ, Wu T, Jacoby DB, Kaliner MA, Rennard SI. NIH conference. Airway inflammation. Ann Intern Med 1995;123(4):288-304.
25. McDonald DM. Neurogenic inflammation in the respiratory tract: actions of sensory nerve mediators on blood vessels and epithelium of the airway mucosa. Am Rev Respir Dis 1987;136(6 Pt 2):S65-72.
26. Trenchard D. Do axon reflexes exist within the lung? Med Hypotheses 1983;12(4):389-98.
27. Coleridge HM, Coleridge JC. Neural regulation of bronchial blood flow. Respiration Physiol 1994;98(1):1-13.
28. Sangwan YP, Coller JA, Schoetz DJ, Roberts PL, Murray JJ. Spectrum of abnormal rectoanal reflex patterns in patients with fecal incontinence. Dis Colon Rectum 1996;39(1):59-65.
29. Kowalski ML, Didier A, Kaliner MA. Neurogenic inflammation in the airways. I. Neurogenic stimulation induces plasma protein extravasation into the rat airway lumen. Am Rev Respir Dis 1989;140(1):101-9.
30. Barnes PJ. Asthma as an axon reflex. Lancet 1986;1:242-5.
31. Barnes PJ. Neuroeffector mechanisms: the interface between inflammation and neuronal responses. J Allergy Clin Immunol 1996;98(5 Pt 2):S73-81, discussion S81-3.
32. Malenka RC. Synaptic plasticity. Mucking up movements. Nature 1994;372(6503):218-19.
33. Vignola AM, Kips J, Bousquet J. Tissue remodeling as a feature of persistent asthma. J Allergy Clin Immunol 2000;105(6 Pt 1):1041-53.
34. Vignola AM, Mirabella F, Costanzo G, et al. Airway remodeling in asthma. Chest 2003;123(90030):417S-a-422.
35. Carter PM, Heinly TL, Yates SW, Lieberman PL. Asthma: the irreversible airways disease. J Investig Allergol Clin Immunol 1997;7(6):566-71.
36. Bockenhauer S, Julliard K, Lo K, Huang E, Sheth A. Quantifiable effects of osteopathic manipulative techniques on patients with chronic asthma. J Am Osteopath Assoc 2002;102(7):371-5.
37. Maitre B, Similowski T, Derenne JP. Physical examination of the adult patient with respiratory diseases: inspection and palpation. Eur Respir J 1995;8(9):1584-93.
38. Gorman RB, McKenzie DK, Pride NB, Tolman JF, Gandevia SC. Diaphragm length during tidal breathing in patients with chronic obstructive pulmonary disease. Am J Respir Crit Care Med 2002;166(11):1461-9.
39. Decramer M. Hyperinflation and respiratory muscle interaction. Eur Respir J 1997;10(4):934-41.
40. Liebermann-Meffert D. The greater omentum. Anatomy, embryology, and surgical applications. Surg Clin North Am 2000;80(1):275-93, xii.
41. Shrager JB, Wain JC, Wright CD, et al. Omentum is highly effective in the management of complex cardiothoracic surgical problems. J Thorac Cardiovasc Surg 2003;125(3):526-32.
42. Agner C, Yeomans D, Dujovny M. The neurochemical basis for the applications of the greater omentum in neurosurgery. Neurol Res 2001;23(1):7-15.
43. Zenilman ME. Origin and control of gastrointestinal motility. Surg Clin North Am 1993;73(6):1081-99.
44. Eslami MH, Richards WG, Sugarbaker DJ. Esophageal physiology. Chest Surg Clin North Am 1994;4(4):635-52.
45. Phillips RJ, Powley TL. Tension and stretch receptors in gastrointestinal smooth muscle: re-evaluating vagal mechanoreceptor electrophysiology. Brain Res Rev 2005;34(1-2):1-26.
46. Grundy D. What activates visceral afferents? Gut 2004;53(Suppl 2):ii5-8.
47. Holzer-Petsche U, Brodacz B. Traction on the mesentery as a model of visceral nociception. Pain 1999;80(1-2):319-28.
48. Blackshaw LA, Grundy D, Scratcherd T. Involvement of gastrointestinal mechano- and intestinal chemoreceptors in vagal reflexes: an electrophysiological study. J Auton Nervous Syst 1987;18(3):225-34.
49. Blackshaw LA, Grundy D, Scratcherd T. Vagal afferent discharge from gastric mechanoreceptors during contraction and relaxation of the ferret corpus. J Auton Nervous Syst 1987;18(1):19-24.
50. Holzer P, Schicho R, Holzer-Petsche U, Lippe IT. The gut as a neurological organ. Wien Klin Wochenschr 2001;113(17-18):647-60.

51. Bohlen HG. Integration of intestinal structure, function, and microvascular regulation. Microcirculation 1998;5(1):27-37.

52. Countee RW. Extrinsic neural influences on gastrointestinal motility. Am Surg 1977;43(9):621-6.

53. Mayer EA, Raybould HE. Role of visceral afferent mechanisms in functional bowel disorders. Gastroenterology 1990;99:1688-704.

54. Sutherland WG. Teachings in the science of osteopathy (ed. Wales A). Fort Worth, TX: Rudra Press; 1990.

55. Chase JW, Homsy Y, Siggaard C, Sit F, Bower WF. Functional constipation in children. J Urol 2004;171(6 Pt 2):2641-3.

56. Camilleri M, Lee JS, Viramontes B, Bharucha AE, Tangalos EG. Insights into the pathophysiology and mechanisms of constipation, irritable bowel syndrome, and diverticulosis in older people. J Am Geriatr Soc 2000;48(9):1142-50.

57. Chitkara DK, Bredenoord AJ, Cremonini F, et al. The role of pelvic floor dysfunction and slow colonic transit in adolescents with refractory constipation. Am J Gastroenterol 2004;99(8):1579-84.

58. Russell G, Abu-Arafeh I, Symon DN. Abdominal migraine: evidence for existence and treatment options. Paediatr Drugs 2002;4(1):1-8.

59. Dignan F, Abu-Arafeh, I, Russell G. The prognosis of childhood abdominal migraine. Arch Dis Child 2001;84(5):415-18.

60. Santicioli P, Maggi CA. Myogenic and neurogenic factors in the control of pyeloureteral motility and ureteral peristalsis. Pharmacol Rev 1998;50(4):683-722.

61. Lammers WJ, Ahmad HR, Arafat K. Spatial and temporal variations in pacemaking and conduction in the isolated renal pelvis. Am J Physiol 1996;270 (4 Pt 2):F567-74.

62. Maggi CA, Giuliani S. Calcitonin gene-related peptide (CGRP) regulates excitability and refractory period of the guinea pig ureter. J Urol 1994;152 (2 Pt 1):520-4.

63. Lawrentschuk N, Russell JM. Ureteric stenting 25 years on: routine or risky? ANZ J Surg 2004; 74(4):243-7.

64. Esbjorner E, Hansson S, Jakobsson B. Management of children with dilating vesico-ureteric reflux in Sweden. Acta Paediatr 2004;93(1):37-42.

65. Leighton DM, Mayne V. Obstruction in the refluxing urinary tract – a common phenomenon. Clin Radiol 1989;40(3):271-3.

66. Buzelin JM. [The symptomatology and consequences of bladder hyperreflectivity (author's transl)]. J Urol (Paris) 1981;87(9):561-86.

67. Petros PE, Ulmsten UI. An integral theory of female urinary incontinence. Experimental and clinical considerations. Acta Obstet Gynecol Scand 1990;153(Suppl):7-31.

68. Landau EH, Churchill BM, Jayanthi VR, et al. The sensitivity of pressure specific bladder volume versus total bladder capacity as a measure of bladder storage dysfunction. J Urol 1994;152(5 Pt 1):1578-81.

69. Petros PE, Ulmsten U. Role of the pelvic floor in bladder neck opening and closure I: muscle forces. Int Urogynecol J Pelvic Floor Dysfunct 1997;8(2):74-80.

70. DeLancey JO, Starr RA. Histology of the connection between the vagina and levator ani muscles. Implications for urinary tract function. J Reprod Med 1990;35:765-71.

71. Baskin L, Howard PS, Macarak E. Effect of physical forces on bladder smooth muscle and urothelium. J Urol 1993;150(2 Pt 2):601-7.

72. Lin AT, Yang CH, Chen CJ, Chen MT, Chiang H, Chang LS. Correlation of contractile function and passive properties of rabbit urinary bladder subjected to outlet obstruction – an in vitro whole bladder study. J Urol 1992;148(3):944-8.

73. Mahony DT, Laferte RO, Blais DJ. Integral storage and voiding reflexes. Neurophysiologic concept of continence and micturition. Urology 1977;9:95-106.

74. Mahony DT, Laferte RO, Blais DJ. Incontinence of urine due to instability of micturition reflexes: Part I. Detrusor reflex instability. Urology 1980;15:229-39.

75. Sato A, Sato RF, Schmidt RF, et al. Somato-vesical reflexes in chronic spinal cats. J Auton Nervous Syst 1983;7:351-62.

76. Sato A. The reflex effects of spinal somatic nerve stimulation on visceral function. J Manipul Physiol Therapeut 1997;15:(1)57-61.

77. Habler H, Hilbers K, Janig W, et al. Viscero-sympathetic reflex responses to mechanical stimulation of pelvic viscera in the cat. J Auton Nervous Syst 1992;38:147-58.

78. FitzGerald MP, Kotarinos R. Rehabilitation of the short pelvic floor. I: Background and patient evaluation. Int Urogynecol J Pelvic Floor Dysfunct 2003;14(4):261-8.

79. FitzGerald MP, Kotarinos R. Rehabilitation of the short pelvic floor. II: Treatment of the patient with the short pelvic floor. Int Urogynecol J Pelvic Floor Dysfunct 2003;14(4):269-75; discussion 275.

80. Beard CJ, Kijewski P, Bussiere M, et al. Analysis of prostate and seminal vesicle motion: implications for treatment planning. In J Radiat Oncol Biol Phys 1996;34(2):451-8.

81. Leigh DA. Prostatitis – an increasing clinical problem for diagnosis and management. J Antimicrob Chemother 1993;32(Suppl A):1-9.

82. Weidner W. Prostatitis – diagnostic criteria, classification of patients and recommendations for therapeutic trials. Infection 1992;20(Suppl 3):S227-31; discussion S235.

83. Gioffre L, Bosco MR, Meloni V. [Role of embryogenesis of the left renal vein and spermatic veins in etiopathogenesis of idiopathic varicocele.] G Chir 2001;22(10):325-32.

84. Barteczko KJ, Jacob MI. The testicular descent in humans. Origin, development and fate of the gubernaculum Hunteri, processus vaginalis peritonei, and gonadal ligaments. Adv Anat Embryol Cell Biol 2000;156:III-X, 1-98.

85. Meares EM, Jr. Prostatitis. Med Clin North Am 1991;75(2):405-24.

86. Shafik A. Pudendal artery syndrome with erectile dysfunction: treatment by pudendal canal decompression. Arch Androl 1995;34(2):83-94.

87. Leibovitch I, Mor Y. The vicious cycling: bicycling related urogenital disorders. Eur Urol 2005;47(3):277-86; discussion 286-7.

88. Umek WH, Morgan DM, Ashton-Miller JA, DeLancey JO. Quantitative analysis of uterosacral ligament origin and insertion points by magnetic resonance imaging. Obstet Gynecol 2004;103(3): 447-51.

89. Petros PP. Severe chronic pelvic pain in women may be caused by ligamentous laxity in the posterior fornix of the vagina. Aust NZ J Obstet Gynaecol 1996;36(3):351-4.

90. Koninckx PR, Renaer M. Pain sensitivity of and pain radiation from the internal female genital organs. Hum Reprod 1997;12(8):1785-8.

91. Mokrzycki ML, Mittal K, Smilen SW, Blechman AN, Porges RF, Demopolous RI. Estrogen and progesterone receptors in the uterosacral ligament. Obstet Gynecol 1997;90(3):402-4.

92. Baker PK. Musculoskeletal origins of chronic pelvic pain. Diagnosis and treatment. Obstet Gynecol Clin North Am 1993;20:719-42.

93. Duleba AJ, Keltz MD, Olive DL. Evaluation and management of chronic pelvic pain. J Am Assoc Gynecol Laparosc 1996;3(2):205-7.

94. Steege JF, Stout AL, Somkuti SG. Chronic pelvic pain in women: toward an integrative model. Obstet Gynecol Surv 1993;48(2):95-110.

95. Robinson JC. Chronic pelvic pain. Curr Opin Obstet Gynecol 1993;5(6):740-3.

96. Hodgkiss AD, Sufraz R, Watson JP, et al. Psychiatric morbidity and illness behaviour in women with chronic pelvic pain. Colpocystodefecography. Dis Colon Rectum 1993;36:1015-21. [Published erratum appears in J Psychosom Res 1994;38(2):167.]

97. Stenchever MA. Management of pelvic pain – give the patient the benefit of the doubt. J Am Assoc Gynecol Laparosc 1995;2(2):113-14.

98. Sichlau MJ, Yao JS, Vogelzang RL. Transcatheter embolotherapy for the treatment of pelvic congestion syndrome. Obstet Gynecol 1994; 83:892-6.

99. Gupta A, McCarthy S. Pelvic varices as a cause for pelvic pain: MRI appearance. Magn Reson Imag 1994;12(4):679-81.

100. Leyendecker G, Kunz G, Wildt L, Beil D, Deininger H. Uterine hyperperistalsis and dysperistalsis as dysfunctions of the mechanism of rapid sperm transport in patients with endometriosis and infertility. Hum Reprod 1996;11(7):1542-51.

101. Propst AM, Storti K, Barbieri RL. Lateral cervical displacement is associated with endometriosis. Fertil Steril 1998;70(3):568-70.

102. Fedele L, Bianchi S, Bocciolone L, Di Nola G, Parazzini F. Pain symptoms associated with endometriosis. Obstet Gynecol 1992;79 (5, Pt 1):767-9.

103. Stovall DW, Bowser LM, Archer DF, Guzick DS. Endometriosis-associated pelvic pain: evidence for an association between the stage of disease and a history of chronic pelvic pain. Fertil Steril 1997;68(1):13-18.

104. Demco L. Mapping the source and character of pain due to endometriosis by patient-assisted laparoscopy. J Am Assoc Gynecol Laparosc 1998;5(3):241-5.

105. Brosens IA. Endometriosis. Current issues in diagnosis and medical management. J Reprod Med 1998;43(3 Suppl):281-6.

106. Kligman I, Drachenberg C, Papadimitriou J, Katz E. Immunohistochemical demonstration of nerve fibers in pelvic adhesions. Obstet Gynecol 1993;82(4, Pt 1):566-8.

107. Balasch J, Creus M, Fabregues F, et al. Visible and non-visible endometriosis at laparoscopy in fertile and infertile women and in patients with chronic pelvic pain: a prospective study. Hum Reprod 1996;11(2):387-91.

108. Nygaard IE, Glowacki C, Saltzman CL. Relationship between foot flexibility and urinary incontinence in nulliparous varsity athletes. Obstet Gynecol 1996;87(6):1049-51.

109. Kunz G, Beil D, Deiniger H, Einspanier A, Mall G, Leyendecker G. The uterine peristaltic pump. Normal and impeded sperm transport within the female genital tract. Adv Exp Med Biol 1997;424:267-77.

110. Bowman MC, Cooke ID, Lenton EA. Investigation of impaired ovarian function as a contributing factor to infertility in women with pelvic adhesions. Hum Reprod 1993;8(10): 1654-6.

111. Matorras R, Rodriguez F, Pijoan JI, et al. Are there any clinical signs and symptoms that are related to endometriosis in infertile women? Am J Obstet Gynecol 1996;174(2):620-3.

112. Shafik A. The role of the levator ani muscle in evacuation, sexual performance and pelvic floor disorders. Int Urogynecol J Pelvic Floor Dysfunct 2000;11(6):361-76.

113. Haney AF, Doty E. The formation of coalescing peritoneal adhesions requires injury to both contacting peritoneal surfaces. Fertil Steril 1994; 61(4):767-5.

114. Barber ED. Osteopathy complete. Virginia Beach: LifeLine Press; 1898.

115. Cathie D. The fascia of the body in relation to function and manipulative therapy. Indianapolis: American Academy of Osteopathy Year Book; 1974: 81-4.

116. Ray NF, Denton WG, Thamer M, Henderson SC, Perry S. Abdominal adhesiolysis: inpatient care and expenditures in the United States in 1994. J Am Coll Surg 1998;186(1):1-9.

117. Holmdahl L, Risberg B. Adhesions: prevention and complications in general surgery. Eur J Surg 1997;163(3):169-74.

118. Chegini N. Peritoneal molecular environment, adhesion formation and clinical implication. Front Biosci 2002;7:e91-115.

119. Liakakos T, Thomakos N, Fine PM, Dervenis C, Young RL. Peritoneal adhesions: etiology, pathophysiology, and clinical significance. Recent advances in prevention and management. Dig Surg 2001;18(4):260-73.

120. Down RH, Whitehead R, Watts JM. Why do surgical packs cause peritoneal adhesions? Aust NZ J Surg 1980;50(1):83-5.

121. Cheong YC, Bajekal N, Li TC. Peritoneal closure – to close or not to close? Hum Reprod 2001;16(8): 1548-52.

122. Jirasek JE, Henzl MR, Uher J. Periovarian peritoneal adhesions in women with endometriosis. Structural patterns. J Reprod Med 1998;43(3 Suppl):276-80.

123. Sulaiman H, Gabella G, Davis MS, et al. Presence and distribution of sensory nerve fibers in human peritoneal adhesions. Ann Surg 2001;234(2):256-61.

124. Herrick SE, Mutsaers SE, Ozua P, et al. Human peritoneal adhesions are highly cellular, innervated, and vascularized. J Pathol 2000;192(1):67-72.

Chapter 10

Osteopathy and obstetrics

OVERVIEW

For many years, osteopaths have been helping women with a variety of complaints associated with pregnancy, with preparation for labour and birth and postpartum recovery. Back pain, for example, need not be one's 'lot' in pregnancy and osteopaths consider that appropriate management of postural and biomechanical factors will either limit or help prevent various aches and pains, and may reduce the risk of more serious mechanical problems such as symphysis pubis dysfunction, sacroiliac pain and sciatica. Keeping an efficient biomechanical balance is also thought to be of value in helping the woman's body adapt effectively to the physical demands of the pregnancy, and minimizing stress on the enlarging uterus and developing baby. Osteopaths contend that efficient mechanics within the body, and especially the pelvis, will have a beneficial impact in the process of labour and birth outcomes, not only for the woman but for the baby as well.

Osteopathic techniques throughout the obstetric period are gentle and designed not to place stress on the tissues. Osteopaths consider that their role is supportive and not intended to replace midwifery or medical obstetric services. Osteopaths feel that in aiding maternal biomechanical fitness, some difficulties experienced during pregnancy, labour and delivery may be reduced. Much work has been done by Renzo Molinari, and also Stephen Sandler, to research, develop and promote the management of pregnant women with osteopathy, whose influence and contribution should be acknowledged.

POSTURAL AND BIOMECHANICAL INFLUENCES

Osteopaths have long considered that posture within pregnancy and maternal position (and the ability to move) in labour are important for maternal and fetal well-being. It is recognized that pregnancy alters the mother's biomechanical balance but this is not something that should automatically create pain and discomfort. Similarly, labour should be a natural event but is often more painful and difficult (leading to a variety of mechanical and physical complications) than it could be.

Anything that will promote physiological adaptation to and compensation for the changing volume of the uterus and the body cavities, shifts in the centre of gravity, consequent alterations in gait and general movement patterns should reduce strain on both the mother and the developing fetus. Ensuring that the spine, pelvis, shoulder and hip girdles are flexible and supple will enable the body to adapt to the changing dynamics that evolve throughout the pregnancy. Limiting restrictions and tensions wherever possible will allow the body to more easily adapt to the pregnancy, therefore placing less stress and strain onto the muscles and ligaments of the back and pelvis, in particular. This should lead to fewer symptoms than might otherwise have been the case.

According to osteopathic philosophy, the torsions and tensions throughout the body may not only affect the biomechanical balance of the mother but may also impact on the developing baby. Osteopaths consider that if the container holding and supporting the uterus (i.e. the mother!) is restricted, inelastic or otherwise in poor mechanical balance, then this transmits 'awkward or abnormal' forces onto the uterine wall and hence to the fetus. This is thought to impact on fetal mobility, positioning and comfort in the later stages of pregnancy when the fetus is no longer able to freely float within the uterine cavity. The idea that external torsion and tension acting on the uterus in this way may affect fetal positioning is somewhat controversial but it plays a role in the osteopathic considerations of neonatal, infant and childhood management.

As stated, many of the pain presentation patterns within pregnancy are thought to be related to poor biomechanical balance. Osteopaths consider that this includes not only somatic biomechanical problems but also tensions and strains in the supporting 'ligaments' of the uterus, such as the round ligaments and the uterosacral ligaments. Tension in these structures is thought to arise for several reasons, such as the uterus not being able to expand 'evenly' or not being supported in a balanced way by surrounding muscles and bony structures. Uneven 'expansion' can arise from particular positions of the baby, especially later in the pregnancy, or as a result of tensions in the maternal body walls and associated bony structures, which can mean the uterus has to bend or twist slightly as it grows. These tensions and constraints either cause tension in the supportive ligaments or arise as a result of tensions within them.

Osteopaths consider that these structures can be influenced by palpation through the abdominal wall and by engaging the bony and soft tissue structures that they are attached or related to. The relationship between uterine tension, uterine ligamentous torsion, maternal pelvic, spinal and body biomechanics and fetal positioning is a reciprocal one. Fetal positioning can influence all the other factors, and those other factors can influence fetal positioning, according to osteopathic philosophy. Hence osteopathic management in obstetrics incorporates optimum fetal positioning, as well as the biomechanical well-being of the mother.

Although pregnancy and birth are natural processes, they do seem to pose a threat to maternal and fetal well-being that is somewhat disproportionate to their 'naturalness'. Pregnancy and birth are not as comfortable in this modern age as many consider acceptable or reasonable, and many people feel that the woman's natural handling of these processes has become disrupted, for a variety of reasons. These include lifestyle, size of babies, medicolegal and fashions of birth practice issues. Consequently, the emphasis on maternal biomechanical factors has perhaps received less attention than it might. The following should serve to highlight the osteopathic approach to pregnancy, labour, and pre- and postnatal issues.

EVOLUTIONARY CHANGES FROM BEING ON ALL FOURS TO STANDING UPRIGHT

Human females have a curved birth canal, which is thought to have arisen during evolution as a consequence of standing upright on two legs. Understanding the changes from four legs to two gives insight into why modern obstetrics is faced with some problems.

Through the eons, the change to standing on two legs rather than four has lead to a more upright orientation of the skeleton, changes to muscle alignments and bony ridges, as well as changes in the shape of the pelvis. Over time, the spine has been held more and more vertically, with the gravitational centres of the head, thorax and abdomen coming to line up vertically one on top of each other rather than side by side as in four-legged creatures.[1] Part of this impetus to stand erect has been associated with load carrying; in other words, the more load you carry, the more vertical your alignment. This could have quite an impact on the way we see spinal alignment in pregnant women. The spine will adapt its pattern of curves as the pregnancy continues, but maintaining good vertical posture throughout the pregnancy may reduce symptoms and problems. Note: spinal curve changes in pregnancy will be discussed later.

Changing from standing on all fours to two legs also impacted on the form and shape of the pelvis. Over time, the birth canal has changed from being a horizontally oriented cylinder to a vertically oriented curved tube, which presents more resistance to the baby as it tries to descend through this passageway. The baby also went through changes, including most significantly an increase to the size of the head. This put more demands upon the pelvic shape and parturition during the evolutionary changes to posture.[2]

The relative sizes of the abdominal and pelvic cavities have also changed over time. The pelvis got bigger as humans developed, and the abdomen relatively smaller. In primates, there was a relatively small pelvis with the reproductive organs being contained in the abdominal cavity; unlike humans, who had a relatively large pelvis that could accommodate the 'shift' of various organs into the pelvic bowl (sigmoid colon, bladder and genital organs). Near term, the pregnancy expands easily in non-humans in view of the relatively small fetus and relatively large abdominal cavity. But, for the opposite reasons (large fetus, small abdomen), the human pregnancy is limited for space during its abdominal expansion. Unlike that of non-humans, human pregnancy is consequently faced with multiple problems. These include 'squeezing' between the anterior abdominal wall and the lordosis of the lumbar spine, compression of the aortocaval vessels, and forward expansion of the abdomen resulting in reorientation of the trunk during erect posture as the pregnant woman approaches term. All these conditions are responsible for numerous pathological entities that occur during human pregnancy and are almost unknown in non-human mammals.[3] As abdominal muscle girdle function is important for spinal stability, it is possible to see how changing the abdominal tensions could adversely impact on spinal support.

Thus, humans not only have a unique way of both standing and moving compared to other mammals, but they have increased abdominal pressures on the expanding uterus and the most complicated birth canal shape and consequent pattern of delivery. As a result, both passages and passenger have to undergo particular mechanical challenges in order for labour and delivery to be successful.

In the light of these changes over time, maintaining biodynamic efficiency throughout the body can be considered essential to reducing their impact and helping to ensure a normal, comfortable pregnancy, labour and birth. If the spine and pelvis in particular do not adapt and compensate for the changes in physical force, then problems and symptoms may result. Osteopaths therefore look at the posture and mechanics of the mother during pregnancy (or before, if possible) and reflect on how the various parts of the body and spine could adapt to the forthcoming changes. A large part of osteopathic management is 'preventive', by trying to maintain sufficient flexibility to ensure smooth adaptation to forces and hence efficient changes in posture and mechanics, lessening development of strain and stress and therefore symptoms. Accordingly, treatment may therefore be directed at currently asymptomatic areas of the back and body, to enable dissipation of forces and increase biomechanical compensatory ability.

SPINAL POSTURAL CHANGES IN PREGNANCY

The normal balance of the spinal curves is that each curve, whether lordosis or kyphosis, is in relative proportion to the others. Thus the cervical and lumbar lordoses are equivalent, and the thoracic kyphosis is in opposite proportion to both the other curves. Changes in the shape of any of the curves, in the position of one section of the trunk relative to another or in the amount of pelvic tilt will all influence the position of other parts of the spine as all the curves have an interdependent biodynamic relationship.[4] Imbalance between the curves and altered muscle coordination patterns may lead to increasing strain on the

spine as pregnancy advances, thereby predisposing to pain and problems.[5]

As Figure 10.1 indicates, there are a number of postural and spinal changes throughout the pregnancy. In the first trimester, there is usually a slight posterior rotation of the pelvis caused by displacement pressures of the other organs. The weight to the uterus is initially taken by the bladder and the pelvic floor and as the uterus increases in size, there is some upward pressure against the small intestine and sigmoid colon. This superior pressure increases and the broad ligaments either side of the uterus will rise up and push against the intestines (as the uterus expands towards the anterior abdominal wall and becomes more vertical).

Initial posterior rotation of the pelvis puts some strain on hip flexors, a little on the lumbar erector spinae and some on the anterior upper abdominals. Towards the end of the first trimester, the abdomen as a whole is beginning to change shape and orientation. The intraperitoneal organs normally move together as a column, easily envisaged when considering the movements of the abdomen caused by diaphragmatic descent and ascent during respiration (whether pregnant or not). As the uterus enlarges, meets the anterior abdominal wall and continues expanding vertically, the visceral column (principally formed by the small and large intestines, and the stomach and liver) will move superiorly. This causes some tension within the abdominal cavity. As the abdominal contents are relatively non-compressible, this can cause some tension onto the diaphragm, leading the dorsolumbar region of the spine to be pulled into relative extension, for example.

Spinal curve changes also occur in the thoracic and cervical curves. The majority of breast changes occur during the first half of the pregnancy and the increased weight of the breasts can cause increased thoracic kyphosis and lower cervical lordosis. Both of these factors can cause mechanical stress at the thoracic inlet.

Near the end of the second trimester, although the pelvis may still be posteriorly rotated in some women, it has more commonly started to rotate anteriorly and consequently the spinal curves reorganize themselves into a different balance. Now there is an increase in lumbar lordosis and tension along the linea alba and anterior abdominal

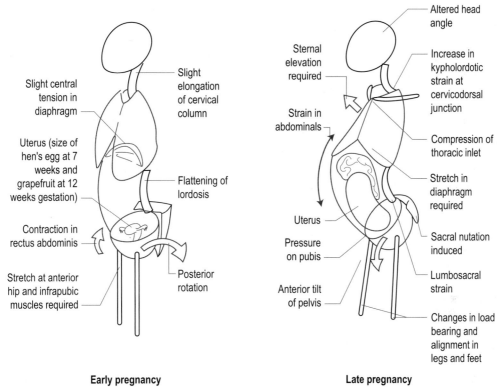

Early pregnancy

Slight central tension in diaphragm

Slight elongation of cervical column

Uterus (size of hen's egg at 7 weeks and grapefruit at 12 weeks gestation)

Flattening of lordosis

Contraction in rectus abdominis

Stretch at anterior hip and infrapubic muscles required

Posterior rotation

Late pregnancy

Altered head angle

Sternal elevation required

Increase in kypholordotic strain at cervicodorsal junction

Strain in abdominals

Compression of thoracic inlet

Stretch in diaphragm required

Uterus

Pressure on pubis

Sacral nutation induced

Lumbosacral strain

Anterior tilt of pelvis

Changes in load bearing and alignment in legs and feet

Figure 10.1   Changes in posture during pregnancy.

muscles as the expanding uterus pushes outwards against them. This can begin to cause strain at the lower end of the sternum and epigastric region, as well as at the symphysis. The (intestinal) visceral column now moves superiorly less and instead starts to distort laterally and posteriorly, and the shape of the abdominal cavity changes by becoming wider in its posterolateral portions. This latter movement requires stretch from the arcuate ligaments of the diaphragm, the rib articulations and intercostal muscles, and other posterior soft tissues like the thoracolumbar fascia and the quadratus lumborum muscles.

In the third trimester (or from midpregnancy), the spine can gradually adopt either a classic lordotic posture or a swayback posture, with associated changes through the rest of the spine. In the lordotic posture, the weight is carried on the pubis and via the abdominal muscles. In the swayback posture, the weight is carried behind the pubis and more on the pelvic floor and pelvic ligaments than the abdominal wall.

In the third trimester, lumbar lordosis usually increases as the lordotic posture is favoured and as a result, head position shifts posteriorly.[6] Although one might think the dorsolumbar region would also remain extended, in fact it may often flatten towards the end of pregnancy, and post partum.[7] This may cause mechanical conflict in the lumbar column. Sacral nutation increases and the posteroinferior pelvis ligaments and coccyx articulations must free off to allow this. The pelvic floor is also being stretched and must elongate whilst remaining toned.

During pregnancy, the fundus of the uterus rises in height until almost the end of pregnancy, when in fact the fundus 'drops' due to relaxation of the abdominal wall; the uterus expands outwards, not upwards, at the end of pregnancy. These volume changes place considerable physical constraints on the thoracoabdominal junction, bounded by the diaphragm. If the thoracic cage is not able to 'lift off' and expand away from the growing uterus, then pressure builds at the upper abdomen, creating strain at the epigastric region and rectus insertions, and onto the stomach and other subdiaphragmatic organs. Increasing pressure at the top of the abdominal cavity may also force the weight of the uterus downwards to press more onto the lower abdominal walls and pubis than otherwise. This could contribute to a variety of painful problems within that region. These changing cavity dynamics are illustrated in Figure 10.2. Many treatments for general spinal and ribcage discomfort involve easing soft tissue and articulatory pressures such that the body can expand and 'give more space' to the developing uterus. This in turn will ease pressure back onto the uterus and associated

ligaments, and should lead to a generally more comfortable pregnancy all round.

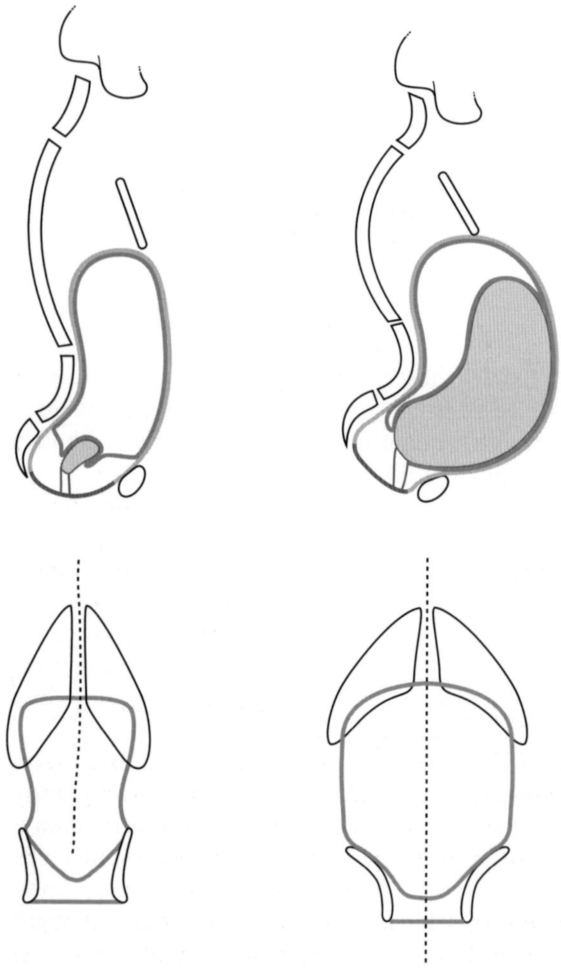

Clinically it is important to view the body as a whole and to understand the relationships between the body cavities and components of the spinal and locomotor systems. Ignorance of this is likely to lead to poor osteopathic diagnosis of problems and less effective treatment protocols and outcomes.

Other curve changes also occur. As normal pregnancy increases, forward flexion and axial rotation, motion of the thoracic segments and the thoracolumbar spine tend to be significantly reduced. However, there is often no significant decrease in the range of side-to-side flexion. The woman can often bend from side to side 'behind' her expanding uterus. Normally the uterus and abdominal cavity will rotate or shift away from the side of compression (i.e. to the left, if the woman bends to the right). This minimizes forces acting upon the uterus and developing fetus. The ease of swing of the uterus can easily be seen when viewed from the front. Poor swing can be an indicator of uneven mechanical balance in the tissues and inelasticity of muscles and other structures, which may require treatment to reduce strain. This is shown in Figure 10.3.

Other changes include an increase in base of support width (how far the feet are apart) during forward flexion and side-to-side flexion. All the above typical late pregnancy strategies (such as increasing the width of the base of support and reducing obstruction from other body parts) are used to minimize the effects of increased trunk mass and girth.[7]

Reviewing the above indicates that the spine (and body) will likely hold itself in several different alignments at different stages of the pregnancy. Each alignment will have a different pattern of curves and tensions. The essence of assessing the spine for its potential to accommodate the pregnancy comfortably centres on considering how well the spine can move into or out of these patterns. Examination consists of assessing the potential for movement from, say, flexion to relative extension in each section of the spine, so that adaptability for the 'next postural alignment' can be evaluated. If the spine can move easily into another alignment, then potential strain to the mechanics should be minimized. If the spine and surrounding tissues do not move easily into another alignment, then stress and strain may

Changing shape of container

Figure 10.2 Changing cavity dynamics during pregnancy. (Adapted from Stone[91], with permission.)

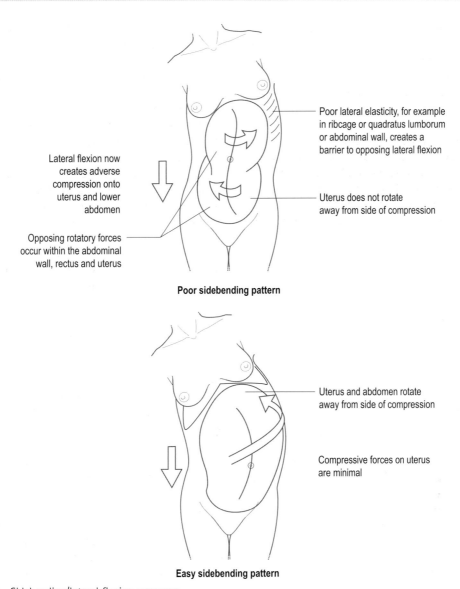

Lateral flexion now creates adverse compression onto uterus and lower abdomen

Opposing rotatory forces occur within the abdominal wall, rectus and uterus

Poor lateral elasticity, for example in ribcage or quadratus lumborum or abdominal wall, creates a barrier to opposing lateral flexion

Uterus does not rotate away from side of compression

Poor sidebending pattern

Uterus and abdomen rotate away from side of compression

Compressive forces on uterus are minimal

Easy sidebending pattern

Figure 10.3   Sidebending/lateral flexion pressures.

ensue at various points, which may lead to symptoms such as pain and reduced mobility. Once poor postural alignment is affecting one part, then the rest of the body's balance is likely to be compromised and so poor mechanical function may spread through the whole body, leading to symptoms in quite distant parts. Box 10.1 gives an introduction to some of the spinal factors that should be examined when gaining an overview of the woman's pregnant posture and potential for change throughout the pregnancy.

CHANGES TO GAIT, HIP AND SHOULDER GIRDLE MECHANICS

With all the spinal changes discussed above, it is easy to appreciate that the shoulder, pelvic girdle and lower limb mechanics would also compensate and adapt throughout pregnancy. Pelvic girdle mechanical problems are thought to contribute to various painful syndromes even though the aetiology of pregnancy-related pain in the pelvis is not completely understood. A better understanding of the gait problems of women with

---

Box 10.1   Spinal changes examination checklist

Are the cervical and lumbar lordoses equivalent and in balance?

If not, which curve is restricted or poorly moving?

If the woman gently rocks her pelvis forwards and backwards when standing, can you see smooth changes to the lumbar lordosis into relative flexion and the dorsolumbar curve into relative extension (with posterior pelvic tilt), and vice versa?

If not, where is the movement block?

In the sitting position, if the shoulders are gently sidebent one way and then the other (inducing a lateral displacement of the spine that passes down to the pelvis), does the coccyx move evenly with that shoulder girdle movement?

Is the coccyx bound from below or is the lateral movement blocked by sidebending restrictions higher up the spine?

In standing sidebending, do the ribs stretch out evenly with the convexity of the curve or do they bind and cause relative reverse sidebending or flat areas on lateral flexion?

How many ribs are involved and are they bound by chest wall soft tissues or at the costovertebral articulations?

---

pregnancy-related pain in the pelvis may contribute to more appropriate treatments which seek to redress some of the mechanical imbalances often found. Individual patients may apply different strategies during walking to cope with underlying problems, so 'one rule does not fit all'. As with spinal change patterns, an individual assessment of coping strategies is essential for effective osteopathic care to be administered.

With gait, there are two main areas of change: in the amounts of rotation between the shoulder girdle and the pelvic girdle, and in foot position or foot orientation (again, the literature suggests that these changes are not uniform).

Coordination between pelvic and thoracic rotations in the transverse plane is important in walking and it seems that one aspect of pelvic pain can arise from poorly coordinated rotation patterns between the thorax/shoulders and the pelvic girdle during the gait cycle.[8] Even in a

healthy (non-painful) pregnancy, there is some slight discoordination between the thoracic and pelvic rotation movement in gait, indicating that this requires considerable compensatory mechanisms to be integrated.[9] Examining the body for ease of rotation in the thoracic cage and in the hip and shoulder girdles would indicate how well the woman is adapting to the pregnancy.

Not all studies find evidence of the typical waddling gait of pregnancy. During walking, there is an increase in the amount the pelvis tips forwards (by around 4°). The general amount of joint 'freedom of movement' significantly increases in the hip and ankle movement patterns. This finding indicates that during pregnancy, there may be an increased demand placed on hip abductor, hip extensor and ankle plantarflexor muscles during walking.[10] In the later stages of pregnancy, there can be a significant increase in the base of gait during walking. This change in gait function is postulated as a compensatory mechanism to improve locomotor stability, and may have important implications for foot function and development of lower extremity dysfunction in pregnant women.[11] There also appears to be a tendency for an increase of load on the lateral side of the foot and the hindfoot. These changes may also be related to the knee laxity often found in later stages of pregnancy. Any of these changes may be responsible for the musculoskeletal complaints of lower limb pain in pregnant women.[12] Changes in lower limb movement patterns will also affect sacral mobility and pelvic balance during walking.

As the gait cycle and lower limb mechanics change, then so too will soft tissue balance through the legs, pelvic and abdominal regions. Foot mechanics may change, which will affect the fibular mechanics and the interosseous membrane, and there will be consequent adaptations through the knee, up the iliotibial tract and adductors, for example, and into the hip and pelvic regions. If tension alters across the symphysis pubis, its stabilizing strength may be compromised. It is possible that adductor muscle tension and alterations in the rectus or oblique muscles of the abdomen may lead to weakening of this joint and contribute to pelvic joint instability. Lower limb torsion patterns could thus be related to pelvic girdle instability and pain, and form part

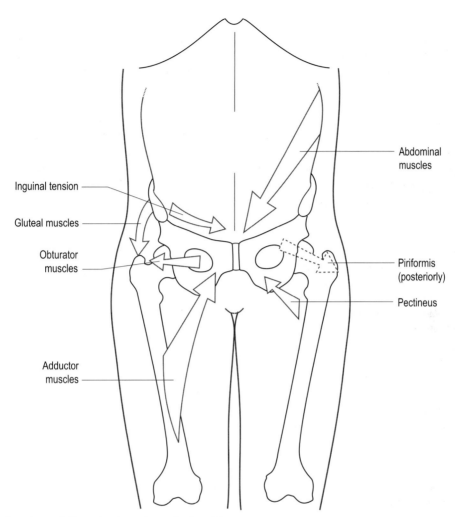

Figure 10.4 Crossing soft tissue tensions at symphysis pubis.

of a global assessment for pelvic dysfunction in pregnancy. Figure 10.4 shows some of the soft tissue crossing the anterior surface of the symphysis pubis, acting as a 'girdle' at the front of the pelvis, and Box 10.2 gives an examination checklist for some of the factors that should be evaluated when exploring the lower limb adaptability for pregnancy.

Summary of gait changes in pregnancy
- Wider stance (base of gait)
- External rotation of hips
- More contact with external border of foot
- More weight bearing on hindfoot
  - All of which makes walking different, the more pregnant you are

- Impacts on lower limb and pelvic joint freedom of movement
- Affects muscle chains up the leg and into the pelvis and back
- Affects fibular movements, foot arch dynamics and iliotibial band/gluteal muscle lateral chains, for example
- Reduces overall spring in the limb
- Criss-cross of tensions across pubis is created. X-shaped 'girdle' of obliques, adductors, pectineus and obturators comes under stress
- Influence of hip joint on ilial movement. External rotation changes this dynamic
- Resultant hip and pubic tensions act to 'pull' pubis apart, contributing to pelvic girdle instability and pain syndromes

CHANGES IN CAVITY DYNAMICS

Some cavity changes have already been introduced, for example the increasing pressures in the abdomen and on the diaphragm muscle as the uterus enlarges.

Developmentally, the abdominal cavity is the most primitive body cavity. Its musculofascial skeleton encompasses the anterior and posterior abdominal walls, the pelvic floor and the diaphragm. Comparative anatomical studies have demonstrated remarkable homology in the muscular and fascial architecture of each of these structures. In addition, all muscular sheets lining the abdominal cavity display a characteristic resting tone enabling them to act as a single functional unit. This has implications for breathing mechanics, and also for other relationships and organ function.[13] For osteopaths, this relationship will be apparent through the shifting fascial torsions that can be felt throughout the abdominal region during pregnancy. Gentle palpation over the abdomen enables the osteopath to 'listen' for the integration between the thorax and abdomen, or within the abdomen itself. If uneven or unbalanced tensions or torsions are felt using this very gentle palpation, the osteopath can 'follow' and release them. Releasing the torsions can alleviate the imbalance between the thoracic and abdominal cavities, and hence improve the space for the uterus and create for it and the fetus a better and more even mechanical supportive framework.

Other changes in this overall relationship influence breathing mechanics. During pregnancy, changes in the thoracic configuration subsequent to progressive increase in the abdominal volume have been found to have a moderate effect on respiratory function, where the cephalic displacement of the diaphragm reduces the expiratory reserve volume and the residual volume.[14] Enhancement of tidal volume is achieved usually by augmentation of ribcage volume displacement (the ribs nearest the diaphragm broaden out). Interestingly, abdominal volume displacement during quiet breathing is not altered in a predictable fashion by being pregnant. Overall, these changes lead to a shallowness of breath and increasing dyspnoea/hyperventilation. The ribcage changes include increased diaphragmatic contraction which leads to a transmission of that force to the lower ribcage via the area of apposition, and that diaphragmatic contraction then accounts for enhancement of the tidal breath. Diminished abdominal compliance might also contribute to the augmentation of ribcage volume displacement.[15] These changes will include adaptations in sternal movements and the biomechanics at the anterior ends of the ribs and of the costal cartilages, as well as through the crural attachments to the lumbar spine and at the posterior rib articulations with the spinal column.

Remember that the respiratory function of pregnant women changes for more than one reason. Gas exchange and alveolar–capillary diffusion are normal or even improved as a consequence of chronic hyperventilation. The latter is the most important functional change, sometimes expressed as a sensation of dyspnoea. The origin of this hyperventilation relates to the decreased threshold of sensibility to carbon dioxide in the respiratory centres, due to the effect of raised progesterone levels.[16]

Clinically, one needs to consider the thoracic cage in its respiratory function, coupled with its rotatory/gait cycle movement patterns, in order to appreciate the integration of function (that adapts over time during the pregnancy) and to understand the biomechanical relationships between the thorax and the pelvis in pregnancy. Many pain patterns could arise from a disintegration of these relationships. Box 10.3 indicates some of the examinations that should be carried out to assess the adaptability of the woman's cavity dynamics to her pregnancy.

SUPPORTS OF THE UTERUS

The anatomy of the uterus and its supporting ligaments has been discussed in Chapters 7 and 9.

Box 10.3   Cavity dynamics examination checklist

Anterior ribcage flexibility
Consider costal cartilage mechanics, pectoral tissue tone, transversus thoracis tension.
  Sternal lift
Do the clavicular articulations and the glenohumoral joints allow this movement?
  Diaphragm elasticity
Consider global lower ribcage elasticity – longitudinally and with AP diameter
  Costal margin elasticity
Subdiaphragmatic relaxation? Rectus abdominis muscle tone? Relationship with pubis and other midline structures?

During pregnancy, the orientation of these ligaments alters somewhat and osteopaths consider that any tension within those ligaments may impact on the even expansion of the uterus, and may possibly influence the process of labour.

The uterine ligaments during pregnancy can be thought of as acting somewhat like the guy-ropes attaching a hot air balloon and its basket. The round ligaments will influence the orientation of the balloon (the uterine body) and the uterosacral ligaments will influence the orientation of the lower segment of the uterus. The fallopian tubes and broad ligaments may influence the lateral walls of the uterus. The normal orientation of the uterus towards the end of the pregnancy is that of sidebending right and rotation right (due to the position of the back of the baby, when it is lying in a left occipitoanterior position). It is thought that uneven tension in the ligaments, resulting from biomechanical imbalance in the somatic structures they attach or relate to, may influence the ability of the uterus to easily expand and accommodate the developing fetus in a position *that is both comfortable for the mother and places the least pressure on the baby*. Adverse tension on the uterus via its ligaments and related structures may adversely influence fetal position.

OPTIMAL FETAL POSITIONING

Optimal fetal positioning is concerned with whether the fetus can align itself within the uterus in the most optimal position for an easy, low-stress vaginal delivery. It is a theory developed by a midwife, Jean Sutton, and an antenatal teacher, Pauline Scott, who found that the mother's position and movement could influence the way her baby lay in the womb in the final weeks of pregnancy. They also noted that the rate of posterior presentation has increased drastically in the last few decades, which they associated with the way women use their bodies, such as sitting in car seats, leaning back on comfortable sofas, together with less physical work. Their advice is to adopt a hands–knees position (kneeling on all fours) and perform pelvic rocking movements. This uses the forces of gravity and the natural fluid-buoyant environment of the uterus to allow the baby's back to settle towards the anterior abdominal wall, leading it to move into a more optimum presentation. The effects of maternal position on presentation and birth outcome are not clear cut,[17] but evidence suggests that optimal presentation may be positively influenced in some women.[18]

The osteopathic interpretation of optimal fetal positioning would concur with the above, but would also consider that biomechanical factors in and around the mother's spine, pelvis and hips, together with mechanical tensions acting on and around the uterus, would also influence the position of the fetus in late pregnancy and leading up to birth. Releasing tensions in the pelvis, hips, back and tissues surrounding the uterus is thought to relieve physical stress around the uterus, making its mechanical environment as accommodating as possible, thereby allowing the fetus to align itself in the most optimal position.

During pregnancy, the uterus changes shape from a sphere to a cylinder, and aligns around the anteroposterior curves of the spine, as well as incorporating lateralizing influences or pressures (uterine ligaments, pelvic shape, scoliosis, abdominal and thoracic wall components and so on). The presence of external factors such as scoliosis can affect uterine positioning, and the position of the mother's spine in relation to the baby's back may influence fetal lie and positioning of the baby's head.[19] Within the uterus, many factors can influence the fetal position, such as placental location.[20,21] Many placentas implant on the right side[22] which may be why most babies prefer to lie 'opposite' the placenta, i.e. with their back to the mother's left (which is considered the optimal vertex lie).

Problems with fetal lie and presentation are most important leading up to and during labour. If a baby is breech or in an occipitoposterior position, then the risk of medical intervention during the birth increases and the chances of an uncomplicated vaginal delivery decrease.[23-26]

Whilst factors such as placental location cannot be influenced by osteopathic treatment, other factors may be amenable to a manual approach, such that the fetus is encouraged to turn or better align itself. Several approaches for helping during labour and for helping babies to turn late in pregnancy to avoid either a posterior or breech presentation have been reported, which include the use of moxibustion,[27] chiropractic[28] and osteopathic care.[29] It should be stressed that the osteopathic approach is not to perform 'external cephalic version'. This is a particular term used to describe the medical approach to turning babies by applying force directly to the pregnant woman's belly. It involves direct manipulation of the fetus into rotation forwards or backwards (after moving the buttocks out of the pelvic brim), to help stimulate cephalic orientation. This is a medical procedure and is performed only by experienced obstetric teams. It has a variable success rate, which is improved in women with low uterine tone, anterior or laterally placed fetal spines, and particular placental locations,[30] but is viewed as a fairly safe obstetric technique which may reduce the prevalence of caesarean sections.[31]

There is risk associated with every procedure, including external cephalic version,[32] and many people working within obstetrics and midwifery, including the pregnant women themselves, are still looking for effective, low-risk and minimal invasive procedures. This is where the osteopathic approach may be of value.

The osteopathic approach would consider the mechanical influences of the following on the overall position of the uterus, on the tensions operating on or within the uterus itself, and upon the fetus directly.

Influence of surrounding structures (some examples)

- Uterine/maternal physical relationship, for example:
  - tension in the diaphragm
  - scoliosis
  - general abdominal organ tension
  - lumbar spine and psoas tensions
  - lumbar spine mobility
- Uterine 'guyropes' or ligaments (some examples):
  - pubic joint and inguinal region influence on round ligaments
  - sacral influence on uterosacral ligament tension
  - pelvic outlet balance on lower uterine segment
  - vaginal and pelvic floor tensions influencing cervix

*Adverse uterine muscular torsions as
a result of the above*

- Affects uterine pressures on fetus (hypothesis)
- Acts via membranous interface

Techniques used to examine and treat any of the above findings are discussed below. They are very gentle, using minimal force, no direct mobilization or attempts to physically rotate the fetus within the uterus. The concept behind the techniques is that they will allow the uterus to be as flexible and accommodating as possible, and will ensure that no adverse mechanical tensions are operating on the uterus from the outside (e.g. from the maternal spine, pelvis, psoas muscles and so on). Ensuring the uterus and its environment are as comfortable as possible allows the fetus more 'space' within which to rotate itself. It will receive different mechanical feedback from its environment, and that may be sufficient for it to be able to reposition itself accordingly.

UTERINE WALL AND MEMBRANOUS TENSIONS

As indicated above, osteopaths consider that the membranes surrounding the fetus in utero are capable of creating adverse tensions that operate on the fetus and on the uterine muscular walls. Gentle unwinding techniques and balanced fascial/'ligamentous' techniques can be used to ease out any torsions, with the idea that this will lead to a more accommodating and comfortable environment for the fetus, helping it align itself into an optimal position (during pregnancy or even during birth). These techniques are subtle, do not include the use of any force and are very minimal in amplitude and vector. They are quite advanced palpatory techniques and are part of an experienced practitioner's technique armoury. These sorts of techniques may be applied in the prepartum or sometimes the intrapartum period, with the consent of the labouring woman and the medical birthing/obstetric team. Again, it should be stressed that these techniques in no way resemble external cephalic version or other manual rotation techniques (where direct pressure is sometimes applied to the fetal head per vaginam, in order to facilitate rotation in labour).

EXAMINATION AND TREATMENT OF UTERINE LIGAMENTS, BODY CAVITY DYNAMICS AND FLEXIBILITY OF POSTERIOR ABDOMINAL WALL

Examination of the uterus and its local environment can be done in a number of ways. This is performed in conjunction with examinations for the low back, pelvis and hips (as well as the more global somatic and visceral components discussed above). The lumbar spine techniques are discussed below, and the standing assessment of the influence of the uterosacral ligaments on lumbosacral mobility is often done right at the beginning of the examination, before the patient sits, and the rest of the examination (including the ligamentous techniques described in a moment) is performed.

One of the standing examinations is that of the round ligaments, as shown in Figure 10.5. In this position, their tension is easily felt and compared from side to side. It is common that one ligament is more prominent than the other (due to the natural rotation of the uterus resulting from the side the baby's back is located). However, neither ligament should be tender or tense. Such findings indicate a problem that could arise from uterine restrictions, pelvic torsion and articulatory problems or lower limb tension, for example. Pubic symphysis movements can also be assessed in this position (for example, when the patient bends first one knee then the other, whilst keeping the feet flat on the floor, thereby creating a lateral tilt of the pelvis). Further general exploration should be performed before making any conclusions.

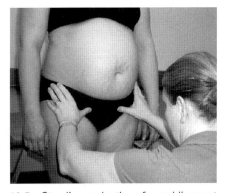

Figure 10.5   Standing evaluation of round ligaments.

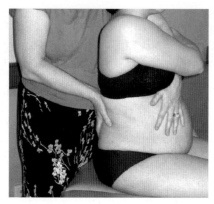

Figure 10.6   Posterior abdominal wall release and balancing with uterus.

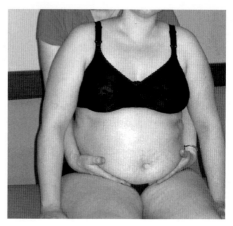

Figure 10.7   Evaluation of the lower segment of the uterus and uterine ligaments.

Another approach can be to examine the posterior abdominal wall and evaluate its general flexibility and its ability to stretch and expand to accommodate the changing shape of the abdominal cavity and the expanding size of the uterus. This is shown in Figure 10.6. The practitioner stands behind the patient and supports along the back with their hip. The anterior arm passes around the shoulder, or under the arm, to reach the abdomen. Care should be taken that this anterior contact is comfortable and unobtrusive. The posterior hand should be placed along the lateral flank of the body and can move slightly inferiorly or superiorly, depending on which posterior abdominal wall structures are being assessed. The elbow of the posterior arm is nestled into the practitioner's side, so as to give support to the forearm and wrist. Now, the practitioner can move their body, with the resultant motion passing through to the patient's posterior abdominal wall with minimal effort. The anterior contact gives some slight counterbalance, to aid in the global movements. It can also assess reactions of the uterus and general mobility of the uterus in combination with the posterior abdominal wall. Where there is a motion barrier, treatment choices can include a gentle articulatory technique or a fascial or functional unwinding approach.

Before treating, the general examination is continued in order to review all the components within the patient's presentation. An idea of the freedom of movement of the uterus within the lower abdominal cavity is of value. This is done by standing behind the patient, as shown in Figure 10.7.

The practitioner gently reaches around the lower abdomen and uterus, and takes a contact either side of the lower uterus. The patient may have to lean slightly to one side and then the other in order for the hands to be placed close to the inguinal region, so as to be close enough to the wall of the lower uterus. For comfort, a small pillow or cushion may be placed between the lumbar region of the patient and the practitioner, for support. The aim of the technique is twofold. One aspect is to evaluate the general tone of the lower uterus and the mobility of the uterus in the pelvic fossae. Very slow and gentle pressure is applied first on one side (towards the midline) and then the other. The practitioner is aiming to very gently ease the uterus out of the fossa and to evaluate any resistance found. The resistance might be as a result of tension in the uterus (from ligamentous restriction, for example) or from the fetus. Tension near the heel of the hand may represent uterosacral ligament restriction, and near the fingers may represent round ligament problems. Even if the fetus is quite laterally placed on one side, both sides of the uterus should still feel flexible and be able to be gently eased away from each iliac fossa. This movement should not be uncomfortable but sometimes the fetus can react to the movement and wriggle a little. In which case, relax the contact and wait for it to resettle before continuing.

The following techniques are not shown in any particular order. Practitioners should plan their

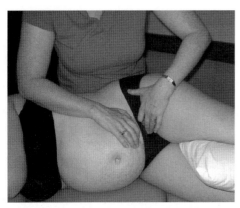

Figure 10.8 Round ligament evaluation and inguinal balancing.

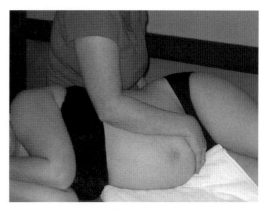

Figure 10.9 Uterosacral ligament balancing.

examination in advance and consider which position to perform each test in (visceral or somatic, or otherwise) before starting, so as to minimize patient handling and reduce the need to continually change the patient's position. This is particularly important with pregnant women, for whom movement is often awkward (especially when they are in pain). The techniques do not show routine somatic examination, which are part of an osteopath's basic skills.

Figure 10.8 shows a sidelying examination of the round ligaments. Here the practitioner is supporting the posterior pelvis and is contacting the inguinal region and lower abdominal/uterine wall, with either hand. The round ligament is palpated either within the inguinal canal or where it exits over the pubis, at the superficial inguinal ring. The ligament is generally palpated and then its stretch and mobility are assessed by gently moving the uterus or the pelvis (via the practitioner's abdominal contact with the patient's posterior pelvis, with the practitioner's wrist contact with the pubic area and upper thigh acting as a counterbalance). Stretch and mobility are evaluated in directions which are mostly caudal-cephalic. Direct lateral (towards the ceiling in this illustration) stretch may be directly applied, if required, or a more global unwinding release may be performed, as the tissue barrier indicates.

The round ligaments may be reacting to many factors, including imbalance at the uterosacral ligaments or posterior pelvic restrictions. The relationship with the uterosacral ligaments can be assessed in a sidelying position, by placing

one hand posteriorly on the patient's sacrum and the other hand over the lower abdomen, to cover the lower uterine area. This is shown in Figure 10.9. The practitioner's posterior hand is longitudinally placed along the midline of the sacrum, with the fingers pointing toward the coccyx. A slight amount of sacral compression can be induced, and small global movement of the sacrum can be added, in order to appreciate the link with the uterosacral ligaments. The sacrum can remain static, if desired, and the necessary motion induced by very gentle mobilization of the uterus. This movement is no more than an 'engagement' or 'taking up of the slack' of the tissues in one direction or another, and there is no need to grossly move the uterus in order to feel the reflection of the movement at the level of the sacrum. This contact can also be used as a very gentle unwinding technique to gradually ease lower abdominal and pelvic restrictions and torsion patterns. By slightly easing the hand contacts inferiorly, the superior components of the pelvic bowl can be assessed, and by moving the posterior contact close to the coccyx and pelvic floor, then the pelvic outlet structures can be addressed in relation to the uterine motion as indicated by the tissue barrier.

The lower uterus and its relations with the pelvis can also be assessed in the supine position. Whilst it may be preferable for some women to avoid lying on their spine, others find this quite acceptable, particularly if they are still sleeping on their back. There should be no problem with uterine circulation if the woman lies on her back for part of the treatment. This position allows

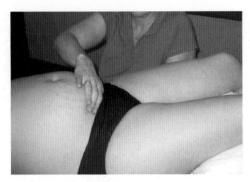

Figure 10.10   Lower uterine and pelvic inlet balancing.

a more global movement of the uterus to be incorporated. The posterior hand is underneath the sacrum and can be placed near to the lumbosacral junction or lower down nearer the coccyx, depending on the focus required at the time. The anterior contact can be adapted in a number of ways. Figure 10.10 shows the practitioner using the index and thenar border of the hand to 'cup' the lower uterus and move it gently from side to side. Placing the anterior hand lower down near the pubic arch can allow bladder and deeper pelvic tissues to be evaluated, for example. This contact is very useful for balancing scar tensions as a result of previous caesarean scars (a topic which is discussed later).

Another useful examination is that of anterior body line integration. This can be done by palpating along the length of the linea alba and feeling for lateralizing or torsional components to any tensions felt, as shown in Figure 10.11. Slight movement or sliding motion can be felt, which

when normally expressed occurs in a longitudinal (caudal-cephalad) direction. Treatment can be applied to follow or 'listen' to these tensions (which are mediated through the fascial systems of the body). Inhibition (or work to trigger points) can also be applied to the fibres of the rectus abdominis muscles running either side of the linear alba, in order to balance forces acting across it. This is useful when there is some discomfort in the abdominal wall, or the lateral body cavity dynamics are not well integrated. Cases of diastasis rectus cannot usually be remedied by these sorts of techniques (and they are usually self-limiting in the short-term postpartum period), but they can make the anterior abdomen more comfortable. The work to the linea alba area may also help reduce stress and irritation at the level of the symphysis pubis, where the rectus inserts, and can be part of a treatment plan for managing symphysis dysfunction. Finally, it can also help relieve upper abdominal or anterior diaphragmatic tension (for example, associated with upper gastrointestinal irritation or breathlessness).

As previously mentioned, much of the osteopathic approach in pregnancy is to enable the woman's body to accommodate to the increasing size of the pregnant uterus as easily as possible. This requires the abdominal cavity to broaden and expand posteriorly, with elasticity in the posterolateral abdominal viscera and tissues being an important prerequisite. The contact shown in Figure 10.12 can be used to evaluate such things as

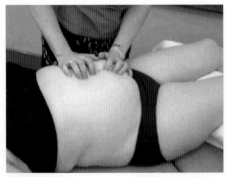

Figure 10.11   Treatment of the linea alba and rectus abdominis tensions.

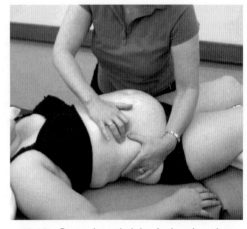

Figure 10.12   Posterolateral abdominal cavity release.

the ascending and descending colons, the kidneys, the quadratus lumborum muscles, Toldt's fascia and so on. One hand can stabilize the uterus and the other can evaluate or mobilize the other organs and associated structures (either individually or generally). Even in late pregnancy, it is possible to mobilize this posterolateral abdominal cavity. A careful contact 'around' the sides and back of the uterus is taken and with small gentle movements, tensions deep into the abdominal cavity can be appreciated. Often a rolling motion is induced between the two hands, in order to mobilize the viscera. Again, if the fetus reacts to any of this movement, then relax the contact and wait for it to resettle. The technique should not be uncomfortable.

This type of examination or treatment technique can also be performed with the patient on her side, as in Figure 10.13. The practitioner can stand behind or in front of the patient. When standing behind as shown, the practitioner's arms form an important part of the technique. They are gently resting on the iliac crest/lateral buttock and the lateral ribcage and lower scapular region. The practitioner can make the pelvic bowl or the shoulder girdle move anteriorly or posteriorly, or they can be stretched apart (by applying caudal and cephalic pressure respectively) to the pelvis and shoulder/rib region. This stretch works through the lateral abdominal region and can relieve stress not only in that cavity but also in the lower ribcage and lateral abdominal muscles, for example. The pelvic and shoulder girdles can also be brought together if required. Usually the shoulder/ribcage and the pelvis are moved independently in a variety of directions, which are determined by the tissue barriers detected in the lateral abdomen. The movement of these parts

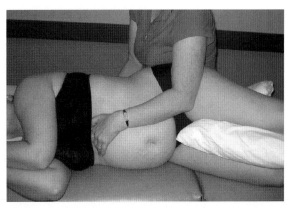

Figure 10.14   Sidelying diaphragmatic and upper abdominal visceral release.

engages the lateral abdomen, allowing the palpating hands to use less pressure and to 'listen' more easily for subtle tensions and torsions.

Having reviewed the inferior and posterolateral abdominopelvic areas, the superior abdominal cavity needs assessing. The upper abdominal contact shown in Figure 10.14 can be adapted to explore a number of factors. The anterior hand is placed above the uterus, near to either the stomach or the diaphragm and costal margin. It can focus on the uterus or the other viscerosomatic structures. The posterior hand can again be placed in a number of positions, depending on the desired focus. Often, it is placed across the lower dorsal spine and associated ribs, in order to appreciate tension in the posterior diaphragmatic components. Through this posterior contact, some indication of the spleen, colonic flexures or cardia of the stomach can also be gained. Diaphragmatic release is performed for a variety of reasons, such as to ease chest mechanics, to improve the functioning of the dorsolumbar spine (where the diaphragmatic crurae insert) or to increase the elasticity and 'spread' of the upper abdominal cavity, for example.

PALPATING FETAL POSITION

The obstetric and/or midwifery team looking after the woman will be formally noting fetal position, and the osteopath makes their own assessment. Whilst all parties are interested in the overall alignment of the fetus, the osteopath considers how comfortably the fetus is placed

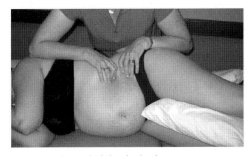

Figure 10.13   Lateral abdominal release.

within its uterine environment, and how much potential for change (movement) there is in its surrounds.

Palpation of fetal parts can be difficult and may be masked by an anteriorly placed placenta, for example. Only very gentle contact should be applied and the walls of the uterus should be soft and accommodating. Sometimes the fetus will respond to the contact and will wriggle and either 'kick' at the palpating hand or move away from it. Make sure that this movement is not blocked. Also, especially in later pregnancy, uterine contractions may be palpable. These are usually natural 'practice' contractions, which are often set off by mechanical changes in the uterine wall, such as fetal movements and palpation. Sometimes, the uterine wall merely 'stiffens' slightly in one section rather than 'contracting' in any large sense. Osteopathic palpation should not be a trigger for labour, and gentle palpation is safe. Any discomfort should mean the contact is changed or stopped. Figure 10.15 shows a bilateral contact over the lower half of the abdomen and uterus, to feel for the hard and soft fetal parts and to gauge some sense of the membranous tensions present.

These sorts of palpations and evaluations can also be performed in the sidelying position, as in Figure 10.16, or sitting, as in Figure 10.17.

Palpating fetal parts and identifying fetal position are not always easy and even very experienced midwives and obstetricians may have some difficulty, without using other aids such as heartbeat position or ultrasound. However, osteopaths can become proficient, and if care is taken, should be able to generally appreciate the basic fetal

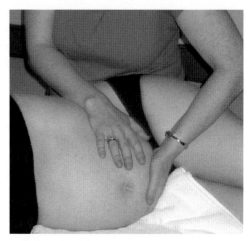

Figure 10.16 Uterine and membranous balancing, sidelying.

position in most cases. It should be stressed that the osteopath does not aim to advise the woman regarding her baby's position; its actual determination is left to the woman's medical care team. As a summary, though, the following is a guide to fetal palpation.

Lie

- Relationship of the long axis of the fetus to the mother. Can be longitudinal (vertex/ cephalic or breech) or oblique (transverse).

Attitude

- Relationship of the fetal parts to each other. Normally in labour all the joints are flexed.

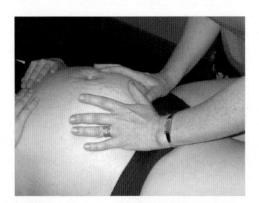

Figure 10.15 Fetal palpation and membrane 'listening'.

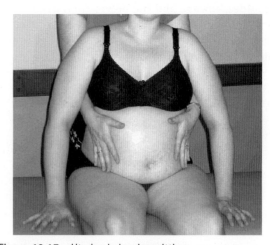

Figure 10.17 Uterine balancing, sitting.

Presentation

- Relates to that part of the fetus which occupies the lower segment of the uterus (head in vertex presentation, buttocks in breech, or shoulders in oblique).

Presenting part

- That portion of the fetus which is bounded by the cervix in the first stage of labour or the vagina in the second stage. In cephalic presentation, the part is the vertex, brow or face. In breech, it is the buttocks or feet.

Position

- Refers to the position of the presenting part to the periphery of the mother's pelvis. In vertex presentation, the occiput is referred to; in breech, it is the sacrum. Note: right or left position (of sacrum or occiput) relates to the mother's right or left.
- In the occipitoposterior presentation, the back is not felt; it is the legs, knees, hands and face that are palpable.
- The baby will be kicking onto the anterior abdominal wall rather than the spine, kidneys and other organs.

PROBLEMS DURING PREGNANCY

BACK PAIN

One of the components related to back pain during pregnancy is the effect on sacral mechanics caused by the physical forces transmitted through the uterosacral ligaments from the developing pregnancy. Even in very early pregnancy, the change in proprioceptive balance caused by the initial enlargement of the uterus and its weight being taken by the pelvic floor complex is considered sufficient to affect sacral (and therefore sacroiliac, coccygeal, pubic and lumbosacral joint movement patterns). As the pregnancy expands, increasing pressure can be mediated through the uterosacral ligaments, and this can contribute to back pain. If standing pelvic movement tests are performed with the weight of the uterus gently supported, this often relieves pain and symptoms and improves movement. This test, illustrated in Figure 10.20, can implicate uneven tension in the uterosacral

ligaments, perhaps from a positional imbalance in the uterus, or tension in other uterine ligaments/attachments, or in relation to a piriformis problem.

Pelvic girdle rotation requires spinal curve changes as discussed above. If these do not occur smoothly, then more mechanical stress will be placed at the low lumbar articulations, causing soft tissue irritation. This can increase in later pregnancy and if extension occurs sharply at the lumbosacral complex, weight bearing can be transferred to the facet articulations, which are not designed to accommodate this for long. Consequently inflammation, muscle spasm and tension build up, leading to painful syndromes and unbalanced movements. Even in the absence of weight-bearing facets, the iliolumbar ligaments can become quite irritated in pregnancy, as they are affected by any adverse sacral or lumbar mechanics which alter the balance between the origin and insertion points of the ligament,[33] creating uneven (symptomatic) tension from one side of the ligament complex to the other.

Lumbar disc herniations are possible in pregnancy, as at other times, and can cause considerable discomfort and pain, with or without associated peripheral neuropathy or cauda equina syndrome. Osteopathic management of this disorder is possible throughout pregnancy, although if severe enough, surgery is considered a safe option.[34]

The influence of the pelvic joint movements, sacral nutation and soft tissue balance in and around the pelvis is also important for lumbar spine mechanics. These factors are discussed below.

SACROILIAC JOINT AND SYMPHYSIS PUBIS DYSFUNCTION

Pelvic pain is one of the most common complaints in pregnancy and is often described differently by different authors/studies. Quite commonly, sufferers are separated into groups relating to symptom areas.[35]

For example, in one study women were divided, according to symptoms, into five subgroups (pelvic girdle syndrome, symphysiolysis, one-sided sacroiliac syndrome, double-sided sacroiliac syndrome, and one miscellaneous). The authors found that the majority of women in the classification groups experienced disappearance of pain within a month after delivery. They also found that the women with pelvic girdle syndrome (pain in all three pelvic joints) had a markedly worse prognosis than the women in the other classification groups.[36] However it is described, pelvic joint/ girdle syndrome is nearly always thought to follow pelvic girdle relaxation due to the pregnancy hormones and is recognized as having prolonged debilitating effects which do not respond well in the long term to current orthodox therapies.

In osteopathic thinking, this separation into syndromes or classification creates confusion, as it implies that the aetiology of problems in each painful area can be separated out and considered in isolation. Osteopaths feel that the biomechanical complex of the pelvis, low back and legs, together with the enlarging uterus and general cavity dynamics, all combine to create unevenness within the pelvis that will focus more or less on certain structures, depending on the unique combination of tensions present in any particular individual. The outcomes of patient management in pelvic pain problems may be improved by a more individually applied analysis.

One aspect of the osteopathic theory about pelvic joint dysfunction was introduced earlier: the influence of lower limb mechanics which become affected by the altered weight bearing during pregnancy. These biomechanical changes are thought to compound any joint instability initiated by the presence of relaxin during pregnancy. When the lower limb is tight or unbalanced for whatever reason and the hip girdle becomes affected, the ilium effectively becomes part of the leg movement complex, rather than part of the pelvis. In other words, the ilium will be influenced by the hip tension, causing adverse stress at the sacroiliacs and/or pubic symphysis. Hence strain at this level will not be relieved unless the lower limb dysfunction is resolved. Also, when the lower limb is tense and its natural elasticity reduced (e.g. within the foot arches and the interosseous membrane) then there will be less shock absorbency acting on the pelvic joints, adding to mechanical distress at those articulations.

Another aspect is the integration of movement dynamics between the pelvic joints themselves and the lumbar spine. There are many theories concerning the axes of movement within the pelvis.[37-40] In osteopathic circles, the following factors are commonly considered, based on sacral

nutation and counternutation movements. In Figure 10.18, sacral movements under vertical load from the lumbar spine/trunk are shown. The sacrum is tipped into a degree of nutation, increasing lumbosacral extension. This movement is balanced by the sacroiliac and iliolumbar ligaments, as well as by various muscles. During gait and other body movements, the load bearing acting on the lumbar column varies, inducing a rhythmic pitching and nodding movement of the sacrum. The orientation of the sacrum and the sacroiliac ligaments creates a 'scissor' shape, as shown. The sacral movements mimic the opening and closing of the scissors. These movements require elasticity and relaxation at different times in the soft tissues of the sacroiliac and low back joints, and those attaching to the sacrum. Too much tension in the pelvic floor can induce sacral counternutation, placing strain at the lumbosacral disc. Too much elasticity in the sacroiliac ligaments and poor tone in the pelvic floor can induce sacral nutation, straining posterior lumbar soft tissues and irritating the facet joints, for example.

The sacrum makes a combined 'pitch, roll and yaw' movement within this scissor action, meaning that the sacral base is constantly changing its orientation, requiring compensatory balancing from the iliolumbar ligaments, and also the long dorsal sacroiliac ligament,[41] to stabilize the lumbar articulations. Increasing cavity pressures and changing dynamics (such as during pregnancy) may distort the pitch, roll and yaw movements in the pelvic and lumbosacral regions, potentially placing increased load on the stabilizing and proprioceptive functions of the iliolumbar ligaments. Hence, iliolumbar ligament strain and pain may be more common, as adaptive patterns will be reduced. Other muscles are involved in this complex balancing act, such as the psoas muscles which are major stabilizers and movers of the lumbar spine and hip joints. Any unevenness in tension in the psoas muscles can lead to increasing lumbar and pelvic instability, causing or aggravating painful problems in those areas. The same is true of the abdominal muscles, including rectus abdominis, which all act to support the thoracolumbar fascia and the lumbar spine.

Treatment directed at the lower limbs and integration of the spinal curve patterns is part of the osteopathic strategy in managing pelvic joint

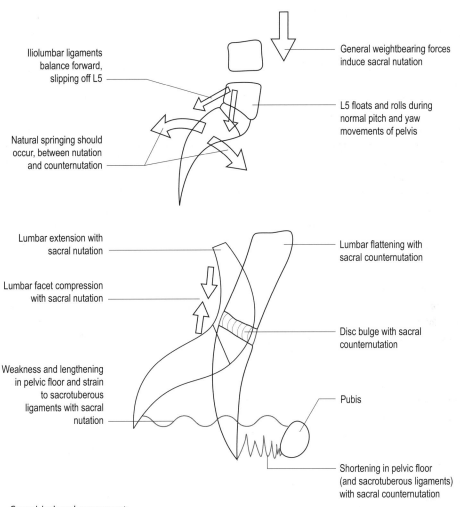

Iliolumbar ligaments balance forward, slipping off L5

General weightbearing forces induce sacral nutation

L5 floats and rolls during normal pitch and yaw movements of pelvis

Natural springing should occur, between nutation and counternutation

Lumbar extension with sacral nutation

Lumbar flattening with sacral counternutation

Lumbar facet compression with sacral nutation

Disc bulge with sacral counternutation

Weakness and lengthening in pelvic floor and strain to sacrotuberous ligaments with sacral nutation

Pubis

Shortening in pelvic floor (and sacrotuberous ligaments) with sacral counternutation

Figure 10.18   Sacral 'scissor' movement.

dysfunction in pregnancy, as is releasing unevenness in uterine ligament balance. Some of these techniques are discussed below.

Sciatica

All these biomechanical adaptations and strains may combine to cause compression or irritation of the sciatic nerve. The nervous system has its own unique biomechanics, moving quite considerably in normal gross body movements.[42,43] Changes in curve patterns and spinal posture will influence the amount of movement of the spinal cord and nerve roots (central and peripheral nervous systems) in and close to the vertebral canal. Movement of head, neck, thoracic cage and lumbar spine can

all influence neural movements, and impart axial torsion onto neural components.[44] Adverse spinal curve mobility may distort normal neural mobility and may contribute to strain within the neural structures. Hence, spinal changes in pregnancy may distort neural biomechanics, giving another reason (apart from direct pressure) why pregnant women get sciatica.

Piriformis syndrome[45] is another cause of posterior pelvic pain and, in some cases, sciatica. Any distortion to sacral and hip mechanics can affect piriformis balance and therefore contribute to sciatic irritation and should be explored in these cases. Pregnant women are also prone to compression of the sciatic nerve within the pelvis before it passes through the greater sciatic notch.

This pressure may be caused by the displacement of other organs or by the enlarging uterus or fetus itself[46,47] and may act to affect the vasa nervorum of the lumbosacral plexus or sciatic nerve and hence its function. Gentle mobilizing of the uterus (to ease its mobility within the pelvis and lower abdomen) may play a role in improving pelvic circulation and relieve pressure effects, thus reducing sciatic irritation. Other mobilizations of the pelvic, hip and low back joints and releasing of associated soft tissue tensions may also be required to relieve sciatic compression from its numerous potential restrictions.

Other maternal palsies are relatively common. Meralgia parasthetica, femoral neuropathy[48] and peripheral facial neuropathy are also associated with pregnancy.[49] Obturator nerve problems are also associated with pregnancy and labour.[50] All these components may be related to soft tissue tensions, mechanical imbalance and pressure from the uterus and fetus due to poor overall cavity dynamics. An osteopathic approach may be useful in all cases.

COCCYX

Changing pelvic tilt, altered mobility at the sacroiliac joints and variations in femoral rotation and motion can all impact on the tension patterns within the sacroiliac, ischiosacral and coccygeal ligaments. These movements can also influence tension within the pelvic floor and levator ani muscles. All these factors can influence coccygeal mechanics and contribute to local pain and irritation. The uterosacral ligaments also attach onto the sacrum, coccyx, coccygeus and piriformis muscles and the ischiosacral ligaments. Increasing weight of the uterus will impact on the uterosacral ligaments, hence affecting the sacral and coccygeal mechanics.

Coccygeal pain and discomfort often cause fear and concern for pregnant women as they feel it might mean a difficult labour or increased stress on the pelvic floor tissues. Figure 10.19 shows some of the muscular and ligamentous attachments of the coccyx. The way the anococcygeal raphe and the levator muscles 'hang off' the bottom of the coccyx is clearly visible. Pelvic floor weakness, tension or scarring may cause uneven tension on the raphe, distorting the coccygeal alignment.

This sort of torsion can also affect the rectal circulation or compound problems of haemorrhoids, which is another source of coccygeal area pain.

Coccygeal pain problems can be eased by pelvic floor work, by per rectal or per vaginal mobilization of the coccyx or stretching and inhibition of the pelvic floor muscles, and can also be helped by various mobilizations or manipulations of the pelvic girdle, hip and low back structures. Osteopaths also theorize that as the top and bottom of the spine work in proprioceptive balance, any restrictions, say, at the lower lumbar spine can affect the upper cervical spine mechanics, and vice versa. They also link embryologically significant structures in a functional way and feel that structures originally arising near the anterior and posterior neuropore would also be functionally linked. This means that, for example, the coccyx and the ethmoid bone are dynamically in balance and restriction in one will lead to dysfunction in the other. Also, in involuntary motion studies and reciprocal tension theories, the coccyx and ethmoid (and other cranial structures) are linked through their mutual attachments to the CNS, dura and meningeal attachments.

Pelvic floor restrictions and coccygeal tension can be important in many painful syndromes of the pelvis and low back, as they can distort the normal functioning and mobility of the articulations in those regions. Although the pelvic floor muscles are not prime movers of the pelvic bones, osteopaths consider that they are prime 'limiters' of pelvic motion, when dysfunctional, hypertonic or weak. For example, tension in the pelvic floor can reduce the ischial tuberosity axes of movement, leading to a relative hypermobility at the sacroiliac joints. This can lead to sacroiliac or low lumbar pain and dysfunction, meaning that the pelvic floor component needs treating in order to resolve the pelvic or low back pain presentation. The ischial tuberosities normally move in a figure of eight/spiral motion during gait, and the pelvic floor tension or weakness leads to uneven spiral dynamics operating at the level of the tuberosities, changing the dynamics of the pelvis as a whole. This seems valid in males as well as females, with many cases of recurrent sacroiliac or iliolumbar strain eased by work to the pelvic floor component.

Considering all the above, treatment of pelvic floor and coccygeal pain can involve work with

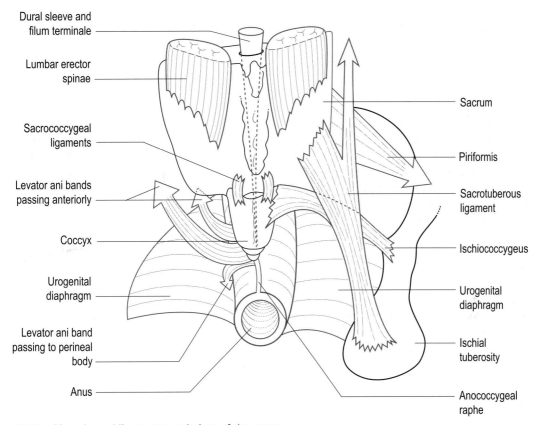

Dural sleeve and filum terminale

Lumbar erector spinae

Sacrococcygeal ligaments

Levator ani bands passing anteriorly

Coccyx

Urogenital diaphragm

Levator ani band passing to perineal body

Anus

Sacrum

Piriformis

Sacrotuberous ligament

Ischiococcygeus

Urogenital diaphragm

Ischial tuberosity

Anococcygeal raphe

Figure 10.19   Muscular and ligamentous relations of the coccyx.

local pelvic factors, local abdominal or pelvic organ balancing, where practicable, or work to the upper cervical spine and head, for example, depending on what is found in the individual patient. It is important to realize that although some mechanical discussions have been separated out to highlight some interesting points in the management of back pain, pelvic pain and so on, it is artificial to do so in practice. Therefore, for all the painful syndromes discussed so far, the biomechanical factors are often interchangeable and integrated, and need to be evaluated as a complete system, not in isolation. This breadth of approach and analysis is one of the key components to osteopathic practice, leading to an individualized approach to treatment and management.

Examination and treatment of the coccyx and pelvic floor has been described in Chapter 7 so only certain techniques will be described below.

EXAMINATION AND TREATMENT TECHNIQUES FOR THE LUMBAR SPINE, PELVIS AND LOWER LIMBS IN PREGNANCY

In this section, a variety of examination techniques are discussed, which can also be adapted as treatment tools, if required.

Figure 10.20 shows a gentle lift to the uterus in order to relieve 'drag' onto the sacrum from the uterosacral ligaments. The patient first performs some simple active movement tasks and the practitioner palpates the local soft tissues, feeling for tissue reactivity to movement. Tissue response and pain levels are noted during these active movements. Now the practitioner gently places one hand under the lower part of the uterus just above the symphysis pubis. (Sometimes the use of the wrist or lower forearm area is helpful.) Applying a gentle upwards lift to the uterus,

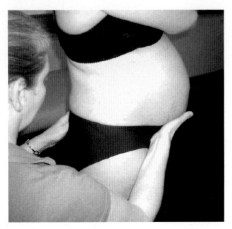

Figure 10.20 Uterine 'lift' to evaluate uterosacral ligament involvement.

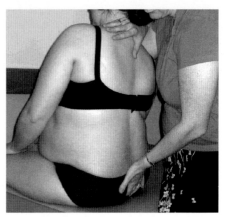

Figure 10.21 Sidebending tests of coccyx.

ensuring this remains comfortable at all times for the patient, the practitioner gets the patient to repeat the painful or awkward movements previously noted, whilst maintaining the lift to the uterus. When there is adverse tension acting on the sacrum from the uterus, this technique will relax those uterosacral ligaments, leading to a reduction in pain or an improvement in movement compared to before (when the uterus was not supported as described). This indicates to the woman and the practitioner that some gentle release of the uterine ligaments may be helpful in that case. If the symptoms do not change, then there is usually a significant restriction or torsion in other structures such as the sacroiliac joint, piriformis muscle or low lumbar spine, for example, which will need to be separately evaluated.

Figure 10.21 shows an evaluation of the spinal column and coccyx. Here the practitioner is carefully palpating at the level of the coccyx, either with one finger near the tip of the coccyx or two fingers resting gently either side of the coccyx. The aim of the technique is to induce a lateral movement into the spinal column and palpate for this movement as it passes through the spine and down to the coccyx. If the spine is translated laterally (sideshifted laterally without much of a curve being introduced) then it is likely that the coccyx will move in the opposite direction to the shoulders. If a curve is introduced in the spine, this not only explores the sinuous movement of the spine more readily but means that a different

motion relationship occurs at the coccyx. This time, the coccyx will move to the same side as the shoulders. This is the case when there is no spinal restriction or no coccyx restriction. When there is a problem, the coccyx cannot move at all, moves unevenly from side to side or moves in a different pattern from that which is expected. All indicate that further examination and treatment are required.

This basic technique can be adapted for therapeutic input. This time, the practitioner is using the shoulder girdle as a guide to 'direct' movement at the level of the sacrum and/or coccyx. Movement can be reflected along the spine to cause small articulatory movements at the sacrum, which can be rhythmically repeated to gradually release the ligamentous restriction. The practitioner 'searches' for the direction of movement in the shoulder girdle which identifies the direction of movement at the level of the coccyx or sacrum which is limited or altered. The practitioner can then apply a direct technique against this tissue barrier or an indirect technique focused in a direction of ease (following the pathway of least resistance, away from the tissue barrier).

Other helpful techniques are those which balance the relationship between the thorax and the abdomen, and between the lower ribcage and the pelvic girdle. These components need to be working in dynamic equilibrium to ensure appropriate adaptation to the pregnant posture. This is shown in Figure 10.22. The practitioner places one hand over the pubis and one hand over the xiphoid/ anterior lower costal margin. This technique is particularly useful for integrating abdominal

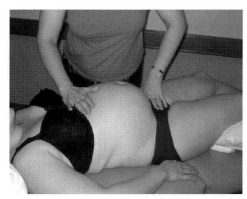

Figure 10.22   Balancing between xiphoid/diaphragm and pubis.

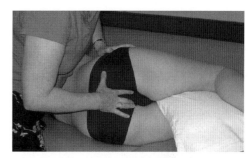

Figure 10.23   Coccyx and posterior pelvic floor release.

wall tensions. The contact can also be slightly adapted, so that the anterior hand contacts the inguinal region on one side (where this has been previously found to be in tension) and the other moves posteriorly to contact over the 12th rib and arcuate ligaments (again, where these have been found to be in tension). Releasing the arcuates and the inguinal ligaments concurrently allows the 'top and bottom' constraining bands of the abdominal cavity to be balanced, which helps many torsions and tensions to settle further. The original contact on the xiphoid and pubis also gives another 'handle' for balancing the thoracic and pelvic floor diaphragms.

Having explored all around the uterus in the previous techniques, an inferior exploration is now useful. The pelvic floor is ideally released after surrounding tensions have been addressed. Where there is stress and tension at the pelvic floor, local work will only have short-term effects if the wide components to that pattern are still in place. Hence, work to the rest of the cavity, the uterus and the rest of the spine or body should often be undertaken prior to specifically focusing on pelvic floor problems. There are some instances where the pelvic tension is very particular and requires local release quite quickly in order to relieve symptoms (such as with coccydynia, haemorrhoids or postpartum episiotomy recovery, for example) but even then, wider factors are also usually needing to be released as a follow-on. In the technique shown in Figure 10.23, the practitioner has one hand stabilizing the pelvis via contact with the lateral buttock or iliac crest. The other hand is placed low on the sacrum, so that the index and middle fingers can pass inferior to the sacral angle. The curve of the fingers will naturally fit around the curve of the lower sacrum and coccyx. The terminal phalanx of each finger should be either side of the coccyx, to allow access to the posterior levator ani tissues. This contact can release tensions in the coccyx articulations as well as the pelvic floor. The other hand contact can mobilize or orient the pelvic bowl in several directions, to aid the tissue response at the pelvic floor level. If required, the other hand can move anteriorly and contact under the belly and onto the pubic arch, again to release through the length of the pelvic floor and to ease torsions that pass along the whole inferior portion of the pelvic bowl.

In Figure 10.24, another adaptation of the above technique is shown. Here the posterior contact is on the sacrum and the anterior hand contact is on the lower belly. This enables a global release of the sacrum to be performed. This contact or position can be 'reversed' if required, so that the practitioner is facing towards the head of the patient. Now, the hand contacting the sacrum will be aligned so that the fingers are pointing towards the lumbar spine, not the coccyx. The other hand

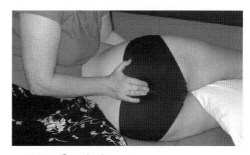

Figure 10.24   Sacral release.

will be supporting the lower belly, usually with the ulnar border of the hand nestled close to the pubic arch and the rest of the hand settling over the lower uterine area.

All the above techniques should have eased sacroiliac, lumbosacral and sacrococcygeal articulatory torsions effectively. A focused exploration of the pubic symphysis can be very useful to 'complete' the examination of the pelvic bowl. Figure 10.25 shows a contact over the symphysis pubis and the superior pubic arch. The fingers can align over the superior pubic arch and the thumbs can contact over the face of the pubis, or even onto the lower pubic arch if required. The aim of this technique is to release torsion over the face of the pubis.

The term 'intraosseous' reveals an interest in the biomechanics of the periosteum and internal bony architecture. Osteopaths consider that the bony trabeculae and periosteal structures can hold torsion and tension, and create stiffness patterns and strain within the bone that effectively reduce its natural springiness and shock absorbency. Small and very focused movements can be used to feel down into the bony tissue to assess these very deep strain patterns. This can be very helpful where there is inflammation, periostitis or tendonitis and where the associated joint is under mechanical stress. In the case of the pubis in particular, the shock-absorbing tendency and natural elasticity of the pubic arch are essential to limit mechanical distress at the joint and to reduce the very debilitating painful syndromes that affect this region. Note: this contact can also be adjusted

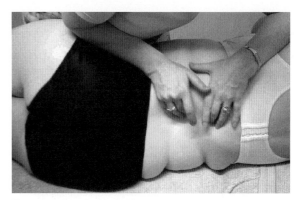

Figure 10.26   Lumbopelvic manipulation.

to turn it into a bilateral release of the inguinal canal and round ligaments, by moving the hand contact a few centimetres higher, above the pubis.

Figure 10.26 shows lumbar spine manipulation, to release muscle tension and reflex tissue irritation and to increase joint mobility in the lumbar spine. There are a number of different components to this technique[51] but the element of iliac contact is particularly important when this technique (or similar) is used in pregnancy (especially late pregnancy). In the third trimester, pelvic pain and lumbar spine irritation are common and restriction in the sacroiliacs or the facet joints in the lumbar region is often found. Care should be taken to avoid pressure on the iliac crest that would close down the space between the two anterosuperior iliac spines of the mother. This could cause unnecessary pressure acting onto the uterus and fetus, which can be avoided by using more upper-level components than lower-level components. The x-ray in Figure 10.27 shows the relative lack of space between the fetal skull and the maternal pelvis in late pregnancy.

Figure 10.28 shows another way of addressing the pelvic bowl and pelvic floor. In this contact, the practitioner is resting their upper abdomen or diaphragm over the anterior iliac crest area. The arms are 'cupping' around the periphery of the ilium. The aim is to have one forearm nestling under the tuberosity and the other wrist nestling under the posterior iliac spines and into the sacroiliac joint sulcus. This allows the practitioner to apply a slightly distracting tension, where the ilium is gently 'floated away' from the sacrum. The practitioner's abdominal contact is not to

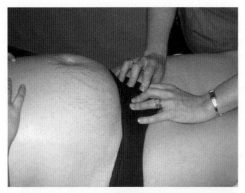

Figure 10.25   Symphysis pubis treatment and 'intraosseous' pubic arch release.

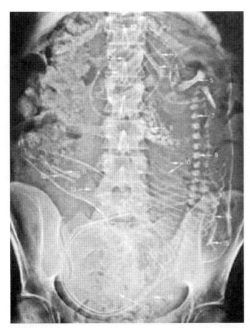

Figure 10.27   X-ray showing fetal head relations to maternal pelvis. Reproduced with permission from Wicke: Atlas der Röntgenanatomie, 7th edn. © Elsevier GmbH, Urban & Fischer Verlag.

compress the sacroiliac joint or to clamp down the space between the two anterior iliac spines, but is there purely to introduce a third point of contact to help turn, rotate or otherwise reorient the alignment of the ilium. The fingers of the two hands can be gently contacting on the sacroiliac ligaments or onto the pelvic floor, if possible. This technique is all about giving space and elasticity to the posterior pelvis, and increasing the body's ability

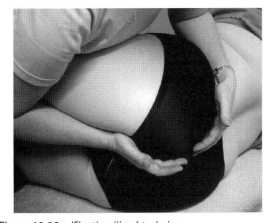

Figure 10.28   'Floating ilium' technique.

to accommodate the pressures of engagement and labour. It would be a very useful technique pre- and intrapartum (and postpartum as well).

Other general techniques which may be useful include:

- hip rotation and traction
- obturator 'muscle energy technique' and inhibition
- ITB/gluteus medius inhibition (a bit like pectoralis minor); feeds into descending lateral stabilizer chain – down the fibula, links with cuboid
- interosseous membrane and tibiofibular joints release, and foot arch/cuboid unwinding
- 12th rib release, sternal mobilization and upper cervical spine articulation and soft tissue release.

INDIGESTION AND REFLUX

Nausea and vomiting occur in 60–70% of pregnancies, usually start at 6–8 weeks and resolve by 16 weeks. Hyperemesis gravidarum is a severe form of vomiting and leads to inadequate hydration, electrolyte imbalance, poor nutrition and weight loss, all of which can compromise maternal and even fetal health and well-being. Hyperemesis occurs in 0.1–1% of pregnancies and must be differentially diagnosed from such things as hepatitis, ulcers, pancreatitis, bowel obstruction, thyrotoxicosis, diabetic ketoacidosis, Addison's disease, hypercalcaemia, urinary tract infection, uraemia and CNS or vestibular disease. It can also be drug induced. Some natural remedies for the normal vomiting or nausea of pregnancy include the use of ginger root for vomiting and avoidance of bananas for heartburn. Separating fluids and solids is also useful, but the use of a nasogastric tube may be required if the problem is very severe.

Reflux, gastric irritation and 'indigestion' in pregnancy are usually considered as hormone related, where sphincter relaxation allows gastric contents to flow in a retrograde manner. Any impact of the 'space-occupying lesion' of the pregnant uterus is mostly dismissed as secondary and, by its very nature, untreatable and also self-limiting over time. However, any inability of the body to accommodate the expanding uterus may impact on the severity of these upper intestinal tract problems, and biomechanical restrictions, especially in the thorax and upper abdomen, may play a role in their aetiology and maintenance. Local biomechanical changes in the diaphragm and thoracic cage/mediastinum may also lead to upper gastrointestinal problems in pregnancy. Cavity changes, spinal curve changes and balancing required between the pelvic and shoulder girdles, for example, may all lead to mechanical distress at the cardiac region of the stomach and the oesophageal hiatus of the diaphragm. Tension in the upper cervical spine may also irritate the vagus nerve, compounding gastric irritation.

Osteopathic treatment can be focused on the diaphragm, thoracic cage, mediastinal tensions (via the sternum, for example), thoracic and abdominal viscera, and rib mechanics to address visceral torsion and compression, which may ease nausea and vomiting symptoms. A variety of techniques can be used to achieve these releases and even late in pregnancy, change can be achieved by working subcostally. Some of these techniques are discussed below and shown in Figure 10.30.

CARPAL TUNNEL AND THORACIC OUTLET SYNDROME

Pregnant women often complain of tingling in the hands and arms, which can have a number of causes. One of the most common is carpal tunnel compression due to fluid retention and increased compartment pressure.[52] Cases often resolve spontaneously within a few weeks of delivery.[53] In the interim period, though, when symptom relief is desired, relieving pressure at the level of the carpal tunnel may be achieved by osteopathic work to the hand and arm structures. Specific treatment of carpal tunnel structures by manipulative, myofascial and stretching techniques can be helpful,[54] and work can also be done to areas relating to fluid drainage in the upper limb, such as the clavicle, thoracic outlet/inlet, upper ribs and lower cervicobrachial region.

Another problem is the thoracic inlet (outlet) syndrome. Neural mobility concepts are also useful here, such as the nerve stretch test.[55] There are several tests to indicate the presence of thoracic outlet syndrome. The Adson Wright test is useful, as is hyperabduction. Using several tests in combination seems to give a clearer indication of the

problem.[56] Thoracic outlet syndrome is associated with scalene or pectoral area myofascial tensions[57] but can also be related to mechanical problems with the cervical spine, anterior chest, clavicle, upper ribs and shoulder girdle complex. Many combinations of tension are possible and a careful global assessment is required to incorporate all components of the movement disorder relevant to the presentation in the individual. In the pregnant woman, the influence of increasing breast size and weight cannot be ignored and this may induce soft tissue tension and irritation in the pectoral tissues that may compound any restriction of movement through the cervicodorsal and thoracic outlet regions, hence aggravating any thoracic outlet syndrome.

EXAMINATION AND TREATMENT OF SHOULDER GIRDLE, BREAST AREA, THORACIC CAGE AND UPPER ABDOMEN IN PREGNANCY

There are many ways to address the shoulder girdle, thoracic inlet and cervicobrachial region, which are standard osteopathic examinations and should be part of an osteopath's basic skills. One method shown here (Fig. 10.29) is useful in pregnancy as it allows contact to the anterior pectoral tissues whilst using the patient's arm as a long lever to help focus the technique.

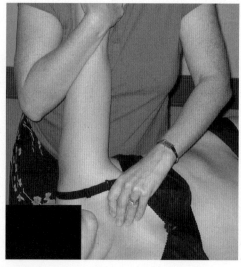

Figure 10.29   Breast, axillary and shoulder girdle release.

The practitioner stands behind the patient and supports her back by ensuring the patient is close to the practitioner's side of the table and that the practitioner's abdomen can support the patient's torso. The practitioner then has one arm guiding the patient's arm as indicated. The practitioner supports the arm near the elbow, to maintain extension at this level, and can use their wrist contact to rotate, traction or compress the arm as a whole. This gives some tissue engagement into the clavicle, the glenohumoral joint or the rotator cuff, depending on the exact arm orientation (and on the particular nature of the tissue barriers presented). The practitioner's other hand is working through the pectoral region. The thumb is eased gently under the pectoral region, to contact next to the pectoralis minor or the upper ribs (or both), or sometimes even near the insertions of serratus anterior. The other part of the hand cups over the pectoral tissues and contacts anteriorly on the muscle and sometimes onto the tail of the breast. The area should not be tender but often is when there is restriction and biomechanical dysfunction present. Inhibition to the soft tissue can be applied, as well as trigger point techniques, if desired. The technique releases a lot of tension in the anterior shoulder which usually releases the clavicle from being dragged inferiorly (and hence clamping down on the thoracic inlet and first rib structures). This relieves pressure on the subclavian vessels, the brachial plexus and the lymphatic thoracic duct. It can also relieve congestion into the axillary fascia and lymph nodes and so help anterior chest and arm drainage. Other contacts directly onto the breast are discussed in the section on mastitis, below.

Figure 10.30 shows another quite global technique which can be adapted to address several different components, depending on the examination findings. The practitioner is supporting the patient's lower torso with their abdomen and one hand is contacting subcostally and the other over the lower ribcage. The abdominal hand gently settles into the softer part of the belly, above the pregnant uterus (even in the third trimester and late pregnancy, sufficient 'space' above the uterus is almost always available for this technique). The abdominal hand uses the side of the index finger as the guiding contact rather than the finger tips as this broader contact is more comfortable. Once

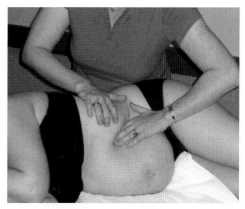

Figure 10.30 Subcostal visceral release and treatment of diaphragm.

the abdominal hand has settled slightly under the costal margin, it rests there a moment whilst the practitioner engages the lower ribcage with their other hand. The ribcage hand gently eases the ribs forwards so as to overlap the costal margin on the abdominal hand. The contact with the ribcage creates the subcostal depth required to begin to assess and treat the upper gastrointestinal tract organs and the diaphragm. With the hands now slightly overlapped, this relationship is maintained throughout the rest of the technique. The two can work in concert, both moving rhythmically and in slightly differing directions as required, in order to relieve tensions found in the area. It is important not to compress the ribcage down onto the abdomen or towards the uterus, as this will block the technique and cause discomfort. Releasing the diaphragm is helpful in cases of breathing problems and upper gastrointestinal irritation and reflux.

Finally in this section, it is important to address any anterior ribcage problems and mediastinal tensions, as these will complicate any cavity dynamics and shoulder girdle and thoracic inlet problems, amongst other things. A general sternal hold for achieving this is shown in Figure 10.31.

PREPARTUM CHECKS

Leading up to the birth, attention can become focused on particular factors. Obviously, if there are other problems still ongoing, they will need to be addressed but if all other things are reasonably balanced, the factors listed in Box 10.4 can be

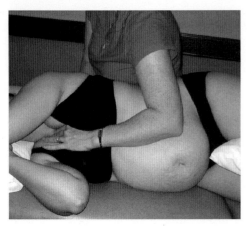

Figure 10.31   Mediastinal, sternal and anterior ribcage release.

useful to consider. The reasons for this are discussed in the next section.

Many of the above techniques are designed to help prepare the woman for labour and to reduce the potential for strain, difficulty and awkward reflex feedback that might inhibit the natural progression of delivery. A closer analysis of the mechanical factors associated with labour and

---

Box 10.4   Prepartum examination checklist

Pelvic floor
Is the woman doing her exercises? Does she need guidance? Is it tender and in need of release and does she need to consider some relaxation prior to the delivery?
    Hip area
Are her hips relatively free and can she stand and rotate her pelvis about without causing discomfort? Can she squat easily? If not, where is the problem and what can be done about it?
    Fetal alignment and uterine tone and torsion
What could be addressed to even the tension in and around the uterus, to help with optimal fetal positioning?
    Upper cervical spine and cranial structures
How are the mechanics of these areas? They are particularly important for the reciprocal relationships with the pelvic bowl, and also for hormonal signals cascading from the hypothalamus and pituitary (according to osteopathic theory).

---

delivery can help focus the practitioner's mind on exactly how they can explore their patients to identify issues that would be important in the intrapartum and postpartum periods.

MECHANICS OF LABOUR AND DELIVERY

The mechanics of labour and delivery have been much investigated over the years, yet there is still much to learn and appreciate. Modern obstetric practice is continuously developing and with the use of epidurals, spinal blocks and almost 'routine' caesarean delivery, the physiological processes of birth are being somewhat influenced through the use of technology.[58] There remains some debate as to whether this is on balance wholly positive or negative.[59] However, the overriding aim for all those involved in obstetric care is to reduce risk, stress and injury to the mother and to the baby; and for delivery to end in the safe arrival of a healthy newborn without unnecessarily harming the mother.

There are five main factors that influence the efficiency of labour: the five 'Ps' of labour.

- Passageway – maternal bony pelvis and soft tissues (including the ability of the cervix to dilate and efface, and the ability of the vaginal canal and the external opening of the vagina (introitus) to distend)
- Passenger – baby
- Powers – primary and secondary
  - Primary/involuntary/uterine contractions
  - Secondary/voluntary/abdominal muscles and diaphragm
- Position – maternal
- Psyche – psychological component of mother

Osteopathic philosophy incorporates views on how to potentially influence all the above factors, making it a very valuable tool not only pre- and postpartum but during the intrapartum period as well.

HARD AND SOFT COMPONENTS OF BIRTH CANAL

There are hard and soft components to the birth canal and both sections must be operating appropriately for the fetal descent and rotation necessary for efficient birth to occur unhindered.

The soft components of the birth canal comprise the fundus of the uterus and the lower segment (which is more fibrous and less elastic than the fundus). The cervix acts as a separate 'gateway' into the hard component area of the birth canal (the bony pelvis) and the other soft component (the vaginal and pelvic outlet soft tissues). The first stage of labour is to help dilate the cervix and to allow full descent and engagement of the presenting parts. The uterus compresses longitudinally to maintain pressure on the cervix and at the lower segment, the walls of the uterus contract so as to pull the cervix open and 'upwards' (as though the cervix will be pulled around the baby's head like pulling on a sweater). At this stage, uterine contractions are quite 'abdominal' and focus on the fundus and body of the uterus. Pain in this stage of labour tends to be around areas segmentally related to L1–2, the lower abdomen and groin area (initially referred through the sympathetic nerves from the uterus). In the second stage of labour, the cervix is fully dilated and the vaginal, pelvic floor and perineal tissues become active. The pain in labour is now more 'perineal', mediated through the sacral plexus of nerves (S2–4). The transition between the first and second stages of labour in particular will engage the bony components of the birth canal.

Osteopathic hypotheses consider that if the fetus is not engaging properly, there might be some tension in the lower segment of the uterus from the uterosacral ligaments (as a result of pelvic restriction or torsion). There might be some reflex discoordination passing between the uterine nerves and the upper lumbar spinal cord as a result of local soft tissue or articulatory tensions. As a result of these or other factors, the cervix might not be gaining sufficient mechanical stimulation from the presenting part, which might interfere with the onset of labour. There is no research into the efficacy of osteopathic care for delayed onset of labour, but approaches to this problem could include stimulation over the upper lumbar region, gentle release and balancing of the tissues in the lower segment area of the uterus, work through the uterosacral ligaments, and balancing of the bony components of the pelvis.

Work could also be addressed to any upper cervical and cranial problems present.

CHANGING SHAPE OF THE BONY BIRTH CANAL

There are many changes in the bony pelvis and the pelvic soft tissues during labour, which need to be appreciated in order to understand the problems that can arise during and after labour (and of course, to help prepare the woman for labour prior to the event). Remember that in humans, the birth canal is a curved tube and consequently the baby needs to rotate to negotiate it. Varying pressures act on the bones and soft tissues of both the mother and the baby at different stages. Osteopaths consider that the bony mechanics of the pelvis during labour may involve the following movements.

- During engagement and early first stage of labour:
  - pelvic inlet opens
  - sacrum tends to counternutate
  - lumbosacral joint flexes
  - ilia flare outwards
- Late first stage:
  - sacrum begins to 'float' as station of head lowers
  - sacroiliac torsion appears as ilia move with initial rotation of baby
- Second stage:
  - pelvic outlet opens
  - sacrum tends to nutate
  - lumbosacral joint moves to extend
  - ilia flare inwards
- Impact of modern birthing practices:
  - lying on back reduces space for sacral movements
  - jams sacrum
  - baby's head contacts posterior pelvic floor
  - lithotomy position strains hips and pubis
  - epidural slows down contractions

Hence, few if any of the above 'ideal' pelvic movements may occur when the mother is weight bearing on the sacrum or is in an otherwise uncomfortable or mechanically restricting position. As will be seen later, osteopaths consider that the pelvic bones should be able to 'float' away from the presenting fetal parts and should offer minimal resistance to descent and rotation movement and share this view with various midwives who support and use natural childbirth practices (Maren Dietze 2001: www.midwifery.org.uk/physiology.htm). Pelvic movements in labour are discussed further below. Changing maternal positions during labour is also thought to ease pressures on the musculoskeletal parts and to enable them to move and better accommodate the descending and rotating fetus, allowing a smoother passage, although there remains some debate about the exact role of maternal position in labour on birth outcomes.[60]

FETAL MOVEMENTS DURING LABOUR

The most 'normal' birth pattern is described in Figure 10.32. Here the baby presents as LOA: 'left occiput anteriorly'. This means the baby's occiput is to the mother's left and it is facing anteriorly rather than posteriorly. The baby engages into the pelvis, facing obliquely (effectively looking at the right sacroiliac joint, were its head not so flexed). Then, the head rotates so the face lines the sacrum (internal rotation). Then, the head extends

around the pubis and once the head is born, the shoulders and body derotate (restitution), to allow the rest of the baby to be born. This is the most physiological direction of movement and if the baby presents differently, this means that the widest parts of the baby do not align to the widest parts of the pelvis during descent and problems can ensue.

PELVIC MOULDING OF MATERNAL PELVIS DURING LABOUR

These rotation movements require quite a lot of physical accommodation by the soft tissues and bony components of the pelvic bowl. The confines of the birth canal are relatively small, with the baby's head only just fitting into the oblique axis of the maternal pelvis during engagement and initial descent. The oblique axis is the broadest at the baby's entrance to the pelvis, and so it is best if the head is aligned this way.

Even so, the descending baby will still stretch out the oblique axis, by pushing on the posterior ilium on one side (the right, if in LOA position) and the anterior ilium on the other (the left, in LOA). This is shown in Figure 10.33. X-ray studies

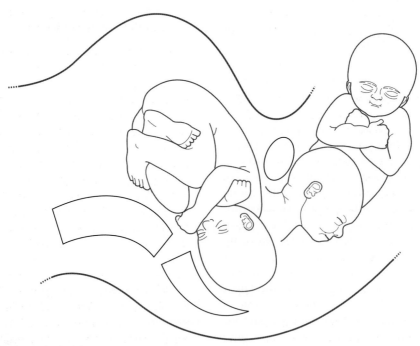

Figure 10.32 Fetal rotation in labour.

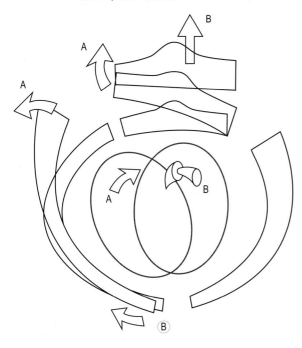

(B) As the face lines the sacrum and the occiput extends around the pubis, the whole sacrum now moves posteriorly and the left sacroiliac joint and pubis have to spread to allow this

(A) As the head rotates internally so that the face lines the sacrum, the right sacroiliac joint (in LOA presentation) has to spread with posterior gapping of ilium. The right sacral alar also begins to move posteriorly

Figure 10.33 Pressures on pelvic joints in labour.

of labour in the 1950s (now unethical, so unable to be reproduced) showed the movements of the sacroiliac joint in relation to the movements of the fetus.[61] These studies showed that the sacroiliac joint moved during labour in relation to the descent of the fetus, and that these movements were not brought about by a change of maternal position. The authors performed many x-ray studies which, although they can be criticized because of the possible disruption they posed to the birth process (the need for the mother to remain still, and repeated examinations during labour), are still of interest (Maren Dietze 2001: www.midwifery. org.uk/physiology.htm).

During birth, hormonal effects on the maternal pelvic tissues are immense and the soft tissue quality changes dramatically to being much more

fluid, elastic and cushioning. This gives some protection to the baby but as the presenting part moves lower, the shape of the pelvis changes and the oblique axis is no longer the broadest, and pressures begin to increase again. Now the head must rotate in order to move into an anteroposterior alignment, which is the broadest part of the pelvis for the baby to exit through. This rotation causes the right sacroiliac joint to bulge further and the right border of the sacrum to move posteriorly. As the head further rotates, the whole sacrum must move posteriorly ('lifting' away from the baby's head).

As the head now extends around the pubis, this stretches the symphysis and the pubic arch (and also the coccyx if the presenting part is too posterior). All this bony pressure stresses the joints and soft tissues and in some cases may also strain directly into the bone itself. In younger mothers, before the pelvic bones have fully ossified, labour and delivery may place additional strain within the bones of the pelvis at the junctions between the individual components of the ilium. This can be assessed with gentle evaluation of the intraosseous components using various osteopathic techniques.

Coupled with these bony movements, a role for the uterosacral ligaments in helping initiate the rotation of the baby's head has been noted.

In a theoretical exploration of the role of the uterine ligaments in the mechanism of labour, Tourne (1985) suggests that the uterosacral ligaments, which connect the uterus with the lower part of the sacrum, bring about the first rotational movement at engagement, aided by the pelvic floor muscles that insert into the coccyx. Tourne believes that it is possible to divide the classical second stage of labour – the stage of expulsion – into two different anatomical and functional parts. The one phase is the intermediate phase where dilatation of the cervix is almost complete and where there is an instinctive reflex that delivery is going to take place and this is very strong, and this is what starts off the oscillation (counter-nutation) of the sacrum and full engagement. Then there is the phase of the delivery itself where the sacrum must slide and rotate, and which cannot be accomplished without perineal relaxation. The uterosacral ligaments take part in the oscillation of the sacrum. Low backache that occurs at the end of pregnancy and in labour is due to strong tension on the uterosacral ligaments, when it is difficult for the head to engage, and can only be relieved when the pelvis tips forward. When delivery is taking place it is important to be rid of all expulsive efforts that may cause contraction of the anterior part of the pelvis. (Maren Dietze 2001: www.midwifery.org.uk/ physiology.htm).

It is essential to consider the ability of the pelvis to absorb these forces and make the required movements, if labour is to be 'unhindered' in this respect. Unfortunately, bony pelvic movements have historically not been considered very much in orthodox obstetric practice and are viewed as less important than, for example, the strength of uterine contractions or rate of cervical dilation. Osteopaths and others contend that if the mother (and her pelvis) cannot move, then the baby is more at risk of becoming stuck and of having problems in rotating fully. This is particularly so if the baby is initially in a posterior presentation. Osteopaths would consider that maintaining and optimizing the movement possibilities in the pelvis are essential for resolution of this difficult obstetrics problem which is responsible for many cases of instrumental intervention and caesarean delivery. As medical technology advances, though, there is increasing interest in the mechanical dynamics between the maternal pelvis and the fetus, and several computer simulations have been developed to explore this relationship, with a view to reducing biomechanical stress and improving birth outcomes.[62,63]

THE PELVIC FLOOR IN LABOUR

The pelvic floor will descend during labour and so needs to be quite pliable. The arrangement of the pelvic floor cradles the baby's head and allows it to help in rotation, whilst descending and elongating – quite a demanding process. The position at which the baby's head can arrive at the perineum can be influential to the stresses (and subsequent trauma) to the pelvic floor as a whole.

The pelvic floor needs to be elastic in order to withstand these pressures and problems can arise if this is not the case. In elongating, the urogenital diaphragm needs to be the most elastic and the distance between the pubis and the perineal body

needs to increase significantly. One study noted that when perineal length and anal position in primigravidae were measured to evaluate their effect on vaginal delivery, women with a short perineum (<4 cm) or a small anal position index had significantly higher rates of episiotomy, perineal tears and instrumented delivery. It was concluded that a short perineum and anterior displacement of the anus were associated with traumatic vaginal delivery in primigravidae.[64] Further factors of the pelvic floor sequelae from childbirth are discussed below.

INTRAPARTUM TECHNIQUES

Osteopathic care in the intrapartum period is not common and most medical practitioners and obstetric teams would be unaware of its existence. The role is supportive and clearly the obstetric team in conjunction with the mother have control of the decision making and clinical actions performed. However, after informed debate, some osteopathic techniques may be acceptable at this time, depending on individual circumstances. The ethics and scope of practice issues within obstetrics and midwifery are already highly contended and osteopaths wishing to work in this field must respect professional boundaries and medicolegal implications.

Most techniques are done in the first stage of labour and include (but are not limited to) the following.

- Balancing ligamentous stabilizing rings of pelvis (as in Figure 10.34).
- Upper lumbar inhibition in first stage and sacral inhibition in second stage.
- Release of diaphragm and upper abdominals – due to the general fatigue and breathing exhaustion of labour, and the expulsive effort straining the abdomen (even without any maternal 'pushing').
- General back massage, to ease thoracolumbar and sacral fascia and erector spinae fatigue
- Gentle articulation of lumbar and sacroiliac joints (more like a very subtle unwinding release rather than any degree of direct mobilization).
- Other techniques such as very gentle uterine and membranous balancing and some pelvic

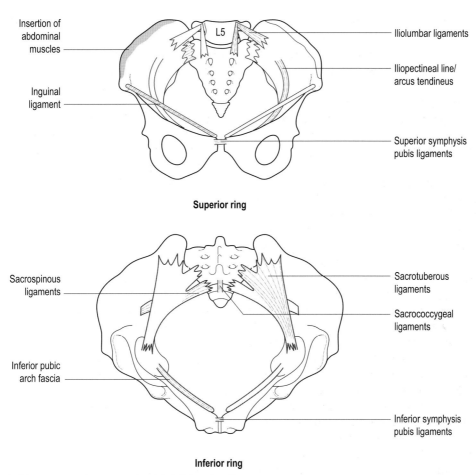

Superior ring

Inferior ring

Figure 10.34 Ligamentous rings around pelvic inlet and outlet.

floor supportive techniques are possible but generally require specialized osteopathic training.

Intrapartum techniques are often performed in between contractions and so the practitioner must work quickly, aiming to release a little at a time.

PAIN IN LABOUR

Every other equivalently painful modern surgical procedure is performed under anaesthesia.

There are three different origins of childbirth pain.

- Visceral pain – early labour, relating to cervical dilation. Visceral pain from the uterus is mediated through L1–2, felt in the back and relevant dermatomes.
- Pressure on surrounding structures, e.g. sciatic nerve, autonomic nervous plexi, bladder and rectum.
- Somatic pain – late labour, caused by lower genital/perineal dilation by fetal presenting part. Somatic pain, from the pelvic floor and perineum, mediated through S2–4, is felt in the vagina, rectum, perineal area and inner thighs. Associated with the urge to push/bear down.

Existing medical approaches to pain relief include nitrous oxide and oxygen. This limits neurone synapse in the CNS and may have a 'distracting' effect. Pethidine is commonly used, which may reduce pain sensation but is more likely just to suppress anxiety and fear. It is recognized as not actually being very effective at pain relief. It is also associated with adverse effects of neonatal respiratory function and feeding patterns. Epidurals are increasingly used and are associated with increased intervention. Here, analgesia is applied into the cord space which can work quickly on unmyelinated fibres, thus reducing visceral pain in labour. It is less effective for somatic pain. There is some concern that, with the pelvic floor muscles being more relaxed (as the mother has reduced sensation), this may reduce rotation of presenting part and create problems with the progression of labour. There is also no, or little, urge to push unless the epidural is allowed to wear off before second stage. It does not prevent actual pushing, though. It often slows down labour so oxytocic drugs may be required to keep contractions going. Its use can control high blood pressure but maternal blood pressure may also drop considerably as a result. On a positive note, women are in less pain and if they need a caesarean, this can be performed immediately (on high dose). Pain relief may also produce relaxation in general, allowing more rapid cervical dilation.

> Osteopaths aim to reduce mechanical and soft tissue stress leading up to labour, and sometimes during it. Their hypothesis is that if the maternal tissues and structures are as accommodating as possible, then this may reduce mechanical resistance to the forces and movements of labour, thereby increasing labour efficiency, reducing the need for instrumental or other intervention, and making the whole process much less painful and uncomfortable.

FETAL HEAD MOULDING

The baby can also dictate the progress of labour and delivery, through its size and presentation. The baby's head is its least compressible part and thus poses the greatest mechanical strain on pelvic mechanics during delivery. Negotiation of the birth canal is aided not only by the strength of uterine contractions but also by the ability of the fetal skull bones to overlap during delivery,

thus reducing head size and aiding descent through the birth canal. Rotatory strains also create stress at various points along the spine, in particular at the upper cervical and cervicodorsal regions. Longitudinal compression may also be present due to the overall effects of contractions.[65] Fetal moulding is more common with primiparous than multiparous women, and with the use of oxytocin and instrumental deliveries.[66]

Osteopaths have many theories concerning the biomechanical effects that labour and delivery have on the fetus, whether born in a vertex or breech presentation, or anterior or posterior alignment. Each type of birth will produce a different strain pattern within the baby, as each will have had its own unique passage through its own individual passageway. There is a large field of work within osteopathic paediatrics that is applied to resolve these strain patterns and to ease various problems that the babies and infants may suffer from, such as restlessness, 'colic' and many other disorders.[67,68]

CAESAREAN SECTION

The controversy over elective caesarean versus vaginal birth with regard to pelvic floor trauma has left many caregivers and patients confused. Caesareans are often performed to minimize pelvic floor injuries, as well as for failure to progress or other complications in labour. The majority of childbirth injuries to the pelvic floor occur after the first vaginal delivery. Caesarean sections performed after the onset of labour may not protect the pelvic floor. Some consider elective caesarean section is the only true primary prevention strategy for childbirth injuries to the pelvic floor.[69]

Sections are increasingly common. They can be an essential procedure but they do have implications for neonatal health. There are three common types of incision: the classical longitudinal incision, the inverted T-scar and the lower uterine transverse scar (LUSCS). This latter is associated with the least risk of rupture in subsequent trial of labour or delivery. Vaginal birth after caesarean section (VBAC) is controversial, and the practice used to be 'once a caesarean, always a caesarean'.

However, VBAC may come back into favour as it is cheaper than another caesarean. It is now cautiously promoted as a trial of labour in a fully staffed hospital, in women with one previous LUSCS.

Planned VBAC has a very high success rate. If the mother has had a previous vaginal delivery, she has the highest rate of success with VBAC; if no prior vaginal birth, she has a low chance of success. When the primary caesarean was for breech, the success rate is cut by half; when the caesarean was performed for failure to progress or dystocia, it is even lower. When the mother has had more than one previous caesarean section (with or without a successful vaginal delivery), her chances of success in a subsequent VBAC are very small.

EXAMINATION AND TREATMENT POST CAESAREAN DELIVERIES

See Figure 10.10 for a general contact for the lower abdomen and caesarean scar area, during pregnancy. Work on caesarean scars can begin within hours or days of delivery. At this stage, the techniques are extremely minimal and utilize very limited pressure and force. The aim is to ease surrounding tissue irritability, leaving the scar area under less strain. Wound hygiene should obviously be respected. Once the staples or stitches are removed, then more direct contact can be applied. After a couple of months, direct stretch and mobilization can be applied within comfort limits. To accompany direct scar management, the following types of approaches are useful.

- Lower abdominal wall release
- Focus on layers from muscle to peritoneum
- Release around inguinal canal and ligament regions
- Relationship of retrovesical pouch and vagina onto uterus should be considered
- Relation of the two pelvic outlets can be reintegrated:
  - from iliolumbar ligaments and iliolumbar fascia, around crests, along inguinal ligament onto pubis
  - from inferior pubis, along rami, along sacrotuberous ligaments, to coccyx

CHILDBIRTH-RELATED PELVIC FLOOR AND PELVIC ORGAN INJURIES

The pelvic floor is a muscular structure, pierced by the urological, genital and distal intestinal tracts. This structure is not a frozen but a functional unit. Normal function can be replaced by dysfunctions of several kinds, overlapping voiding, sexual, genital and defaecatory behaviour. For instance, vaginismus is akin to anismus and vesicourethral dyssynergia. Many urological, genital and digestive dysfunctions are a sort of 'body signature' of the trauma, which must be dealt with if the symptom is to disappear. Urologists, gynaecologists, gastroenterologists and colorectal surgeons should not only exchange ideas but should be aware of the pathologies of neighbouring specialties: there should be a more holistic vision of pelvic floor function, including sexuality, if disorders in this region are to be fully appreciated.[70] This is not only true in urogynaecology and gastroenterology, but also in relation to obstetrics and, in particular, the consequences of labour and postpartum pelvic function.

As indicated above, vaginal delivery is associated with the risk of pelvic floor damage. The pelvic floor sequelae of childbirth include anal incontinence, urinary incontinence and pelvic organ prolapse.[71] The birthing process is recognized to be clearly traumatic to the pelvic floor.[72] Five factors are known to affect perineal integrity (either positively or negatively): episiotomy, third-trimester perineal massage, mother's position in second-stage labour, method of pushing, and administration of epidural analgesia.[73] Some studies have looked at how the use of forceps affects the pelvic floor. Some authors consider that advanced degrees of forceps rotations do not result in any clinically significant increase in infant or maternal morbidity relative to that encountered with lesser degrees of forceps rotation.[74] Others consider that forceps delivery is not responsible for a higher incidence of pelvic floor complaints or greater changes in bladder neck behaviour or urethral sphincter functions. However, others have found that patients with forceps delivery have a significantly greater decrease in intraanal pressure and a greater incidence of a weak pelvic floor.[75]

There is huge debate as to whether episiotomies are beneficial or not. They are performed to ease pressures on the fetal head, to reduce fetal distress and to 'prevent' more serious tears of the pelvic floor. However, there is no certainty that their routine use is reasonable and that the woman is consequently assured of better long-term pelvic floor and continence function than if she had had no incision.[76] Performing the episiotomy is one thing, and repairing it is another. It is not comforting to discover that studies reveal that medical residents attending births are often undertrained with respect to pelvic floor anatomy and repair procedures. One study found that residents from 47% of obstetric programmes indicated that the majority of residents received no formal training in pelvic floor anatomy, episiotomy or perineal repair and, when engaged in such activities, had limited supervision.[77]

This is clearly not in the woman's best interests and for osteopaths, the aim would be to help maintain optimum pelvic floor function so that the birthing process is as uninterrupted and stress free as possible, so ensuring a possibly lower injury rate to the pelvic floor. Another method of possible prevention is to focus on antenatal pelvic floor exercises, which are thought to be effective in reducing the risk of postpartum stress incontinence in primigravidae with bladder neck mobility.[78] Prepartum pelvic floor exercises are also associated with fewer incidences of prolonged second-stage pushing, which in itself is a stress to the pelvic floor.[79]

BLADDER AND BOWEL FUNCTION

There are many consequences to the pelvis post partum, not only to the pelvic floor but to pelvic organ mobility and support in general. After both spontaneous and instrumental deliveries, stress urinary incontinence is relatively common and, to a lesser degree, faecal incontinence. Substantial bladder neck hypermobility and urethral length changes can occur and intravaginal and intraanal pressures may be altered postmpartum.[80] Pelvic organ prolapse is partially responsible for these problems and is thought to be related as much to the first stage of labour as the second.[81] Obstetric injury may take the form of direct muscular damage to the anal sphincter, as occurs during a

third-degree tear, and/or may be the result of cumulative damage to the pudendal nerves. Mechanical, neural and endocrine factors may all play a causative role in faecal incontinence.[82]

EXAMINATION AND TREATMENT OF THE PELVIC FLOOR, BLADDER AND BOWEL

Whether the woman has had an uneventful vaginal delivery, has torn or had an episiotomy, or has had various instrumental interventions, she is likely to be suffering some degree of perineal and pelvic floor stress. The pelvic floor problems can be treated directly, with an external contact or per vaginally, for example. Internal pelvic floor assessment would not be done for a minimum of 6 weeks post partum but external pelvic floor work can be done within hours or days of the delivery, if the type of technique applied is suitably adjusted. Most women will not present for treatment until at least a few weeks after delivery when their postpartum bleeding has ceased, they are more generally recovered and they can arrange for someone to look after the baby! Usually women receive care for their pelvic floor from midwives or physiotherapists, who give advice, exercises or such things as electrical stimulation. Osteopaths can be uniquely helpful as their awareness of soft tissue reactions, complex pelvic mechanics and specific palpatory skills make them well placed to address scarring and spasm sequelae that others are not trained for. Examination and treatment of the pelvic floor and other pelvic organs have been described in previous chapters.

MASTITIS

Around 3–11% of women with mastitis can go on to develop a breast abscess.[83] Any delay in treatment can lead to the development of breast abscesses[84] and antibiotics are the usual therapy, along with aspiration and incision and drainage techniques, and the continuation of breastfeeding. Manual stripping of pus from the breast has been identified as reducing the incidence of abscess formation.[85] Osteopaths would not perform that technique but can offer a general treatment approach that would be supportive of the orthodox or medical management of mastitis/breast abscess.

General cases of 'sore breasts' and nipple irritation can be helped with osteopathic treatment to the breast, shoulder girdle, anterior ribcage and axillary regions, as part of a general osteopathic approach. Again, this would be an adjunct to the orthodox management, which usually centres around breastfeeding instruction and the use of nipple shields and lanolin.[86] The osteopathic techniques are aimed at improving breast drainage, release of connective tissue and duct tension within the breast, and reducing neural irritation that may be affecting breast tissues. Each breast has around 5–9 ducts terminating at the nipple, which are separate from each other.[87] Release around the breast can involve unwinding/relaxing along each general area of the breast or can be focused at the nipple, where the terminal duct can be 'unwound' together. Note: the terms 'unwind' and 'unwound' relate to an osteopathic manoeuvre which aims to move the tissues very gently and subtly into a direction of 'ease', in other words, away from any tissue barrier. The woman should always be advised to seek medical advice when suffering from mastitis.

The techniques for releasing the breast can also be aimed at the nerves and vessels supplying the breast. The suspensory ligament of the nipple runs transversely along the fifth rib and links into the lateral border of pectoralis minor and also the sternum. The neurovascular bundle for the nipple runs along the suspensory ligament/lateral border of pectoralis minor,[88] making treatment to this structure very relevant to breast symptoms, as well as techniques to the axillary tissue in general. The internal mammary artery and vein run along the internal surface of the costal cartilages and chondrosternal junctions. Restrictions in these articulations can impact on breast drainage.

BREAST UNWINDING AND RELEASE

Figure 10.35 shows direct treatment to the breast. This can be done during pregnancy or post partum, depending on symptoms. Contact can be taken with both hands cupping the breast, feeling for areas of tension, inconsistency, congestion and irritation. The practitioner can unwind the breast using gentle small movements of the hands that slightly mobilize within the breast tissue or simply 'follow' tensions as dictated by the tissue

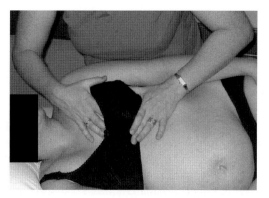

Figure 10.35   Treatment of the breast.

barriers present. A contact can also be taken directly onto the nipple and associated tensions can be treated as well. The woman's consent will be required and after careful discussion and guidance, the technique is often performed easily without discomfort. Hygiene issues should be respected when working directly onto the nipple.

SUCKLING ISSUES

There are particular actions required of the breast during feeding[89] and if these cannot be performed appropriately (for example, as a result of breast tension or torsion within the ducts/nipple area) then suckling issues in the infant may be complicated. Osteopaths can treat the breast component (as above) and also the baby (around the head, throat, jaw and neck, for example) to ease tensions there that might be interfering with suckling and breast-latching actions.[90]

OBSTETRIC CAUTIONS

There are many medical disorders that need to be carefully monitored in pregnancy, including diabetes, iron deficiency, hydramnios, blood pressure and hypertension, and pre-eclampsia. Thrombolytic disease is a major cause of maternal morbidity, and pulmonary embolus can occur post partum as well as during pregnancy. Other bleeding disorders in pregnancy include placenta praevia. It is important to be aware of all these disorders, their medical management and the risks they pose to the mother and fetus. Although pregnancy is not an illness, osteopaths should continually bear in mind that pregnant women can become ill and care should be taken when monitoring the progress of such things as headache, leg pain and any abdominal or pelvic discomfort, in case the cause is not musculoskeletal but systemic.

There seems to be no evidence of osteopathically induced miscarriage or of success in osteopathic induction of labour. However, it may be prudent to avoid certain types of treatment such as manipulation during risk times for miscarriage (for example, around weeks 12 and 16) or late in pregnancy to avoid too much direct stimulation

to the coccyx, cervix and lower uterine segment (although it is still possible to treat the patient generally at these times, and some work from experienced practitioners may be performed locally on some occasions). This is not so much because techniques are known to cause problems or trigger uterine contractions but that these things can occur concurrently and coincidentally. This may reduce maternal concern or confusion.

There is a massive field of research waiting to be done on the osteopathic management of pregnant patients and as knowledge and evidence are gained, they should continue to inform and refine practice.

References

1. Romano M. Bipedal verticality, social behaviour, environmental adaptation and human evolutionary development. Ann Ig 1989;1(6):1351-75.
2. Rosenberg KR, Trevathan WR. The evolution of human birth. Sci Am 2001;285(5):72-7.
3. Abitbol MM. Growth of the fetus in the abdominal cavity. Am J Phys Anthropol 1993;91(3):367-78.
4. Harrison DE, Cailliet R, Harrison DD, Janik TJ. How do anterior/posterior translations of the thoracic cage affect the sagittal lumbar spine, pelvic tilt, and thoracic kyphosis? Eur Spine J 2002;11(3):287-93.
5. Sihvonen T, Huttunen M, Makkonen M, Airaksinen O. Functional changes in back muscle activity correlate with pain intensity and prediction of low back pain during pregnancy. Arch Phys Med Rehabil 1998;79(10):1210-12.
6. Franklin ME, Conner-Kerr T. An analysis of posture and back pain in the first and third trimesters of pregnancy. J Orthop Sports Phys Ther 1998;28(3):133-8.
7. Gilleard WL, Crosbie J, Smith R. Static trunk posture in sitting and standing during pregnancy and early postpartum. Arch Phys Med Rehabil 2002;83(12):1739-44.
8. Wu W, Meijer OG, Jutte PC, et al. Gait in patients with pregnancy-related pain in the pelvis: an emphasis on the coordination of transverse pelvic and thoracic rotations. Clin Biomech (Bristol, Avon) 2002;17(9-10):678-86.
9. Wu W, Meijer OG, Lamoth CJ, et al. Gait coordination in pregnancy: transverse pelvic and thoracic rotations and their relative phase. Clin Biomech (Bristol, Avon) 2004;19(5):480-8.
10. Foti T, Davids JR, Bagley A. A biomechanical analysis of gait during pregnancy. J Bone Joint Surg Am 2000;82(5):625-32.
11. Bird AR, Menz HB, Hyde CC. The effect of pregnancy on footprint parameters. A prospective investigation. J Am Podiatr Med Assoc 1999;89(8):405-9.
12. Nyska M, Sofer D, Porat A, Howard CB, Levi A, Meizner I. Planter foot pressures in pregnant women. Isr J Med Sci 1997;33(2):139-46.
13. Stelzner F. [Fascia skeleton of the abdominal cavity – hernia and anorectal incontinence]. Langenbecks Arch Chir 1991;376(2):108-20.
14. Clerici C. [Modifications of respiratory function during pregnancy]. Rev Pneumol Clin 1999;55(5):307-11.
15. Gilroy RJ, Mangura BT, Lavietes MH. Rib cage and abdominal volume displacements during breathing in pregnancy. Am Rev Respir Dis 1988;137(3):668-72.
16. Le Merre C, Prefaut C. [Pregnancy and the respiratory function]. Rev Mal Respir 1988;5(3):249-54.
17. Kariminia A, Chamberlain ME, Keogh J, Shea A. Randomised controlled trial of effect of hands and knees posturing on incidence of occiput posterior position at birth. BMJ 2004;328:490.
18. Andrews CM, Andrews EC. Physical theory as a basis for successful rotation of fetal malpositions and conversion of fetal malpresentations. Biol Res Nurs 2004;6(2):126-40.
19. Ververs IA, de Vries JI, van Geijn HP, Hopkins B. Prenatal head position from 12–38 weeks. II. The effects of fetal orientation and placental localization. Early Hum Dev 1994;39(2):93-100.

20. Fianu S, Vaclavinkova V. The site of placental attachment as a factor in the aetiology of breech presentation. Acta Obstet Gynecol Scand 1978; 57(4):371-2.

21. Gardberg M, Tuppurainen M. Anterior placental location predisposes for occiput posterior presentation near term. Acta Obstet Gynecol Scand 1994;73(2):151-2.

22. Hoogland HJ, de Haan J. Ultrasonographic placental localization with respect to fetal position in utero. Eur J Obstet Gynecol Reprod Biol 1980;11(1):9-15.

23. Ponkey SE, Cohen AP, Heffner LJ, Lieberman E. Persistent fetal occiput posterior position: obstetric outcomes. Obstet Gynecol 2003;101(5 Pt 1):915-20.

24. Fitzpatrick M, McQuillan K, O'Herlihy C. Influence of persistent occiput posterior position on delivery outcome. Obstet Gynecol 2001;98(6):1027-31.

25. Roman J, Bakos O, Cnattingius S. Pregnancy outcomes by mode of delivery among term breech births: Swedish experience 1987–1993. Obstet Gynecol 1998;92(6):945-50.

26. Rietberg CC, Elferink-Stinkens PM, Visser GH. The effect of the Term Breech Trial on medical intervention behaviour and neonatal outcome in The Netherlands: an analysis of 35,453 term breech infants. Br J Obstet Gynaecol 2005;112(2):205-9.

27. Coyle ME, Smith CA, Peat B. Cephalic version by moxibustion for breech presentation. Cochrane Database Syst Rev 2005;(2):CD003928.

28. Pistolese RA. The Webster Technique: a chiropractic technique with obstetric implications. J Manipul Physiol Ther 2002;25(6):E1-9.

29. King HH, Tettambel MA, Lockwood MD, Johnson KH, Arsenault DA, Quist R. Osteopathic manipulative treatment in prenatal care: a retrospective case control design study. J Am Osteopath Assoc 2003;103(12):577-82.

30. Aisenbrey GA, Catanzarite VA, Nelson C. External cephalic version: predictors of success. Obstet Gynecol 1999;94(5 Pt 1):783-6.

31. Collaris RJ, Oei SG. External cephalic version: a safe procedure? A systematic review of version-related risks. Acta Obstet Gynecol Scand; 83(6):511-18.

32. Lau TK, Lo KW, Rogers M. Pregnancy outcome after successful external cephalic version for breech presentation at term. Am J Obstet Gynecol 1997; 176(1 Pt 1):218-23.

33. Pool-Goudzwaard AL, Kleinrensink GJ, Snijders CJ, Entius C, Stoeckart R. The sacroiliac part of the iliolumbar ligament. J Anat 2001;199(Pt 4):457-63.

34. Brown MD, Levi AD. Surgery for lumbar disc herniation during pregnancy. Spine 2001;26(4):440-3.

35. Nilsson-Wikmar L, Harms-Ringdahl K, Pilo C, Pahlback M. Back pain in women post-partum is not a unitary concept. Physiother Res Int 1999; 4(3):201-13.

36. Albert H, Godskesen M, Westergaard J. Prognosis in four syndromes of pregnancy-related pelvic pain. Acta Obstet Gynecol Scand 2001;80(6):505-10.

37. Wang M, Dumas GA. Mechanical behavior of the female sacroiliac joint and influence of the anterior and posterior sacroiliac ligaments under sagittal loads. Clin Biomech (Bristol, Avon) 1998;13(4-5): 293-9.

38. Sturesson B, Uden A, Vleeming A. A radiostereo-metric analysis of movements of the sacroiliac joints during the standing hip flexion test. Spine 2000;25(3):364-8.

39. Kissling RO, Jacob HA. The mobility of the sacroiliac joint in healthy subjects. Bull Hosp Jt Dis 1996; 54(3):158-64.

40. Jacob HA, Kissling RO. The mobility of the sacroiliac joints in healthy volunteers between 20 and 50 years of age. Clin Biomech (Bristol, Avon) 1995;10(7):352-61.

41. Vleeming A, Pool-Goudzwaard AL, Hammudoghlu D, Stoeckart R, Snijders CJ, Mens JM. The function of the long dorsal sacroiliac ligament: its implication for understanding low back pain. Spine 1996;21(5):556-62.

42. Kleinrensink GJ, Stoeckart R, Mulder PG, et al. Upper limb tension tests as tools in the diagnosis of nerve and plexus lesions. Anatomical and bio-mechanical aspects. Clin Biomech (Bristol, Avon) 2000;15(1):9-14.

43. Harrison DE, Cailliet R, Harrison DD, Troyanovich SJ, Harrison SO. A review of biomechanics of the central nervous system. Part II: spinal cord strains from postural loads. J Manipul Physiol Ther 1999;22(5):322.

44. Harrison DE, Cailliet R, Harrison DD, Troyanovich SJ, Harrison SO. A review of biomechanics of the central nervous system. Part III: spinal cord stresses from postural loads and their neurologic effects. J Manipul Physiol Ther 1999;22(6):399-410.

45. Papadopoulos EC, Khan SN. Piriformis syndrome and low back pain: a new classification and review of the literature. Orthop Clin North Am 2004;35(1):65-71.

46. Delarue MW, Vles JS, Hasaart TH. Lumbosacral plexopathy in the third trimester of pregnancy: a report of three cases. Eur J Obstet Gynecol Reprod Biol 1994;53(1):67-8.

47. Turgut F, Turgut M, Mentes E. Lumbosacral plexus compression by fetus: an unusual cause of radiculopathy during teenage pregnancy. Eur J Obstet Gynecol Reprod Biol 1997;73(2):203-4.

48. Pildner von Steinburg S, Kuhler A, Herrmann N, Fischer T, Schneider KT. [Pregnancy-associated femoral nerve affection.] Zentralbl Gynakol 2004;126(5):328.

49. Danielides V, Skevas A, van Cauwenberge P, Vinck B, Tsanades G, Plachouras N. Facial nerve palsy during pregnancy. Acta Otorhinolaryngol Belg 1996;50(2):131-5.

50. Lindner A, Schulte-Mattler W, Zierz S. [Postpartum obturator nerve syndrome: case report and review of the nerve compression syndrome during pregnancy and delivery.] Zentralbl Gynakol 1997;119(3):93.

51. Hartman L. Handbook of osteopathic technique, 3rd edn. London: Chapman and Hall; 1997.

52. Bahrami MH, Rayegani SM, Fereidouni M, Baghbani M. Prevalence and severity of carpal tunnel syndrome (CTS) during pregnancy. Electromyogr Clin Neurophysiol 2005;45(2): 123-5.

53. Wand JS. Carpal tunnel syndrome in pregnancy and lactation. J Hand Surg [Br] 1990;15(1):93-5.

54. Sucher BM. Myofascial manipulative release of carpal tunnel syndrome: documentation with magnetic resonance imaging [see comments]. J Am Osteopath Assoc 1993;93(12):1273-8.

55. Walsh MT. Upper limb neural tension testing and mobilization. Fact, fiction, and a practical approach. J Hand Ther 2005;18(2):241-58.

56. Gillard J, Perez-Cousin M, Hachulla E, et al. Diagnosing thoracic outlet syndrome: contribution of provocative tests, ultrasonography, electrophysiology, and helical computed tomography in 48 patients. Joint Bone Spine 2001;68(5):416-24.

57. Sucher BM. Thoracic outlet syndrome – a myofascial variant: Part 1. Pathology and diagnosis. J Am Osteopath Assoc 1990;90(8):686-96, 703-4.

58. Kozak LJ, Weeks JD. U.S. trends in obstetric procedures, 1990–2000. Birth 2002;29(3):157-61.

59. Sizer AR, Nirmal DM. Occipitoposterior position: associated factors and obstetric outcome in nulliparas. Obstet Gynecol 2000;96(5 Pt 1):749-52.

60. Gupta JK, Hofmeyr GJ. Position for women during second stage of labour. Cochrane Database Syst Rev 2004;(1):CD002006.

61. Borell U, Fernstrom I. The movements at the sacro-iliac joints and their importance to changes in the pelvic dimensions during parturtion. Acta Obstet Gynecol Scand 1957;36(1):42-57.

62. Melchert F, Wischnik A, Nalepa E. The prevention of mechanical birth trauma by means of computer aided simulation of delivery by means of nuclear magnetic resonance imaging and finite element analysis. J Obstet Gynaecol 1995;21(2):195-207.

63. Liu Y, Scudder M, Gimovsky ML. CAD modeling of the birth process. Part II. Stud Health Technol Inform 1996;29:652-66.

64. Rizk DE, Thomas L. Relationship between the length of the perineum and position of the anus and vaginal delivery in primigravidae. Int Urogynecol J Pelvic Floor Dysfunct 2000;11(2):79-83.

65. Carreiro J. An osteopathic approach to children. Edinburgh: Churchill Livingstone; 2003.

66. Sorbe B, Dahlgren S. Some important factors in the molding of the fetal head during vaginal delivery – a photographic study. Int J Gynaecol Obstet 1983;21(3):205-12.

67. Magoun HI. Infants and children. In: Osteopathy in the cranial field, 3rd edn. Kirksville, MO: Cranial Academy; 1976.

68. Frymann VM. Relation of disturbances of craniosacral mechanism to symptomatology of the newborn. J Am Osteopath Assoc 1966;65:1059-75.

69. Heit M, Mudd K, Culligan P. Prevention of childbirth injuries to the pelvic floor. Curr Womens Health Rep 2001;1(1):72-80.

70. Devroede G. Front and rear: the pelvic floor is an integrated functional structure. Med Hypotheses 1999;52(2):147-53.

71. Dannecker C, Anthuber C. The effects of childbirth on the pelvic-floor. J Perinat Med 2000;28(3):175-84.

72. Dainer MJ. Vaginal birth and natural outcome. Curr Opin Obstet Gynecol 1999;11(5):499-502.

73. Flynn P, Franiek J, Janssen P, Hannah WJ, Klein MC. How can second-stage management prevent perineal trauma? Critical review. Can Fam Physician 1997;43:73-84.

74. Hankins GD, Leicht T, Van Hook J, Uckan EM. The role of forceps rotation in maternal and neonatal injury. Am J Obstet Gynecol 1999;180 (1 Pt 1):231-4.

75. Meyer S, Hohlfeld P, Achtari C, Russolo A, De Grandi P. Birth trauma: short and long term effects of forceps delivery compared with spontaneous delivery on various pelvic floor parameters. Br J Obstet Gynaecol 2000;107(11):1360-5.

76. Hartmann K, Viswanathan M, Palmieri R, Gartlehner G, Thorp J Jr, Lohr KN. Outcomes of routine episiotomy: a systematic review. JAMA 2005;293(17):2141-8.

77. McLennan MT, Melick CF, Clancy SL, Artal R. Episiotomy and perineal repair. An evaluation of resident education and experience. J Reprod Med 2002;47(12):1025-30.

78. Reilly ET, Freeman RM, Waterfield MR, Waterfield AE, Steggles P, Pedlar F. Prevention of postpartum stress incontinence in primigravidae with increased bladder neck mobility: a randomised controlled

trial of antenatal pelvic floor exercises. Br J Obstet Gynaecol 2002;109(1):68-76.

79. Salvesen KA, Morkved S. Randomised controlled trial of pelvic floor muscle training during pregnancy. BMJ 2004;329(7462):378-80.

80. Meyer S, Schreyer A, De Grandi P, Hohlfeld P. The effects of birth on urinary continence mechanisms and other pelvic-floor characteristics. Obstet Gynecol 1998;92(4 Pt 1):613-18.

81. Sze EH, Sherard GB 3rd, Dolezal JM. Pregnancy, labor, delivery, and pelvic organ prolapse. Obstet Gynecol 2002;100(5 Pt 1):981-6.

82. Fitzpatrick M, O'Herlihy C. The effects of labour and delivery on the pelvic floor. Best Pract Res Clin Obstet Gynaecol 2001;15(1):63-79.

83. Amir LH, Forster D, McLachlan H, Lumley J. Incidence of breast abscess in lactating women: report from an Australian cohort. Br J Obstet Gynaecol 2004;111(12):1378-81.

84. Dener C, Inan A. Breast abscesses in lactating women. World J Surg 2003;27(2):130-3.

85. Bertrand H, Rosenblood LK. Stripping out pus in lactational mastitis: a means of preventing breast abscess. Can Med Assoc J 1991;145(4):299-306.

86. Brent N, Rudy SJ, Redd B, Rudy TE, Roth LA. Sore nipples in breast-feeding women: a clinical trial of wound dressings vs conventional care. Arch Pediatr Adolesc Med 1998;152(11):1077-82.

87. Love SM, Barsky SH. Anatomy of the nipple and breast ducts revisited. Cancer 2004;101(9):1947-57.

88. Wueringer E, Tschabitscher M. New aspects of the topographical anatomy of the mammary gland regarding its neurovascular supply along a regular ligamentous suspension. Eur J Morphol 2002;40(3):181-9.

89. Smith WL, Erenberg A, Nowak A. Imaging evaluation of the human nipple during breast-feeding. Am J Dis Child 1988;142(1):76-8.

90. Fraval M. Osteoapthic treatment of infants with a sucking dysfunction. J Am Acad Osteopathy 1998;8(2):25-33.

91. Stone C. Science in the art of osteopathy: osteopathic principles and practice. Cheltenham: Nelson Thornes; 1999.

Appendix

CHAPTER CONTENTS

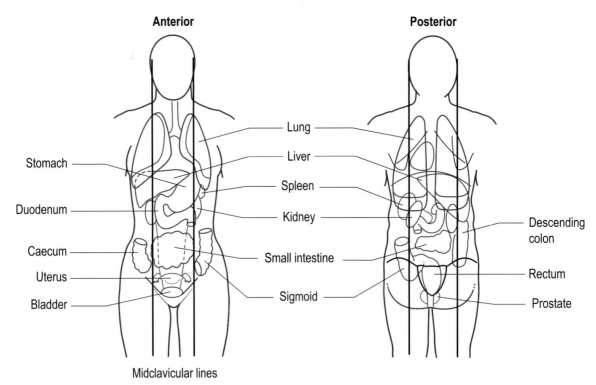

Anterior   Posterior

Stomach

Duodenum

Caecum

Uterus

Bladder

Lung

Liver

Spleen

Kidney

Small intestine

Sigmoid

Descending colon

Rectum

Prostate

Midclavicular lines

Figure A1   Anterior, posterior and lateral views of the body, indicating which visceral structures are generally related to which skeletal structure.

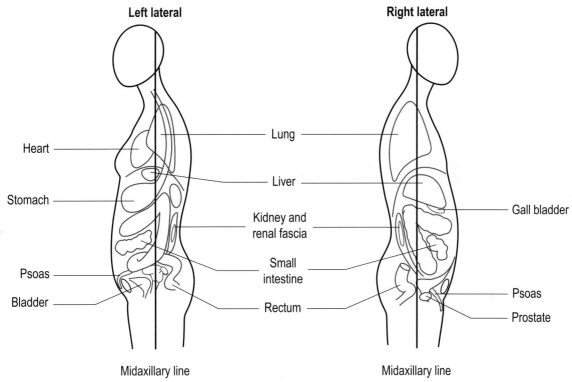

Figure A1   continued.

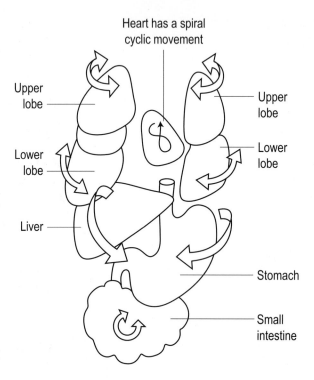

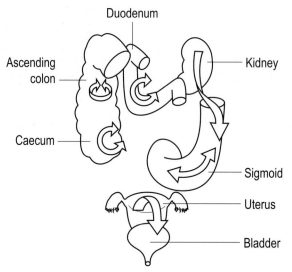

Figure A2 Basic visceral motility.

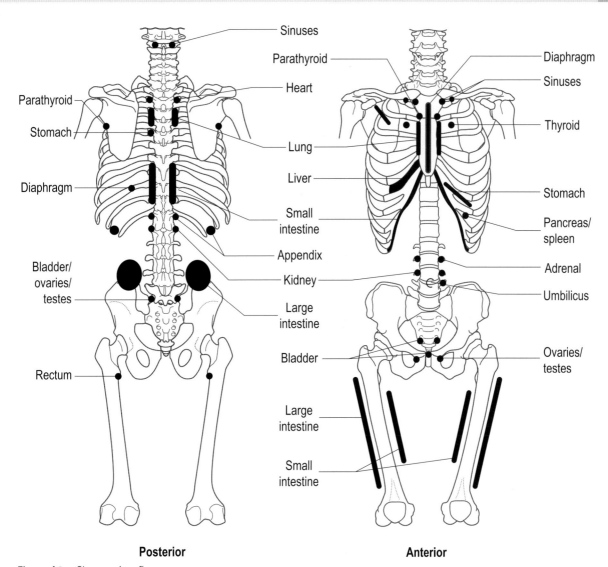

Posterior   **Anterior**

Figure A3   Chapman's reflexes.

Index